The Early Course
of Schizophrenia

The Early Course of Schizophrenia

Edited by

Tonmoy Sharma
Clinical Neuroscience Research Centre
Kent, UK
and

Philip D. Harvey
Department of Psychiatry
Mount Sinai School of Medicine
New York, NY, USA

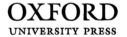
OXFORD
UNIVERSITY PRESS

OXFORD

UNIVERSITY PRESS

Great Clarendon Street, Oxford OX2 6DP

Oxford University Press is a department of the University of Oxford.
It furthers the University's objective of excellence in research, scholarship,
and education by publishing worldwide in

Oxford New York

Auckland Cape Town Dar es Salaam Hong Kong Karachi
Kuala Lumpur Madrid Melbourne Mexico City Nairobi
New Delhi Shanghai Taipei Toronto

With offices in

Argentina Austria Brazil Chile Czech Republic France Greece
Guatemala Hungary Italy Japan South Korea Poland Portugal
Singapore Switzerland Thailand Turkey Ukraine Vietnam

Oxford is a registered trade mark of Oxford University Press
in the UK and in certain other countries

Published in the United States
by Oxford University Press Inc., New York

A catalogue record for this title is available from the British Library

Library of Congress Cataloging in Publication Data

(Data available)

ISBN 0-19-8510845 (Hbk)   978-0-19-851084-0
0-19-8568959 (Pbk)   978-0-19-856895-7

10 9 8 7 6 5 4 3 2 1

Typeset by Cepha Imaging Pvt. Ltd., Bangalore, India.
Printed in Great Britain
on acid-free paper by Biddles Ltd, King's Lynn

Contents

Section 1

Schizophrenia in the premorbid period

Chapter 1

Prenatal events that influence schizophrenia

Ezra Susser and Mark G. Opler

Introduction

The past decade has witnessed a dramatic increase in research on hypothesized fetal origins of schizophrenia. Much of this research has been motivated by the 'neurodevelopmental hypothesis' articulated during the 1980s. This theory proposed that the developing brain is vulnerable to genetic and environmental insults that yield subtle alterations in structure and function and elevate the risk of psychosis later in life (Murray and Lewis 1987, Waddington *et al.* 1999, Weinberger 1987). Although there is ongoing debate as to the nature of the developmental antecedents and their relationship to subsequent events, the neurodevelopmental hypothesis has become widely accepted and has significantly reshaped the field of schizophrenia research over the last several decades.

This chapter first discusses some of the key evidence supporting the neurodevelopmental hypothesis of schizophrenia. We then review some of the findings on obstetric complications, which until recently was the principal focus of many studies in the field. Next, we present recent evidence for the role of specific prenatal exposures as risk factors for schizophrenia. The chapter concludes with an overview of ongoing studies and future directions in which this work may proceed.

Throughout, we will emphasize findings from prospective cohorts followed across the lifecourse. These studies have provided some of the strongest evidence to date and hold the potential to transform this field of study.

Evidence for the neurodevelopmental hypothesis

At one point, schizophrenia was commonly believed to be a 'functional' psychosis, with no apparent organic or structural basis (Gallagher 1977). During the 1960s and 1970s, research on its physical basis was not in vogue, despite ongoing efforts.

This era was marked by Plum's declaration that such work was 'the graveyard of neuropathologists', implying that many a career had been spent in futile search of a non-existent structural defect (Plum 1972). However, in the 1980s, research on schizophrenia as a brain disorder expanded dramatically. Neuroimaging techniques suggested that subtle structural changes could be measured in the brains of patients with schizophrenia, such as increased ventricular volume (Kelsoe *et al.* 1988). In addition, a number of retrospective studies revealed that patients who developed schizophrenia seemed to be developmentally different from the general population with respect to childhood behavior and neuromotor function, suggesting early life origins of the illness (reviewed by McDonald and Murray 2000).

Over the last decade, as evidence for some early disturbance in brain development has accumulated and been refined, the neurodevelopmental focus has come to predominate. Below, we highlight some of the key findings on which the hypothesis rests.

Structural evidence of developmental disruption

Patients with schizophrenia do not demonstrate the gross pathology observed in other central nervous system disorders, such as the clear degeneration of the substantia nigra seen in Parkinson's disease. However, more subtle findings on schizophrenia have been reported in postmortem and other studies, indicating structural disarray at the cellular level. Histopathology and cytoarchitectural studies have shown increased neural density and decreased neuropil in patients with schizophrenia as compared to controls (Roberts *et al.* 1996). Several reviews and meta-analyses support the view of somewhat reduced volume overall without marked changes in the number of neurons, accompanied by volumetric changes and altered connectivity between and within different regions (Harrison 1999). Studies using imaging and volume visualization techniques suggest increased ventricular volume and reductions in the volume of the cortex and hippocampus (Halliday 2001). It is difficult, however, to determine whether postmortem evidence and other measurements collected during late life occurred prior to disease onset as a part of the etiologic process, rather than subsequent to illness as a result of a degenerative process or treatment.

A complementary set of findings localized to early life are beginning to form and lend support to the neurodevelopmental hypothesis. Patients with schizophrenia appear to exhibit a greater number of minor physical anomalies than the general population. Minor physical anomalies include measurable alterations in the development of the feet, hands, mouth, eyes, and head. Often taken as evidence of developmental disruption, notable excesses occur following exposure to certain teratogens, such as those characteristic patterns of anomalies used to diagnose fetal alcohol syndrome (McGrath *et al.* 1995). Minor physical anomalies are linked to early fetal brain development, because they arise from the same ectodermal tissue that develops into the central nervous system. Studies by McNeil, Waddington and colleagues, and several others have suggested that the average number of minor physical anomalies in an individual with schizophrenia is approximately doubled, and significant numbers of minor physical anomalies may be found in as many as 60 per cent of patients (McNeil and Cantor-Graae 2000, Waddington and Youssef 1987). A number of potential prenatal disruptors that might cause increases in minor physical anomalies and also increase the risk of schizophrenia and related disorders have been investigated using epidemiologic approaches (Murphy and Owen 1996).

Developmental antecedents

In addition to physical findings, neurobehavioral differences observed prior to the onset of symptomatic disease are a second line of evidence for the role of early developmental processes in schizophrenia. These developmental antecedents have been studied as continuously distributed variables, including social functioning, academic performance, and IQ. A number of different study designs have been employed in efforts to measure these factors in individuals who go on to develop schizophrenia. These designs have included historical cohorts and case-control studies utilizing various retrospective and records-based approaches. However, prospectively collected cohorts where subjects are identified at birth, followed by data collection at several timepoints during childhood and adolescence benefit from more accurate exposure and outcome classification, as well as the capacity to study a greater range of factors in depth.

Several birth cohorts established at the middle of the twentieh century have been adapted to study psychotic disorders as the samples they have followed have passed into the age of risk. The longest running study of note in this category is the 1946 Medical Research Council National Survey of Health and Development, which enrolled all 13,687 births in England, Scotland, and Wales between 3 March and 9 March, 1946. A random subset of 5,936 subjects was assessed over the lifecourse. Followed from birth into adulthood, this group represents a socially stratified sample that has had 20 assessments since birth, and is still being followed as the cohort progresses into its 57th year (Wadsworth 1987).

The Medical Research Council Survey has investigated events throughout childhood. These have included assessments made at eleven points prior to the age of 16. Interviews conducted at age 36 using the Present State Examination and a register of psychiatric hospital admissions identified 30 cases of schizophrenia. Findings from the Medical Research Council National Survey have shown increased risk for schizophrenia in subjects with delayed development during the first two years of life, such as increased time to learning to walk. Observations throughout development demonstrated relationships to schizophrenia, including impaired educational attainment as measured by standardized test scores at ages 8, 11, and 15, altered social functioning in the form of social isolation at ages 4 and 6 and increased social anxiety throughout adolescence (Jones *et al.* 1994).

A second birth cohort study, the 1958 National Child Development Study composed of 98 per cent of the live births in one week in March 1958 in Great Britain, gave similar results for education, isolation, social anxiety, and schizophrenia. Particularly, from age 7 to 16, poorer educational attainment was found in the group that would later develop schizophrenia, with no relative change in the degree of impairment over time when compared to controls (Done *et al.* 1991). Gender differences were noted among those who would later develop schizophrenia, specifically that boys were more likely to exhibit violent and antisocial behavior, while girls were more likely to be withdrawn and isolated (Sigurdson *et al.* 2002).

Complemented by others, the major conclusions of such studies of childhood and adolescence are that behavioral differences and motor anomalies in people who will later develop schizophrenia are evident throughout early life. This suggests that at least some of the factors that contribute to the emergence of symptomatic disease must have been present in early life, prior to the emergence of these observed differences.

Epidemiologic evidence for obstetric complications

Investigations of obstetric complications have been conducted for decades, producing both positive and negative findings. Several reviews and meta-analyses have noted that the exposure definitions employed in these studies are quite variable, including reports of overall maternal health as well as more discrete sets of maternal conditions. In some instances, studies of the same underlying mechanism use divergent methods to assess exposure. For example, several studies hypothesize that hypoxic conditions are the primary mechanism through which obstetric complications increase the risk for schizophrenia, but they differ on the basis of the measures used to assess hypoxia, variable including or excluding cyanosis, low Apgar scores, meconium in amniotic fluid, or uterine bleeding (Cannon *et al.* 2002). Even in studies that attempt to focus on a specific factor, insufficient standardization of exposure definitions may continue to hinder the interpretation of results. For example, studies of uterine bleeding may utilize any recorded report or evidence of bleeding due to any cause as exposure (Scott 1972). Without quantifying the extent of bleeding, identifying the conditions associated with bleeding, or specifying the time point in pregnancy during which the bleeding occurred, there may be a great deal of variety in exposure definitions.

In addition to the lack of standard exposure definitions within and between studies, many meta-analyses and reviews of the area fail to account for the role of study design, and several include results from both cohort and case-control studies. This presents difficulties, as case-control studies employing retrospective approaches are prone to various forms of error. Studies demonstrate that accuracy of maternal recall is highly varied with respect to the events of pregnancy, although not necessarily systematically biased between cases and controls (Buka *et al.* 2000). McIntosh and colleagues have shown that recall bias in studies of obstetric complication may be based on other factors, such as childhood behavioral abnormalities (McIntosh *et al.* 2002).

Despite these limitations, several well-designed population-based studies have been conducted. These are exemplified by a study conducted in Sweden by Dalman and colleagues that has demonstrated a positive relationship to obstetric complications (Dalman *et al.* 2001). Using a National Birth Registry containing all births in Sweden between 1973 and 1977, a sample of 507,516 births was linked to a National Inpatient Registry and 238 subjects in the sample with an inpatient record of ICD-9 defined schizophrenia recorded between 1987 and 1995 were defined as cases. A number of reported complications were grouped under three etiologic mechanisms of obstetric complications, (1) hypoxic stress, (2) extreme prematurity, and (3) fetal malnutrition. While all three contribute to the risk, after the results are controlled for potential confounders, only fetal malnutrition as assessed by pre-eclampsia is reported as being related to schizophrenia.

In summary, the role of obstetric complications has been difficult to assess, and most meta-analyses have been equivocal. Inconsistent findings and a lack of construct validity have hampered efforts to draw definitive conclusions. However, this work has played a critical role in the field, providing important support for the feasibility of research into early influences on schizophrenia, and suggesting avenues for research on specific exposures. In an effort to avoid the difficulties of recall bias, construct validity, and measurement error, recent investigations of prenatal insult have generally used more specific exposure definitions in prospectively collected samples.

Epidemiologic evidence for specific prenatal exposures

In keeping with the neurodevelopmental hypothesis, recent investigations have often been focused on known neurodevelopmental disruptors. Many hypotheses have been advanced and a number of studies have produced suggestive results. However, the methods employed have been extremely variable. Thus, the strength of each result can only be assessed in light of the methodology employed, including sampling, diagnostic criteria, and exposure ascertainment. At this point in the field, a systematic approach is required to evaluate the relative merits and validity of the flood of new findings that is beginning to emerge. In this context, rather than survey a miscellany of reports, we choose to focus on some very recent findings from ongoing studies that exemplify three classes of prenatal exposure: nutritional deprivation, infection, and chemical exposure. Using these examples, we will also demonstrate an approach to critiquing findings.

Collecting data on the prenatal environment is a challenging task. Investigators may take advantage of natural experiments in which a notable event exposes a population to an identifiable ecological disaster (e.g. studies of the atomic bombings in Hiroshima and Nagasaki). A second method is the use of prenatal or birth cohorts established in the past during early development and identifiable in the present day. Several of the studies referred to in this section are based on prenatal rather than birth cohorts. Prenatal cohorts are preferable when studying processes that begin prior to birth, beginning data collection with the mothers during pregnancy and continuing follow up of the offspring after birth. Two large prenatal cohorts were founded in the United States during the 1950s. While birth and prenatal cohort studies are often initiated in order to study infant and child health, rather than later life onset disorders such as schizophrenia, the methodological strength and flexibility of such cohort studies permits their use in investigations of many exposure-disease combinations beyond those for which they were originally designed (Susser and Terry, 2003).

Prenatal nutritional deprivation

A series of studies on the effects of prenatal nutritional deprivation on the neurodevelopment of offspring were conducted within the framework of a unique historic event (Susser *et al.* 1998). The Dutch Famine Study has its roots in the Nazi occupation of Holland during the Second World War. During the occupation, food supplies were limited through destruction of farmland to build airfields and fortifications and appropriation of existing supplies and food stores. In the later stages of the war, anticipating an Allied invasion, a strike by railroad workers brought transportation to a halt. The Nazis retaliated by blockading all shipments, including food supplies into the western part of the country. At the time, western Holland was one of the most densely populated parts of the world, with the majority living in urban areas. With resources already strained, the blockade precipitated a severe famine. It is important to note the strength of the 'natural experiment' that this tragic confluence of events afforded; a famine that was well defined in time and space in a large, urban society that was otherwise well fed, had widespread access to health care, and extensive record keeping.

The studies that were conducted on the effects of prenatal exposure to the famine illustrate the longitudinal approach, crossing from conception to birth and into adulthood, using observational data across the lifespan and requiring the efforts of multiple generations of researchers. The original studies by Stein and colleagues were designed to assess the effects of prenatal famine on neurodevelopmental outcomes, particularly mental retardation and reduced IQ. Although a series of studies found no effect on either IQ or other measures of mental performance, indices of the presence of central nervous system anomalies at birth, such as spina bifida and anencephaly, were related to conception during the most severe stages of the famine (Stein and Susser 1975). This study set the stage for a generational succession wherein the son of the two primary investigators of the original study (E. Susser) extended observations of the Dutch Famine cohorts into adulthood in order to study early prenatal exposure to the famine as a risk factor for schizophrenia.

Using data collected from national psychiatric registries, rates of schizophrenia were found to be approximately doubled for individuals conceived at the height of the famine, similar to findings on central nervous system anomalies. Nutrient deprivation for the mothers of this group fell below 1,000 kCal/day during early gestation (Susser *et al.* 1996). Early gestational exposure to famine conferred risk for schizophrenia, whereas late gestational exposure did not. Other studies extending these findings to schizophrenia spectrum personality disorders also showed a twofold increase in risk for early gestational exposure to famine (Hoek *et al.* 1998).

The Dutch Famine studies are notable for the use of a natural experiment, and improved timing and classification of exposure as compared to previous work. However, it is important to note that the natural experiment is not equivalent to a controlled trial. Many subjects may have altered the degree to which they were exposed to famine through several mechanisms, including the purchase of extra rations on the black market. Alternative explanations for the effects of the famine must be considered beyond caloric restriction. For example, the consumption of unusual foods and potentially toxic items such as tulip bulbs was documented during the famine. Moreover, the degree to which specific underlying mechanisms can be further investigated in this population is limited. The role of micronutrient levels during development, particularly folic acid and retinoids, have been suggested as an etiologic factor in schizophrenia, but these hypotheses cannot be further tested in this population.

Prenatal infection

Torrey, Crow, and others began suggesting a link between exposure to viral agents and schizophrenia during the 1970s (Torrey and Peterson 1973, Crow 1978). Theories on viral infection and schizophrenia received renewed attention in the neurodevelopmental hypothesis, suggesting that *prenatal* infection may predispose to adult schizophrenia. A wide variety of infectious diseases have been studied, with primary interest focusing on viral agents. Of the various forms that have been investigated, the most convincing evidence exists for the roles of rubella and influenza.

Rubella

Rubella infection has long been associated with a number of central nervous system birth defects in the offspring of women infected during pregnancy, particularly cataracts, deafness, and minor physical anomalies. Congenital rubella shares certain characteristics with schizophrenia, such as impaired social functioning in childhood, increased CSF volume, and larger lateral ventricles (Stevens 1997). Similar to the Dutch Famine studies, observations on the neurodevelopmental aspects of congenital rubella motivated epidemiologic studies to examine associations to schizophrenia and related disorders.

In 1964, a rubella epidemic in the United States resulted in an estimated 20,000 cases of congenital malformations. The Rubella Birth Defects Evaluation Project was founded at New York University Medical Center to evaluate and manage congenital malformations and other sequelae in the offspring of mothers exposed to rubella during pregnancy. A total of 243 infants were enrolled. Their exposures were documented serologically or via viral isolation, rather than by report. In 1967, Stella Chess initiated a behavioral study to evaluate the psychological effects of congenital rubella and assist parents in the treatment and education of their children. The study detected high rates of developmental abnormalities previously associated with rubella exposure, but also noted high rates of autism and separation anxiety disorder. These observations led Chess to propose several important theories, including viral teratogens as a possible causal agent in neuropsychiatric disorders (Chess *et al.* 1971).

Chess and co-authors concluded their review of the original study by noting 'uncertainty about their future', and stressing the importance of follow-up assessments. This statement proved to be prophetic, as continued studies of the same cohort were conducted at two other points, including one evaluation of 66 subjects between the ages of 21–23 and a second conducted ten years later. While the first study occurred before most subjects would have passed through the age of risk for schizophrenia, the second study captured 53 subjects ranging in age between 31–33 (Brown *et al.* 2000). Most had been documented as being exposed to rubella in the first trimester. Eleven cases were diagnosed with schizophrenia or other non-affective psychotic disorders (20.4 per cent), a very high proportion when compared to general population rates of approximately 1 per cent. This result suggests that some feature of viral infection confers an increase in risk. Several mechanisms have been proposed, such as physiologic responses to infection (hyperthermia and elevated cytokines), neurotoxic effects of the infectious agent itself, and potential teratogenic side effects of antibiotics and other medication.

This study is one of the first to use serologically documented cases of infection, and is therefore an important example of direct measurement of a prenatal exposure. Nonetheless, there are several limitations that should be noted. The number of total subjects is relatively small, as is the number of cases. In addition, the subjects followed up represent a small proportion ($\approx$25 per cent) of the original group defined by Chess in 1964 and may not be a representative sample. Another concern is that of disease definition, i.e. that rubella-induced developmental disability constitutes a condition similar to, but distinct from schizophrenia. Therefore, despite the many strengths of the study, it should not be considered definitive.

Influenza

The current interest in prenatal influenza exposure and schizophrenia can be traced to a study by Mednick and colleagues in 1988. They examined hospitalization rates for schizophrenia in offspring of women resident in and around Helsinki, comparing those whose mothers were pregnant during the 1957 influenza A_2 epidemic with those whose pregnancies did not coincide with the epidemic. Their findings suggest that rates of schizophrenia among offspring whose mothers were resident in the city during the epidemic in the second trimester of pregnancy were approximately doubled in the offspring of women not pregnant during the epidemic. This ecological design does not use individual level documentation of influenza infection, relying on comparisons of population-wide rates of disease between exposed and unexposed populations, defined on the basis of place of residence during the epidemic. As such, it is susceptible to confounding with other factors that cannot be accounted for, such as medication or elevated body temperature. Another concern is the 'ecologic fallacy' whereby it cannot be determined whether the individuals within the exposed or unexposed populations are the same who are later diagnosed with schizophrenia.

Other studies of similar design have reported comparable findings. On the other hand, there have been several failures to replicate. Currently, rather than accumulating more equivocal results, researchers have begun to employ different study designs. In an effort to avoid the particular errors to which ecological approaches are prone, cohort studies have been conducted, assessing influenza exposure at the individual level.

Two early cohort studies examined influenza with individual exposure data. The first, a study by Crow et al., was conducted using the previously described 1958 National Child Development Study cohort in Great Britain. This study reported no association between prenatal influenza and schizophrenia (Crow and Done 1992). However, exposure to the 1957 epidemic was assessed retrospectively by asking mothers after birth if they had had influenza during their pregnancy. As demonstrated in studies of obstetric complication, retrospective measures utilizing maternal recall or midwife report may be inaccurate. Additionally, this study had only 945 subjects in the group exposed to influenza during the second trimester.

A later study conducted by Cannon and colleagues used prospectively collected reports of influenza in a cohort in Dublin that had been exposed to the same epidemic (Cannon et al. 1996). This cohort had been designed specifically to study the effects of early life exposure to influenza, though not originally designed to extend to adult health outcomes. Cannon et al. evaluated adult psychiatric status by conducting maternal interviews and through review of psychiatric records. This study also failed to show a relationship to schizophrenia. Again, there were too few subjects in the cohort for a reliable test of the hypothesis, with 238 exposed and 287 unexposed. It should also be noted that clinical records of exposure, while preferable to the use of maternal recall, do not always contain desired information, such as the identity of the infectious agent. Such records also tend to miss less symptomatic cases of influenza.

In order for the field to advance beyond marginal or equivocal findings, future work must ascertain prenatal exposure to influenza through quantifiable measurements, e.g. archived biological samples collected prior to diagnosis. In addition, large numbers of subjects are required to be able to accurately assess the relatively modest increases in risk that any single factor is likely to contribute to a multifactorial disease such as schizophrenia. To provide a prototype, we will describe one ongoing study that has examined prenatal influenza and other exposures.

The Prenatal Determinants of Schizophrenia Study, initiated in 1996, is based on a cohort of approximately 20,000 pregnant women, established in Northern California between 1959–1966 as part of the Childhood Health and Development Study (Susser *et al.* 2000). This study includes a precious resource, maternal sera drawn during prenatal visits. These samples were stored and maintained at NIH facilities, frozen at –20° C in anticipation of future studies. They have been used in combination with hospital records and new diagnostic data to examine the effects of several exposures, including prenatal influenza exposure (Brown *et al.* 2001).

Cases of schizophrenia and other spectrum disorders were identified from a database of inpatient, outpatient, and pharmacy records. Records for cohort members with diagnoses indicative of psychosis or prescriptions for antipsychotic medication were reviewed, abstracted, and rated by two psychiatrists for the presence or absence of psychosis. These ratings were then used to identify potential cases to be sought for a thorough diagnostic interview. Ultimately, seventy-one cases of schizophrenia and related spectrum disorders were identified. Controls were selected from the cohort and matched to cases on the basis of several factors, including date of membership in the cohort, date of birth, gender, timing of first maternal blood draw, and the number of available serum samples.

For the analysis of influenza exposure, the stored maternal serum from cases and matched controls, the hemeagglutination inhibition test was performed on four antigens of influenza strains known to be prevalent between 1959–1966 in northern California, including A/H2N2/Japan/57, A/H2N2/Japan/62, A/H2N2/Taiwan/64, and B/Massachusetts/66. Exposure to influenza usually results in a rise in antibody titers, referred to as seroconversion. Typically, seroconversion is characterized as a fourfold rise in antibody titers taken in serial samples. As most subjects in this study had single samples taken within each trimester, a single cut-off level was sought as a proxy of influenza exposure during pregnancy. Validity studies demonstrated that levels of >1:20 in a single serum sample were highly specific and sensitive.

First trimester exposure was associated a sevenfold increase in risk of schizophrenia spectrum disorder, while second and third trimester exposure showed no increase in risk. However, while first trimester is usually defined as the period between zero and ninety days following the last menstrual period (post-LMP), the blood draws taken in this study only occur as early as 46 days post-LMP. Therefore, first trimester here signifies, in effect, the latter part of first trimester. Additional analyses were conducted analyzing exposure during the first and second halves of pregnancy defined as 0–142 days (in effect, 40–142 days post-LMP) and from 143 days post-LMP until termination of pregnancy, respectively. Exposure between the midpoints of first trimester and second trimester of pregnancy conferred a threefold increase in risk, while no increase was seen following exposure during the second half of pregnancy or when second trimester exposure was considered.

While clearly an advance over previous work, this study has three key limitations. First, the number of cases of schizophrenia and related spectrum disorders with the required prenatal sera was fairly small, totaling 64 cases and two matched controls per case. Although the study found a substantial association between prenatal influenza exposure and schizophrenia, the confidence limits of this association are quite wide. Second, influenza infection is typically documented by noting an increase in titers over time, and the measure used in this study represents a proxy of the established standard. Third, the increase in risk does not exactly correspond with previous findings with respect to timing of exposure. Prior reports have indicated that second trimester exposure is associated with increases in risk, while exposure during first trimester and first half of pregnancy confers risk in this study. Further investigation is required to explain this difference.

Biological markers of lead exposure

Another potential risk factor being measured in the Prenatal Determinants of Schizophrenia study is lead. Lead represents the first chemical exposure to be studied as a prenatal antecedent of schizophrenia in a birth cohort. Lead has been known as a toxic agent for centuries, and has been shown to be a neurodevelopmental disruptor associated with deficits in intelligence, impaired attention, and juvenile delinquency. Some studies have followed samples with prenatal exposures into adolescence; however, there is a dearth of literature on long-term effects, particularly on the subsequent risk of mental disorders during adulthood.

While there are several techniques for assessing lead exposure in biological samples, the principal one is studies of prenatal exposure through direct measurements on maternal blood. The Prenatal Determinants of Schizophrenia Study has stored sera, not whole blood containing the lead-sequestering erythrocytes required for direct measurements in small volumes. Techniques for direct measurement of lead could not be employed. However, a biological marker of lead exposure, δ-aminolevulinic acid (δ-ALA) may be detected in urine, plasma, and serum using high-pressure liquid chromatography with fluorescence detection.

Feasibility studies were conducted to assess the utility of this technique in small volumes of stored maternal serum. It was determined that second trimester serum was likely to be the best indicator of prenatal exposure, as both lead and corresponding δ-ALA levels are believed to be relatively stable at midpregnancy. Second trimester samples were available for 44 cases and 75 matched controls (one to two controls per case).

A single 100 μL aliquot of second trimester serum was made available for each subject. A concentration of 9.5 ng/mL of δ-ALA, corresponding to a blood lead level of 15 μg/dL was used as a cutoff value to divide the sample into exposed and unexposed subjects. Samples were coded and blinded with respect to case status. Using this approach, lead exposure as measured by elevated δ-ALA was associated with about a twofold increase in risk of schizophrenia spectrum disorders in this sample (OR = 2.3, p = 0.5). The small numbers of subjects contribute to the wide confidence limits.

As in the previously described influenza study, some limitations should be noted. First, the use of a biological marker rather than direct measurements means that the observed increase in risk cannot be conclusively ascribed to lead exposure. Serum δ-ALA itself may be the exposure of interest. In experimental models, δ-ALA has been shown to be neurotoxic, interfering with GABA neurotransmission (Cory-Slechta 1995). Second, the findings of this study are also difficult to interpret conclusively, since the sample size is relatively small and the result has a wide confidence interval.

Future directions

Among the principles that have been illustrated in this field are the use of prospectively collected cohorts in combination with archived biological samples. This method has allowed research to move from broad 'catch-all' definitions of exposure toward the investigation of more specific mechanisms. Each of the recent studies that this chapter described has utilized a longitudinal approach, made possible by the foresight of early generations of researchers in combination with the efforts of those who succeed them. The conduct of future studies in this vein requires the current generation of investigators to emulate their approach.

The initial results from prenatal cohort studies are suggestive, but the process they represent is still in its early days. Every area of inquiry described in this chapter will benefit from further refinements in technique and method. Nutritional deprivation might be explored in greater detail, requiring researchers to develop methods to measure the effects of individual micronutrients. In the case of infectious agents, the strains that cause the greatest increases in risk, the molecular components of infection that affect the developing brain, and the timing of exposure may be further specified. A wider variety of chemical exposures could eventually be examined and the proximal effects of exposure eventually teased apart and differentiated from consequent physiologic responses.

Preventive approaches to treatment are the ultimate goal of epidemiology and the study of the developmental antecedents of schizophrenia. At the present time, the available evidence is insufficient for preventive action. Nonetheless, the growing evidence is motivating discussion of interventions that might in the future be employed at the level of the general population. Several recent reviews of the area discuss the potential impact of decreasing exposure to risk factors and increasing the use of protective factors (McGrath 2000, Mojitabai *et al.* 2003). For example, optimized prenatal care may decrease exposure to hypoxic events while nutritional supplementation known to help protect against other neurodevelopmental conditions might also reduce the risk of schizophrenia.

We believe that in order to reach the goal of effective prevention, the functional integration of clinical findings, genetic data, and molecular neurobiology is critical, along with the development of appropriate technologies and statistical methods. Investigators with interdisciplinary training, comfortable with the language and concepts of study design at the population level and at the level of the neuron will play a crucial role in the future of the field.

References

Brown AS, Cohen P, Harkavy-Friedman J *et al.* (2001). A.E. Bennett Research Award. Prenatal rubella, premorbid abnormalities, and adult schizophrenia. *Biological Psychiatry*, 49, 473–86.

Brown AS, Schaefer CA, Wyatt RJ *et al.* (2000). Maternal exposure to respiratory infections and adult schizophrenia spectrum disorders: a prospective birth cohort study. *Schizophrenia Bulletin*, 26, 287–95.

Buka SL, Goldstein JM, Seidman LJ and Tsuang MT (2000). Maternal recall of pregnancy history: accuracy and bias in schizophrenia research. *Schizophrenia Bulletin*, 26, 335–50.

Cannon M, Cotter D, Coffey VP *et al.* (1996). Prenatal exposure to the 1957 influenza epidemic and adult schizophrenia: a follow-up study. *British Journal of Psychiatry*, 168, 368–71.

Cannon M, Jones PB and Murray RM (2002). Obstetric complications and schizophrenia: historical and meta-analytic review. *American Journal of Psychiatry*, 159, 1080–92.

Chess S, Fernandez P, and Korn S (1971). Psychiatric disorders of children with congenital rubella. Brunner/Mazel, New York, NY.

Cory-Slechta DA (1995). Relationships between lead-induced learning impairments and changes in dopamergic, cholinergic, and glutamatergic neurotransmitter system functions. *Annual Review of Pharmacology and Toxicology*, 35, 391–415.

Crow, TJ (1978). Viral causes of psychiatric disease. *Postgraduate Medical Journal*, 54, 763–7.

Crow TJ and Done DJ (1992). Prenatal exposure to influenza does not cause schizophrenia. *British Journal of Psychiatry*, 161, 390–3.

Dalman C, Thomas HV, David AS, Gentz J, Lewis G and Allebeck P (2001). Signs of asphyxia at birth and risk of schizophrenia. Population-based case-control study. *British Journal of Psychiatry*, 179, 403–8.

Done DJ, Crow TJ, Johnstone EC *et al.* (1991). Childhood antecedents of schizophrenia and affective illness: social adjustment at ages 7 and 11. *British Medical Journal*, 302, 1576–80.

Gallagher BJ (1977). The attitudes of psychiatrists toward etiological theories of schizophrenia. *Journal of Clinical Psychology*, 33, 99–104.

Halliday GM (2001). A review of the neuropathology of schizophrenia. *Clinical and Experimental Pharmacology and Physiology*, 28, 64–5.

Harrison PJ (1999). The neuropathology of schizophrenia. A critical review of the data and their interpretation. *Brain*, 122, 593–624.

Hoek HW, Brown AS and Susser E (1998). The Dutch famine and schizophrenia spectrum disorders. *Social Psychiatry and Psychiatric Epidemiology*, 33, 373–9.

Jones P, Rodgers B, Murray R and Marmot M (1994). Child development risk factors for adult schizophrenia in the British 1946 birth cohort. *Lancet*, 344, 1398–402.

Kelsoe JR Jr, Cadet JL, Pickar D and Weinberger DR (1988). Quantitative neuroanatomy in schizophrenia. A controlled magnetic resonance imaging study. *Archives of General Psychiatry*, 45, 533–41.

McDonald C and Murray R (2000). Early and late environmental risk factors for schizophrenia. *Brain Res Brain Res Rev*, 31(2-3), 130–7.

McGrath, JJ (2000). Universal interventions for the primary prevention of schizophrenia. *Australian & New Zealand Journal of Psychiatry*. 34, S58–64.

McGrath JJ, van Os J, Hoyos C, Jones PB, Harvey I and Murray RM (1995). Minor physical anomalies in psychoses: associations with clinical and putative aetiological variables. *Schizophrenia Research*, 18, 9–20.

McIntosh AM, Holmes S, Gleeson S *et al.* (2002). Maternal recall bias, obstetric history and schizophrenia. *British Journal of Psychiatry*, 181, 520–5.

McNeil TF and Cantor-Graae E (2000). Minor physical anomalies and obstetric complications in schizophrenia. *Australia & New Zealand Journal of Psychiatry*, 34, S65–73.

Mednick SA, Machon RA, Huttunen MO and Bonett D (1988). Adult schizophrenia following prenatal exposure to an influenza epidemic. *Archives of General Psychiatry*, 45, 189–92.

Mojtabai R, Malaspina D and Susser E (2003). The concept of population prevention: application to schizophrenia. *Schizophr Bull*, 29(4), 791–801.

Murphy KC and Owen MJ (1996). Minor physical anomalies and their relationship to the aetiology of schizophrenia. *British Journal of Psychiatry*, 168, 139–42.

Murray RM and Lewis SW (1987). Is schizophrenia a neurodevelopmental disorder? *British Medical Journal (Clinical Research Edition)*, 295, 681–2.

Plum F (1972). Prospects for research on schizophrenia. Neurophysiology. Neuropathological findings. *Neuroscience Research Program Bulletin*, 10, 384–8.

Roberts RC, Conley R, Kung L, Peretti FJ and Chute DJ (1996). Reduced striatal spine size in schizophrenia: a postmortem ultrastructural study. *Neuroreport*, 7, 1214–8.

Sigurdsson E, Van Os J and Fombonne E. Are impaired childhood motor skills a risk factor for adolescent anxiety? Results from the 1958 U.K. birth cohort and the National Child Development Study (2002). *American Journal Psychiatry*, 159, 1044–6.

Scott JR (1972). Vaginal bleeding in the midtrimester of pregnancy. *American Journal of Obstetrics and Gynecology*, 113, 329–334.

Stein Z and Susser M (1975). The Dutch famine, 1944–1945, and the reproductive process. I. Effects or six indices at birth. *Pediatric Research*, 9, 70–6.

Stevens JR (1997). Anatomy of schizophrenia revisited. *Schizophrenia Bulletin*, 23, 373–83.

Susser E and Terry MB (2003). A conception-to-death cohort. *Lancet*, 361, 797–8.

Susser ES, Hoek HW and Brown AS (1998). Neurodevelopmental disorders after prenatal famine: The story of the Dutch Famine Study. *American Journal of Epidemiology*, 147, 213–6.

Susser ES, Neugebauer R, Hoek HW *et al.* (1996). Schizophrenia after prenatal famine. Further evidence. *Archives of General Psychiatry*, 53, 25–31.

Susser ES, Schaefer CA, Brown AS, Begg MD and Wyatt RJ (2000). The design of the prenatal determinants of schizophrenia study. *Schizophrenia Bulletin*, 26, 257–73.

Torrey EF and Peterson MR (1973). Slow and latent viruses in schizophrenia. *Lancet*, 2, 22–4.

Waddington JL *et al.* (1999). Schizophrenia: Evidence for a 'cascade' process with neurodevelopmental origins. In Susser E, Brown A, and Gorman J (eds) *Prenatal Exposures in Schizophrenia*, pp. 3–34. American Psychiatric Press, Washington, DC.

Waddington JL and Youssef HA (1987). Is schizophrenia a neurodevelopmental disorder? *British Medical Journal (Clinical Research Edition)*, 295, 997–8.

Wadworth, ME (1987). Follow-up of the first national birth cohort: findings from the Medical Research Council National Survey of Health and Development. *Paediatric & Perinatal Epidemiology*, 1, 95–117.

Weinberger DR (1987). Implications of normal brain development for the pathogenesis of schizophrenia. *Archives of General Psychiatry*, 44, 660–9.

Chapter 2

Interactions of genetic predisposition and intrauterine events in the etiology of schizophrenia

Lauren M. Ellman and Tyrone D. Cannon

Genetic influences contribute substantially to the risk for developing schizophrenia, accounting for approximately 83 per cent of the variance (Cannon *et al.* 1998). Of the putative environmental contributors to the disorder, obstetric complications (OCs) are the most robust predictors of schizophrenia (McNeil 1988). There is still some controversy over whether the effects of OCs depend on (Cannon *et al.* 1990), covary with (Fish *et al.* 1992) or are independent of (Lewis and Murray 1987) genetic influences. Which of these models is correct is critical for efforts to locate predisposing genes for this disorder and could have significant implications for primary prevention. If obstetric risk factors are capable of producing schizophrenia by themselves, without the contribution of a genetic liability for schizophrenia (phenocopy model), then exposure to these risk factors (with a given degree of severity and in a specified time window) would be expected to lead to expression of the disorder reliably, and limiting exposure to such factors could constitute effective primary prevention. If obstetric risk factors are associated with the genes for schizophrenia (gene-environment covariation model), then one would expect a relative increase in the number of OCs in individuals carrying the genes for the disorder, regardless of whether they express the illness phenotypically. In this case, the influences of genetic and obstetric factors would be confounded, and it would not be clear whether the obstetric influences exert an etiologic effect that is independent of the effect exerted by genetic influences in schizophrenia, or vice versa. If an obstetric influence depends on the presence of genetic diathesis for schizophrenia (gene-environment interaction model), then the occurrence of an OC in a genetically vulnerable individual would increase the probability of the individual developing the disorder. Of course, it is also possible that genetic and obstetric risk factors for schizophrenia occur independently of each other but aggregate additively in influencing risk for disease expression (additive influences model). In practical terms, it is difficult to differentiate the gene-environment interaction model from the additive influences model, because both predict a relative increase in the rate of OCs among individuals who develop schizophrenia compared to their relatives who do not develop schizophrenia and compared to the general population.

This chapter summarizes recent work from our laboratory evaluating the manner in which pre- and perinatal events are linked to increased risk for developing schizophrenia, focusing in particular on hypoxia-associated OCs. Such complications are relatively common, occurring in the histories of approximately 30–40 per cent of cases of schizophrenia and approximately 5–10 per cent of the population overall (Cannon 1997; Buka *et al.* 1993). A series of OCs have been linked to schizophrenic outcome, such as fetal malnourishment, maternal infection during pregnancy, maternal stress during pregnancy, and rhesus incompatibility (Cannon 1997; Selten 1998, Buka *et al.* 2001, Brown and Susser 2002, Palmer *et al.* 2002, Verdoux, 2004). Nevertheless, it remains to be determined whether such factors increase risk for schizophrenia through a non-hypoxic mechanism. We will also discuss another class of OCs–maternal psychosocial stress during pregnancy–that has been evaluated as a risk factor for schizophrenia in only a small number of studies but which has the potential to explain a relatively large share of the non-genetic component of schizophrenia, given the relatively high base rate of psychosocial stress, particularly among mothers with schizophrenia.

Epidemiological studies of hypoxia-associated OCs as risk factors for schizophrenia

We have examined whether a history of OCs differentiated schizophrenic patients from their unaffected siblings in two epidemiological samples. The first sample consisted of the Philadelphia birth cohort from the National Collaborative Perinatal Project (NCPP). This project prospectively studied over 50,000 women and offspring from the prenatal period until 7 years after birth at multiple sites throughout the United States from 1959 to 1966. The Philadelphia cohort consisted of 9,236 offspring of 6,753 mothers who delivered at two inner-city hospitals; the offspring represented 90 per cent of all of the deliveries at these hospitals (Niswader and Gordon 1972). Forty six per cent of the children (n = 4,280) were from families with two or more children participating in the study.

In 1996, we conducted a search using the Penn Longitudinal Database (Rothbard *et al.* 1990), a database documenting contacts with public mental health facilities in Philadelphia from 1985 to 1995, to identify individuals from the NCPP cohort who had previous contact with a mental health professional. Our search yielded 1,197 individuals and of these individuals 339 (3.7 per cent of birth cohort) had a previous diagnosis of a psychotic disorder (194 with schizophrenia or schizoaffective disorder and 145 with affective or drug-induced psychosis). The remaining 858 individuals (9.3 per cent of birth cohort) received a psychiatric diagnosis without psychotic symptomatology, such as affective, anxiety, adjustment, developmental, and substance abuse disorders. The diagnoses obtained from this register were assigned by hundreds of mental health professionals, who likely used a variety of techniques in diagnostic assessments. As an attempt to validate the diagnoses from the register, we conducted a diagnostic validation study using the psychiatric medical records from the patients with a psychotic disorder. In total, we were able to access the medical records for 144 patients who had been treated at 15 mental health facilities. Chart reviews were conducted by 6 diagnosticians using a standard coding form based on DSM-IV criteria. Following chart reviews, 72 patients received a diagnosis of schizophrenia or schizoaffective disorder, 41 were diagnosed with a psychotic form of major depression or bipolar disorder, and 31 received a diagnosis of substance abuse, anxiety disorder, atypical psychosis, psychotic disorder due to a general medical condition, personality disorder or adjustment disorder. Of the 72 schizophrenia spectrum patients, 56 had siblings without a history of a psychiatric treatment who also participated in the NCCP study. Controls were individuals without a sibling with schizophrenia and who had not had contact with a mental health facility in the greater Philadelphia area as an adult (n = 7,914).

Extensive pre- and perinatal medical data were gathered on the participants in the NCPP study. Given previous findings linking hypoxia-associated obstetric complications to schizophrenic outcome (Cannon 1997), we were interested in exploring the relationship between the number and severity of hypoxia-associated complications and risk for schizophrenic outcome. A scale was developed to combine a series of complications associated with fetal and perinatal hypoxia. This scale included both indirect and direct indices of hypoxia. Direct hypoxia-associated complications included the following variables: blue at birth, required resuscitation, neonatal cyanosis, and neonatal apnea. Indirect complications were selected based on validation with direct measures of hypoxia from previous studies (Low *et al.* 1992; Arabin *et al.* 1993; Maier *et al.* 1994; Low *et al.* 1995; Adamson *et al.* 1995; Salafia *et al.* 1995). These included abnormalities of fetal heart rate or rhythm, umbilical cord knotted or wrapped tightly around neck, third trimester bleeding, placental hemorrhaging or infarcts, polyhydramnios, meconium in amniotic fluid, and breech presentation. Complications were each assigned 1 point on the scale.

Results from this study indicated that mother's age, baby's sex, birth order, sociol economic status (SES), and hypoxia-associated OCs significantly predicted schizophrenic outcome, whereas there were no significant effects of season of birth, birth weight and prenatal OCs unrelated to hypoxia, such as maternal infection during pregnancy. Risk for schizophrenia increased by 1.41 times for each 1-unit increase on the hypoxia-associated OC scale. Individuals with a history of three or more hypoxia-associated OCs were 3.84 times more likely to develop schizophrenia or schizoaffective disorder compared with individuals without such a history (see Figure 2.1). Moreover, we found no association between hypoxia-associated OCs and unaffected sibling status (see Figure 2.2), suggesting that this obstetric event differentiated unaffected and affected siblings.

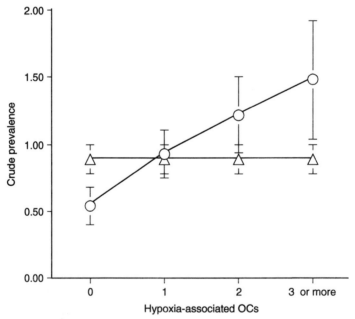

Figure 2.1 Prevalence (± standard errors) of schizophrenia as a function of the number of hypoxia-associated obstetric complications in their histories. Lines indicated by circles gives the observed prevalence of the psychotic outcome at each degree of hypoxia exposure. The line indicated by triangles gives the prevalence expected of no association between hypoxia and psychotic outcome. For every 1 unit increase on the hypoxia severity scale, there was a 1.41 increased likelihood of being schizophrenic ($p = 0.001$).

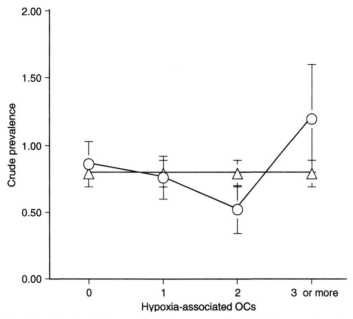

Figure 2.2 Prevalence (± standard errors) of being an unaffected sibling as a function of the number of hypoxia-associated obstetric complications in their histories. Lines indicated by circles gives the observed prevalence of sibling status at each degree of hypoxia exposure. The line indicated by triangles gives the prevalence expected of no association between hypoxia and sibling status. No significant relationship was found between hypoxia and unaffected sibling status.

Interestingly, the relationship between hypoxia-associated OCs and schizophrenic outcome was confined to patients who exhibited an early age at first treatment contact. Patients were separated into early and late ages of first treatment contact (median age = 27.1 years) and hypoxic pre- and perinatal events only predicted the psychotic status for individuals with an early age at first treatment. Conversely, hypoxia-associated OCs were not associated with psychotic status for those individuals with a later age at first treatment (see Table 2.1).

We followed up this study by examining the strength and generalizability of the aforementioned results, by examining the role of fetal hypoxia on schizophrenic outcome using an epidemiologically ascertained sample from a 1955 Finnish birth cohort. In this study we were able to verify psychiatric morbidity by interviewing all participants with the Structured Clinical Interview for DSM-III-R, Patient or Non-Patient edition (SCID) (Spitzer *et al.* 1987). Similar to the results from the Philadelphia Birth Cohort, we found that

Table 2.1 Frequencies (and percentages) of hypoxia-associated obstetric complications by adult psychiatric outcome

Obstetric variable	No diagnosis	Schizophrenia Early-onset	Later-onset	Non-schizophrenic siblings
Abnormal heart rate/rhythm	732 (10.6)	6 (17.6)	3 (8.3)	2 (3.2)
Blue at birth	1,360 (19.9)	13 (38.2)	7 (20.0)	19 (30.7)
Required resuscitation	50 (0.8)	1 (3.0)	1 (2.9)	0 (0)
Neonatal apnea	111 (1.6)	0 (0)	1 (2.8)	1 (1.6)
Cyanosis	53 (0.8)	1 (2.9)	0 (0)	1 (1.6)
Cord knotted/wrapped around neck	1,748 (25.6)	14 (41.2)	9 (25.7)	17 (27.0)
Third trimester bleeding	1,182 (17.4)	12 (35.3)	5 (14.7)	8 (12.7)
Placental hemorrhaging/infarcts	354 (5.1)	0 (0)	1 (2.8)	1 (1.6)
Polyhydramnios	58 (0.9)	0 (0)	2 (5.9)	1 (1.6)
Meconium in amniotic fluid	1,581 (23.6)	15 (45.5)	10 (28.6)	15 (24.6)
Breech presentation	136 (1.7)	0 (0)	1 (2.6)	1 (1.6)
Hypoxia scale (sum of above items)				
0	2777 (35.0)	5 (14.7)	10 (26.3)	24 (38.1)
1	2,885 (36.3)	9 (26.5)	18 (47.4)	22 (34.9)
2	1,544 (19.5)	11 (32.4)	8 (21.1)	8 (12.7)
3 or more	734 (9.2)	9 (26.5)	2 (5.3)	9 (14.3)

hypoxia-associated obstetric complications significantly predicted schizophrenic status for patients with an early age of first onset (see Table 2.2). We also found no association between prenatal exposure to infection or fetal growth retardation and schizophrenic status, suggesting that other possible teratogens did not equally portend psychotic status. Moreover, there was no relationship between a history of hypoxia-associated OCs and non-affected sibling status. Of particular note was that the rates of exposure to hypoxia-associated obstetric complications or other complications were comparable between patients with later-onset schizophrenia, non-schizophrenic siblings of patients, and demographically similar comparison subjects. This finding is important because it weakens the gene-environment covariation model, which asserts that fetal hypoxia may be associated with a genetic risk for schizophrenia. Given that the unaffected siblings likely carry genes for the disorder, if the gene-environment covariation was correct, we would expect an increased rate of OCs in siblings of schizophrenic patients, which we did not observe.

Table 2.2 Obstetric characteristics by adult diagnostic outcome (Mean ± SD or N (%))

Characteristics	Early-onset schizophrenia (N = 36)[b]	Later-onset schizophrenia (N = 44)[b]	Siblings (N = 61)[b]	Comparison subjects (N = 56)[b]	Analysis F, df	Analysis X², df
Birthweight (g)[a]	3401.5 ± 594.3	3605.0 ± 465.5	3467.4 ± 516.2	3598.1 ± 516.0	1.4, 3	
Birth length (cm)[a]	49.9 ± 2.0	50.5 ± 1.9	50.2 ± 1.9	50.4 ± 2.4	0.5, 3	
Placental weight (g)[a]	651.8 ± 107.3	662.3 ± 131.6	635.3 ± 104.5	661.0 ± 110.3	0.5, 3	
Placental size (cm²)[a]	329.3 ± 81.9	329.9 ± 77.6	328.3 ± 81.1	355.7 ± 91.6	0.7, 3	
Head circumference (cm)[a]	349.3 ± 12.1	352.4 ± 14.5	349.2 ± 12.9	345.0 ± 14.3	0.9, 3	
Gestational age (wks)	37.6 ± 2.7	37.9 ± 1.3	37.8 ± 1.9	37.5 ± 2.5	0.3, 3	
Fetal growth retardation	7 (19.4)	8 (18.2)	14 (22.9)	7 (12.5)		2.2, 3
Fetal infection	1 (6.3)	5 (20.0)	5 (16.7)	3 (5.7)		4.8, 3
Birth asphyxia[c]	8 (34.8)	3 (9.1)	7 (16.3)	3 (6.1)		9.4, 1*

[a] Adjusted for gestational age, gender, and social class.

[b] Note: because not all obstetric data were available for every subject, percent values are sometimes based on a smaller sample size.

[c] Later-onset schizophrenics, unaffected siblings, and non-psychiatric comparison subjects were collapsed into an overall comparison group for analyses of individual hypoxia-associated OCs, as none of the three groups were associated with hypoxia at the multivariate level.

* p < 0.01.

In addition, the majority of subjects with a history of hypoxia-associated obstetric complications did not become schizophrenic; therefore it is unlikely that this obstetric event independently causes schizophrenia, weakening support for the phenocopy model. Further, 33 per cent of the patients with schizophrenia (22 per cent of those with early-onset schizophrenia) had no history of hypoxia-associated obstetric complications, therefore it appears that contrary to our earlier findings fetal asphyxia does not necessitate an earlier form of the disorder, but still increases the likelihood of it.

Results from these studies support the gene-environment interaction model, because a history of hypoxia-associated OCs significantly differentiated schizophrenic patients from their unaffected siblings, suggesting that this obstetric event interacted with a genetic diathesis for the disorder that, in turn, led to one sibling developing the disorder. Further, findings from these studies suggest that hypoxia-associated OCs are not a necessary condition for developing the disorder, since OCs did not predict schizophrenia with a later age of onset. It seems as if schizophrenic patients with a history of hypoxia-associated OCs may represent a unique group of individuals, characterized by an earlier age of onset and possibly a worsened clinical picture. Despite these findings, it also appears that there are multiple etiological pathways for the emergence of schizophrenic symptomatology, some of which do not rely on the occurrence of an early hypoxia-related neuronal injury, since not all schizophrenic patients have a history of hypoxia-associated OCs.

Animal models of fetal hypoxia

Animal studies have linked early hypoxic events to alterations in neuronal substrate implicated in schizophrenia. Hypoxia-associated OCs have been found to affect many areas of the brain and often the results depend on the severity, duration, and timing of the hypoxic event. A complete review of this literature is beyond the scope of this chapter; thus we will focus primarily on animal findings most relevant to proposed models of brain abnormalities found in schizophrenic patients (Nayakas *et al.* 1996).

Rees *et al.* (1998) examined the effects of hypoxemia, secondary to prolonged placental insufficiency, on fetal brain development in sheep. The results indicated that hypoxemia disrupted neuronal development and connections in the hippocampus, cerebellum, and visual cortex. When the duration of the hypoxia was increased to twenty days during late gestation, abnormalities were found in the cerebellum and white matter lesions were found in the cortex. Shorter periods of hypoxia during mid-gestation were associated with reductions in the cortical white matter, as well as hippocampal density reductions.

In addition, findings from rat studies have linked perinatal oxygen insufficiency (induced by caesarian section) with dopamine hypofunction in the prefrontal cortex, increased dopamine (DA) levels in the nucleus accumbens and striatum, and increased dopamine D1 receptor binding in the nucleus accumbens (El-Khodor and Boksa 1997; Boksa *et al.* 2002; Brake *et al.* 2000). Similarly, rats exposed to hypoxic events between postnatal days 7 and 11 (similar to weeks 32–36 of gestation for humans) exhibited deficits in working memory, increased sleep, locomotor hyperactivity, and increased D1 and VMAT2 protein expression in the striatum (Decker *et al.* 2003).

Effects of OCs on brain function and structure in schizophrenia patients

Similar to findings from animal studies, a history of fetal hypoxia has been associated with structural brain abnormalities in schizophrenic patients. Using a 1955 birth cohort from Helsinki Finland (Cannon *et al.* 2002), magnetic resonance imaging (MRI) scans were conducted with 64 schizophrenic and schizoaffective patients, 51 non-psychotic siblings, and 54 demographically matched controls without a family history of psychosis. Results from this study indicated that a history of fetal hypoxia was significantly associated with reduced gray matter and increased cerebrospinal fluid (CSF) throughout the cortex in psychotic patients and their unaffected siblings (see Figures 2.3 and 2.4). These reductions were greatest in the temporal lobe and when the hypoxia occurred in cases who were born small for their gestational age (defined as birth weight at or below the tenth percentile for a given gestational age; see Table 2.3). Further, fetal hypoxia predicted enlarged ventricles among patients, but not among unaffected siblings. Moreover, fetal hypoxia was not related to any reductions in regional brain volumes among control participants and was unrelated to reductions in white matter among any of the comparison groups. Finally, there were main effects of small for gestational age status and prenatal infection status on reduced gray matter volumes and sulcal CSF.

There are multiple explanations that could account for the aforementioned findings. First, one could make the argument that OCs other than hypoxia, such as fetal growth retardation and prenatal infection, contribute to or account for the structural brain abnormalities found in this study. This explanation is unlikely, since neither variable was significantly associated with fetal hypoxia or adult psychotic status. Furthermore, controlling for fetal growth retardation and prenatal infection did not modify the significance of the fetal hypoxia results. Another interpretation is that a neurally disruptive mechanism other

Table 2.3 Regional gray (GM) and white matter (WM) and sulcal (SCSF) and ventricular cerebrospinal fluid (VCSF) brain ratios by risk group and fetal hypoxia*

Tissue	Region	Patients No Hypoxia	Hypoxia	ES	Siblings No Hypoxia	Hypoxia	ES	Controls No Hypoxia	Hypoxia	ES
		(N = 49)	(N = 15)		(N = 38)	(N = 13)		(N = 42)	(N = 12)	
GM	Frontal	52.8 + 0.5	49.9 + 0.8	−0.384†	53.8 + 0.6	51.7 + 0.8	−0.332‡	53.8 + 0.7	54.3 + 0.9	0.071
	Temporal	62.1 + 0.5	58.0 + 0.8	−0.555†	62.5 + 0.6	59.4 + 0.8	−0.472†	63.2 + 0.7	63.5 + 0.9	0.052
	Posterior	53.2 + 0.5	50.9 + 0.8	−0.308‡	52.2 + 0.6	49.8 + 0.8	−0.372‡	52.1 + 0.7	52.5 + 0.9	0.064
WM		35.0 + 0.4	34.5 + 0.6	−0.109	35.1 + 0.4	35.7 + 0.5	−0.151	35.8 + 0.4	35.7 + 0.6	−.025
SCSF	Frontal	12.1 + 0.7	16.1 + 1.0	0.451†	11.3 + 0.8	12.7 + 1.0	0.171	10.1 + 0.8	10.3 + 1.1	−0.026
	Temporal	7.1 + 0.7	11.3 + 1.0	0.471†	6.4 + 0.8	8.9 + 1.0	0.331‡	5.3 + 0.8	5.2 + 1.1	−0.006
	Posterior	7.6 + 0.7	9.8 + 1.0	0.245§	7.8 + 0.8	9.7 + 1.0	0.245	7.4 + 0.8	7.3 + 1.1	−0.015
VCSF		1.7 + 0.2	2.5 + 0.3	0.314‡	1.5 + 0.2	1.8 + 0.3	0.114	1.6 + 0.2	1.3 + 0.3	−0.109

*Values are least square means + SEM adjusted for total brain volume, age, gender, substance abuse, maternal infection during pregnancy, prematurity/small-for-gestational-age status, and family membership; ES refers to effect size, defined as the difference in the means of the group with hypoxia compared to the group without, divided by their pooled standard deviation.

† $p < 0.001$; ‡ $p < 0.01$; § $p < 0.05$.

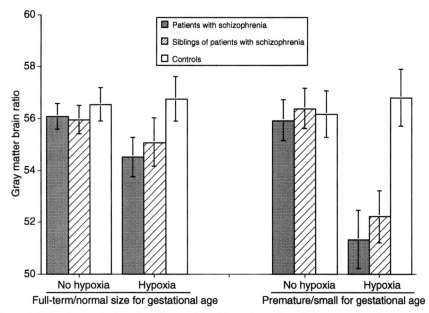

Figure 2.3 The figure depicts the effects of fetal hypoxia and small for gestational age status on least square mean ± standard errors) gray matter–brain ratios of schizophrenic patients, siblings, and controls. Out of 64 schizophrenic patients, 51 were normal size at birth (10 with and 41 without a history of fetal hypoxia) and 13 were small for their gestational ages (5 with and 8 without a history of fetal hypoxia). Among the 51 siblings, 37 were normal size at birth (8 with and 29 without a history of fetal hypoxia) and 14 were small for gestational age (5 with and 9 without a history of fetal hypoxia). Among the 54 controls, 42 were normal size at birth (8 with and 34 without a history of fetal hypoxia) and 12 were small for gestational age (4 with and 8 without a history of fetal hypoxia).

than oxygen insufficiency accounts for the neuronal abnormalities found in this study, since we found no significant reductions in white matter volumes typically associated with hypoxia. However, as mentioned previously, the effects of hypoxia on the brain depend on the time, duration, and severity of the hypoxic event. These effects can range from abnormalities in dendritic aborization and neurite outgrowth to cell death, whereby reductions in both white and gray matter would be expected primarily in the extreme cases (Nayakas *et al.* 1996). Further, data from fetal sheep studies suggest that hypoxia (secondary to placental insufficiency) resulted in significant reductions in the thickness of cortical structures, without any damage to cortical white matter, which was due to increases in the density of neurons due to reduced synaptogenesis and neuropil development (Rees *et al.* 1998). The structural brain abnormalities found in this study conform to the aforementioned findings,

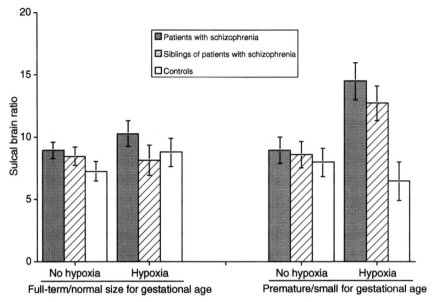

Figure 2.4 This figure depicts the effects of fetal hypoxia and small for gestational age states on least square mean (± standard errors) overall sulcal cerebrospinal fluid–brain ratios of schizophrenic patients, siblings, and controls. Sample sizes are provided in Figure 2.3.

since reductions in neuropil outgrowth would result in reductions in gray matter volume, but not white matter, suggesting that the synaptic contacts between neurons, rather than cell bodies and their axons, are disrupted.

This study lends further support to the gene-environment interaction model for multiple reasons. First, these data weaken support for the phenocopy model that supposes that the OCs act independently of a genetic vulnerability to cause the disorder. The phenocopy model would predict that all of the individuals exposed to hypoxia-associated OCs should exhibit brain abnormalities associated with schizophrenia, which was not supported by our data. Our results found structural brain abnormalities only in individuals at heightened genetic risk for the disorder (schizophrenic patients and non-affected siblings) and not in controls at low genetic risk for the disorder, thus providing evidence for the gene-environment interaction model. Moreover, the effects of hypoxia on gray matter and sulcal CSF were greater among patients than their siblings, and the effects of hypoxia on ventricular CSF were only present among patients. These findings suggest that hypoxia differentially affected brain structures in patients who presumably carry a greater genetic vulnerability to schizophrenia compared with their non-psychotic siblings.

Using the same Finnish birth cohort, high-resolution MRIs were conducted to measure hippocampal volumes in the three comparison groups (see Van Erp *et al.* 2002 for more details pertaining to this methodology). Results indicated that as the degree of genetic liability for schizophrenia increased, hippocampal volumes decreased (see Figure 2.5). Specifically, psychotic patients had smaller hippocampal volumes than their non-psychotic siblings and non-psychotic siblings had smaller hippocampal volumes than healthy comparison subjects. In addition, when comparing patients with and without a history of hypoxia to healthy controls combined with unaffected siblings (groups were combined for added power), there were marginal group-by-hypoxia interaction effects (see Figure 2.6); however, these results appeared to be influenced primarily by a small effect of hypoxia in the psychotic cohort. To explore this finding further, the effects of hypoxia were analyzed within the psychotic cohort. Results indicated that patients exposed to a hypoxia-associated OCs had significantly smaller hippocampal volumes than those who were not exposed to hypoxia.

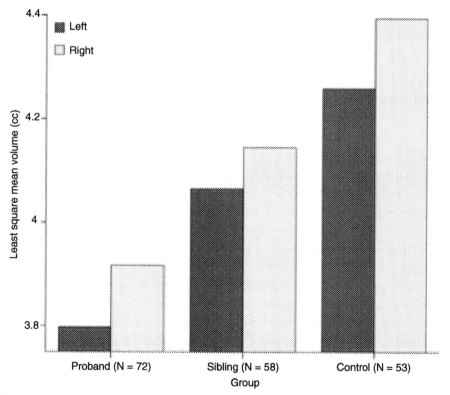

Figure 2.5 Hippocampal volumes in patients with schizophrenia or schizoaffective disorder, their unaffected siblings, and healthy comparison subjects with no family history of psychosis.

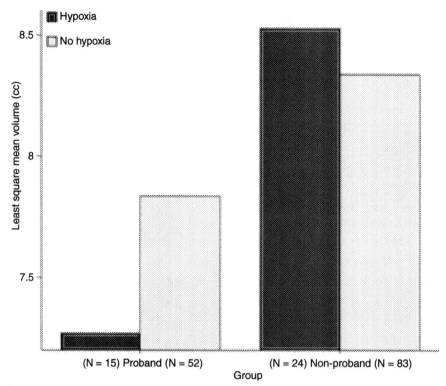

Figure 2.6 Relation of fetal hypoxia to hippocampal volumes in patients with schizophrenia or schizoaffective disorder and in unaffected subjects (unaffected siblings and healthy controls combined to increase power).

Additional analyses were conducted to corroborate the aforementioned findings, exploring the relationship between fetal hypoxia and hippocampal volume differences between patients and their unaffected siblings. The findings revealed a marginal main effect of hypoxia. Moreover, the differences in volumes were significantly larger for the groups exposed to hypoxia compared with the groups without such a history (see Figure 2.7). Finally, within the schizophrenic/schizoaffective disorder patients, smaller hippocampal volumes correlated positively with age at onset independent of duration of illness.

These findings likely suggest that genes associated with schizophrenia are responsible for reductions in hippocampal volumes found in patients and non-psychotic siblings, evidenced by a step-wise decrease in hippocampal volumes with increased genetic liability for the disorder. Based on twin and adoption studies that have found little to no association with shared familial environments and risk for schizophrenia, it is unlikely that shared environmental influences account for these hippocampal reductions (Cannon *et al.* 1998).

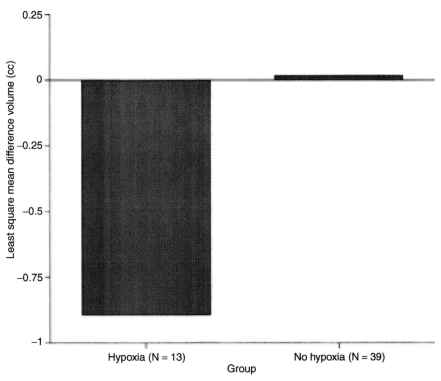

Figure 2.7 Relation of fetal hypoxia to hippocampal volume differences between patients with schizophrenia or schizoaffective disorder and their unaffected siblings.

In addition, smaller hippocampal volumes were found in patients and non-psychotic siblings exposed to fetal hypoxia compared to those without such a history, which lends support to the interaction model.

The two studies discussed above linking fetal hypoxia to structural brain abnormalities in schizophrenic patients add to a body of research suggesting that the neural abnormalities in schizophrenia may have a developmental origin. At the end of this chapter, we describe a neurodevelopmental model of schizophrenia that helps to explain the role of these early environmental insults within the context of the developing human brain.

Psychosocial stress during pregnancy and schizophrenia

Findings such as the ones mentioned above have provoked an interest in exploring the relationship between pre- and perinatal factors and the development of schizophrenia. One focus of these investigations has been on examining how psychosocial stress during pregnancy is related to the risk for developing schizophrenia in offspring. There is considerable debate over the term 'stress'. Despite this ambiguity, researchers have attempted to explore whether maternal stress experienced during pregnancy can adversely affect fetal development and create an additional vulnerability for disorders such as schizophrenia. Huttunen and Niskanen (1978) found an association between the loss of a father during months 3–5 and 9–10 of pregnancy and increased risk for schizophrenic outcome, as well as the likelihood of committing crimes in adulthood. Another study (van Os and Selten 1998) suggested that first trimester exposure to the May 1940 invasion of the Netherlands by the German army significantly predicted adult schizophrenic outcome, whereas exposure to another type of stressor (the 1953 Dutch flood) only marginally increased the risk of non-affective psychosis and schizophrenia during all three trimesters of pregnancy (Selten *et al.* 1999). Despite accumulating data suggestive of a link between psychosocial stress during pregnancy and increased risk for schizophrenia in offspring, no studies have systemically explored the inter-action between psychological functioning during pregnancy and a genetic diathesis for schizophrenia in a prospective design. Moreover, in all of the above studies, pertaining to schizophrenic outcome, stress was not directly measured, but rather assumed based on events that were presumed to be stressful for an entire population.

Despite the apparent limitations of the available studies linking maternal psychosocial stress during pregnancy to schizophrenic outcome of offspring, hormones associated with psychological stress have been hypothesized to affect much of the same neuronal changes implicated in schizophrenia. Animal studies suggest that exposure to chronic stress can lead to dendritic atrophy, suppressed neurogenesis, and cell death in the hippocampus (McEwen 1999; Sapolsky 1992). Similarly, some findings have indicated that corticotropin-releasing hormone (CRH)–a hormone released during stress–produces sensitivity to dopamine (DA) agonists, suggesting that the hypothalamic-pituitary-adrenal axis (HPA axis) may modify DA receptor sensitivity; and likewise, DA/D2 agonism leads to increased cortisol release (reviewed in Walker *et al.* 1996). In human and animal studies, DA neuronal systems have been implicated in memory functioning, particularly working memory (Cannon *et al.* 2000; Muller *et al.* 1998; Glickstein *et al.* 2002) which is especially relevant for understanding schizophrenia given consistent findings of abnormalities in DA functioning and working memory deficits in schizophrenic patients (Saykin *et al.* 1994; Grace and Moore 1998). Given the aforementioned findings, how could maternal stress during pregnancy affect fetal development? If the mother experienced heightened stress during pregnancy, we could expect there to be elevated levels of cortisol (and other stress hormones) that could travel across the placenta and lead to dopaminergic receptor sensitivity in the fetal brain, abnormal fetal HPA-axis functioning, and structural changes in the hippocampus. In turn, these changes in fetal neuronal development could lead to learning and memory deficits in offspring, as well as changes in reactivity to stimuli because of altered HPA-axis functioning.

This proposed model is supported by data from rat studies, which suggests that prenatal stress leads to a reduction in hippocampal cell proliferation, altered HPA-axis functioning, and deficits in spatial learning in offspring (Lemaire *et al.* 2000). Moreover, studies with rhesus monkeys demonstrate that norepinepherine and epinepherine may be related to decrease blood flow to the uterus, hypotension in the mother, and bradycardia (slow heart rate, usually defined as less than 60 beats per minute) in fetuses, which suggests a reduction in oxygen levels in blood traversing the placenta (Paarlberg *et al.* 1995). Other animal studies have found that elevated cortisol levels resulted in decreases in utero-placental blood flow, which lead to decreased oxygen to the fetal brain; therefore maternal psychosocial stress during pregnancy is likely an alternative pathway by which the effects of hypoxia could alter neuronal development (Bocking *et al.* 1986). As mentioned earlier in this chapter, there are many effects of decreased oxygen to the fetal brain, some of which are damage in temporal and subcortical brain regions, including the hippocampus (Rees *et al.* 1998).

The neurodevelopmental model of schizophrenia

The neurodevelopmental model of schizophrenia helps to explain further how early environmental insults, such as stress during pregnancy and OCs, fit within the structural and functional development of the central nervous system (Feinberg 1982). In normal development, synaptic density increases until approximately two years of age, slowly declining during childhood, and then declining steeply during late childhood and early adolescence (Huttenlocher 1979). Early in development there is an excess of axons in the cortex, as well as superfluous axonal projections to neuronal sites, which dramatically changes in the mature brain (Owen *et al.* 1988). During adolescence, there is a sharp decrease in synaptic density, as well as axon retraction and neuronal fallout, which coincides with an emergence of abilities to solve highly abstract and complex problems. According to the neurodevelopmental model, schizophrenic patients may have too many, too few, or unnecessary synaptic connections that are eliminated during adolescence, which results in the onset of psychotic symptomatology. Essentially, according to this view, schizophrenia would occur due to an abnormally aggressive synaptic pruning process, leading to a reduction in synaptic connectivity beyond a psychosis threshold (Feinberg 1982; Cannon *et al.* 1999; McGlashan and Hoffman, 2000).

Early environmental insults during the pre- or perinatal periods would fit within this neurodevelopmental model by reducing the amount of synaptic pruning necessary to cause psychotic symptomatology, which would lead to an earlier age of onset, and possibly portend a worsened clinical outcome. During the synaptic pruning process in adolescence, neurons will compete to form connections with target areas of the brain; however, if the target site is lesioned or the process is interrupted, neuronal cell death can occur. In addition, there can be a fall out rate from competing neurons in adjacent neuronal substrates. Axonal elimination during development, as well as programmed cell death, is thought to be controlled by a feedback system from the target cell, whereby the innervating neurons competes for a tropic factor necessary to maintain the connection, and when there is a neurobiological lesion this leads to asynchronous input to the target, and axonal eliminations occurs (Purves and Lichtmann 1980).

Summary

In conclusion, the preponderance of data linking intrauterine events to schizophrenic outcome supports the gene-environment interaction model. If this model is correct, we should be able to find genes that render the brain more vulnerable to the effects of hypoxia and other early environmental insults, such as maternal stress during pregnancy. Additional studies are needed to identify more precisely the specific changes in neuronal connectivity that are associated with the onset of psychotic symptoms and determine the mechanisms by which early insults such as fetal hypoxia contribute to determining the timing of onset (e.g. by interacting with later maturation events such as synaptic pruning). In addition, most of the research has focused on links between perinatal complications and schizophrenic outcome, while there have been fewer studies exploring the role of the prenatal period in the etiology of schizophrenia. As mentioned previously, research investigating the role of maternal stress during pregnancy as a risk factor for schizophrenia in offspring has been limited to retrospective studies with no direct psychological or neuroendocrine measures of stress. Prospective investigations are necessary to parse apart the putative roles of events during the prenatal period and the subsequent neurodevelopmental sequelae. More importantly, in a prospective design it would be more feasible to directly examine the interactions between intrauterine events, such as maternal stress during pregnancy, a genetic liability for schizophrenia. Further exploration into the aforementioned areas will ultimately aid in the development of early intervention strategies during the pre- and perinatal periods.

References

Adamson, S.J., Alessandri, L.M., Badawi, N., Burton, P.R., Pemberton, P.J. and Stanley, F. (1995) Predictors of neonatal encephalopathy in full-term infants. *BMJ*, 311, 598–602.

Arabin, B., Snyjders, R., Mohnhaupt, A., Ragosch, V. and Nicolaides, K. (1993) Evaluation of the fetal assessment score in pregnancies at risk for intrauterine hypoxia. *Am J Obstet Gynecol*, 169, 549–54.

Bocking, A.D., McMillen, I.C., Harding, R. and Thorburn, G.D. (1986) Effect of reduced uterine blood flow on fetal and maternal cortisol. *J Dev Physiol*, 8, 237–45.

Boksa, P., Zhang, Y. and Bestawros, A. (2002) Dopamine D1 receptor changes due to caesarean section birth: effects of anesthesia, developmental time course, and functional consequences. *Exp Neurol*, 175, 388–97.

Brake, W.G., Sullivan, R.M. and Gratton, A. (2000) Perinatal distress leads to lateralized medial prefrontal cortical dopamine hypofunction in adult rats. *J Neurosci*, 20, 5538–43.

Brown, A.S., and Susser, E.S. (2002). In utero infection and adult schizophrenia. *Ment Retard Dev Disabil Res Rev* 8(1), 51–7.

Buka, S.L., Tsuang, M.T. and Lipsitt, L.P. (1993) Pregnancy/delivery complications and psychiatric diagnosis. A prospective study. *Arch Gen Psychiatry*, 50, 151–6.

Buka, S.L., Tsuang, M.T., Torrey, E.F., Klebanoff, M.A., Bernstein, D., and Yolken, R.H. (2001). Maternal infections and subsequent psychosis among offspring. *Arch Gen Psychiatry*, 58(11), 1032–7.

Cannon, T.D., Mednick, S.A. and Parnas, J. (1990) Antecedents of predominantly negative- and predominantly positive-symptom schizophrenia in a high-risk population. *Arch Gen Psychiatry*, 47, 622–32.

Cannon, T.D. (1997) On the nature and mechanisms of obstetric influences in schizophrenia: A review and synthesis of epidemilogic studies. *International Review of Psychiatry*, 9, 387–397.

Cannon, T.D., Kapiro, J., Lonnqvist, J., Huttunen, M. and Koskenvuo, M. (1998) The genetic epidemiology of schizophrenia in a Finnish twin cohort: a population-based modeling study. *Archives of General Psychiatry*, 55, 67–74.

Cannon, T.D., Rosso, I.M., Bearden, C.E., Sanchez, L.E. and Hadley, T. (1999) A prospective cohort study of neurodevelopmental processes in the genesis and epigenesis of schizophrenia. *Development and Psychopathology*, 11, 467–485.

Cannon, T.D., Rosso, I.M., Hollister, J.M., Bearden, C.E., Sanchez, L.E. and Hadley, T. (2000) A prospective cohort study of genetic and perinatal influences in the etiology of schizophrenia. *Schizophr Bull*, 26, 351–66.

Cannon, T.D., van Erp, T.G., Rosso, I.M., Huttunen, M., Lonnqvist, J., Pirkola, T., Salonen, O., Valanne, L., Poutanen, V.P. and Standertskjold-Nordenstam, C.G. (2002) Fetal hypoxia and structural brain abnormalities in schizophrenic patients, their siblings, and controls. *Arch Gen Psychiatry*, 59, 35–41.

Decker, M.J., Hue, G.E., Caudle, W.M., Miller, G.W., Keating, G.L. and Rye, D.B. (2003) Episodic neonatal hypoxia evokes executive dysfunction and regionally specific alterations in markers of dopamine signaling. *Neuroscience*, 117, 417–25.

El-Khodor, B.F. and Boksa, P. (1997) Long-term reciprocal changes in dopamine levels in prefrontal cortex versus nucleus accumbens in rats born by Caesarean section compared to vaginal birth. *Exp Neurol*, 145, 118–29.

Feinberg, I. (1982) Schizophrenia: caused by a fault in programmed synaptic elimination during adolescence? *J Psychiatr Res*, 17, 319–34.

Fish, B., Marcus, J., Hans, S.L., Auerbach, J.G. and Perdue, S. (1992) Infants at risk for schizophrenia: sequelae of a genetic neurointegrative defect. A review and replication analysis of pandysmaturation in the Jerusalem Infant Development Study. *Arch Gen Psychiatry*, 49, 221–35.

Glickstein, S.B., Hof, P.R. and Schmauss, C. (2002) Mice lacking dopamine D2 and D3 receptors have spatial working memory deficits. *J Neurosci*, 22, 5619–29.

Grace, A.A. and Moore, H. (1998) Regulation of information flow in the nucleus accumbens: A model for the pathophysiology of schizophrenia. In M.F. Lezenweger, and R.H. Dworkin (eds) *Origins and Development of Schizophrenia*. American Psychological Association, Washington D.C., pp. 123–57.

Huttenlocher, P.R. (1979) Synaptic density in human frontal cortex–developmental changes and effects of aging. *Brain Res*, 163, 195–205.

Huttunen, M.O. and Niskanen, P. (1978) Prenatal loss of father and psychiatric disorders. *Arch Gen Psychiatry*, 35, 429–31.

Lemaire, V., Koehl, M., Le Moal, M. and Abrous, D.N. (2000) Prenatal stress produces learning deficits associated with an inhibition of neurogenesis in the hippocampus. *Proc Natl Acad Sci USA*, 97, 11032–7.

Lewis, S.W. and Murray, R.M. (1987) Obstetric complications, neurodevelopmental deviance, and risk of schizophrenia. *J Psychiatr Res*, 21, 413–21.

Low, J.A., Simpson, L.L. and Ramsey, D.A. (1992) The clinical diagnosis of asphyxia responsible for brain damage in the human fetus. *Am J Obstet Gynecol*, 167, 11–15.

Low, J.A., Simpson, L.L., Tonni, G. and Chamberlain, S. (1995) Limitations in the clinical prediction of intrapartum fetal asphyxia. *Am J Obstet Gynecol*, 172, 801–4.

Maier, R.F., Gunther, A., Vogel, M., Dudenhausen, J.W. and Obladen, M. (1994) Umbilical venous erythropoietin and umbilical arterial pH in relation to morphologic placental abnormalities. *Obstet Gynecol*, 84, 81–7.

McEwen, B.S. (1999) Stress and hippocampal plasticity. *Annu Rev Neurosci*, 22, 105–22.

Sapolsky, R. (1992) *Stress, the Aging Brain, and the Mechanisms of Neuronal Death*. MIT Press, Cambridge, MA.

McGlashan, T.H. and Hoffman, R.E. (2000) Schizophrenia as a disorder of developmentally reduced synaptic connectivity. *Archives of General Psychiatry*, 57, 637–47.

McNeil, T.F. (1988) Obstetric factors and perinatal injuries. In M.T. Tsaung and J.C. Simpson (eds) *Handbook of Schizophrenia*, vol. 3: Nosology, epidemiology and genetics, pp. 319–43. Elsevier Science Pub. Co.; New York.

Muller, U., von Cramon, D.Y. and Pollmann, S. (1998) D1- versus D2-receptor modulation of visuospatial working memory in humans. *J Neurosci*, 18, 2720–8.

Niswader, K.R. and Gordon, M. (1972) *The collaborative perinatal study of the National Institute of Neurological Diseases and Stroke: The women and their pregnancies*. W.B. Saunders, Philadelphia.

Nyakas, C., Buwalda, B. and Luiten, P.G. (1996) Hypoxia and brain development. *Prog Neurobiol*, 49, 1–51.

Owen, M.J., Lewis, S.W. and Murray, R.M. (1988) Obstetric complications and schizophrenia: a computed tomographic study. *Psychol Med*, 18, 331–9.

Paarlberg, K.M., Vingerhoets, J.J.M., Passchier, J., Dekker, G.A. and Van Geijn, H.P. (1995) Psychosocial factors and pregnancy outcome: A review with emphasis on methodological issues. *Journal of Psychosomatic Research*, 39, 563–95.

Palmer, C.G., Turunen, J.A., Sinsheimer, J.S., Minassian, S., Paunio, T., Lonnqvist, J. *et al.* (2002). RHD maternal-fetal genotype incompatibility increases schizophrenia susceptibility. *Am J Hum Genet,* 71(6), 1312–9.

Purves, D. and Lichtman, J.W. (1980) Elimination of synapses in the developing nervous system. *Science,* 210, 153–7.

Rees, S., Mallard, C., Breen, S., Stringer, M., Cock, M. and Harding, R. (1998) Fetal brain injury following prolonged hypoxemia and placental insufficiency: a review. *Comp Biochem Physiol A Mol Integr Physiol,* 119, 653–60.

Rothbard, A.B., Schinnar, A.P., Hadley, T.R. and Rovi, J.I. (1990) Integration of mental health data on hospital and community services. *Administrative and Policy in Mental Health,* 18, 91–9.

Salafia, C.M., Minior, V.K., Lopez-Zeno, J.A., Whittington, S.S., Pezzullo, J.C. and Vintzileos, A.M. (1995) Relationship between placental histologic features and umbilical cord blood gases in preterm gestations. *Am J Obstet Gynecol,* 173, 1058–64.

Saykin, A.J., Shtasel, D.L., Gur, R.E., Kester, D.B., Mozley, L.H., Stafiniak, P. and Gur, R.C. (1994) Neuropsychological deficits in neuroleptic naive patients with first-episode schizophrenia. *Arch Gen Psychiatry,* 51, 124–31.

Sapolsky, R. (1992). *Stress, the aging brain, and the mechanisms of neuronal death.* MIT Press; Cambridge.

Selten, J.P., van der Graaf, Y., van Duursen, R., Gispen-de Wied, C.C. and Kahn, R.S. (1999) Psychotic illness after prenatal exposure to the 1953 Dutch Flood Disaster. *Schizophr Res,* 35, 243–5.

Spitzer, R.L., Williams, J.B.W. and Gibbon, M. (1987) *Structured Clinical Interview for DSM-III-R (SCID).* Biometrics Research.

Van Erp, T.G., Saleh, P.A., Rosso, I.M., Huttunen, M., Lonnqvist, J., Pirkola, T., Salonen, O., Valanne, L., Poutanen, V.P., Standertskjold-Nordenstam, C.G. and Cannon, T.D. (2002) Contributions of genetic risk and fetal hypoxia to hippocampal volume in patients with schizophrenia or schizoaffective disorder, their unaffected siblings, and healthy unrelated volunteers. *Am J Psychiatry,* 159, 1514–20.

van Os, J. and Selten, J.P. (1998) Prenatal exposure to maternal stress and subsequent schizophrenia. The May 1940 invasion of The Netherlands. *Br J Psychiatry,* 172, 324–6.

Verdoux, H. (2004). Perinatal risk factors for schizophrenia: how specific are they? *Curr Psychiatry Rep,* 6(3), 162–7.

Walker, E.F., Neumann, C.C., Baum, K., Davis, D.M., DiForio, D. and Bergman, A. (1996) The developmental pathways to schizophrenia: Potential moderating effects of stress. *Development and Psychopathology,* 8, 647–65.

Chapter 3

Cognitive functioning before or at the onset of the first episode

Abraham Reichenberg and Michael Davidson

Introduction

A great deal of speculation and research has been devoted to determining whether a relationship exists between intellectual performance and schizophrenia. Since Kraepelin (1919) it has been recognized that deterioration in intellectual performance is a characteristic of schizophrenia patients. Bleuler (1950) described deterioration in school performance as a premorbid or prodromal sign in schizophrenia. However, despite decades of research, the developmental course of intellectual functioning in schizophrenia has been widely debated. Some studies have suggested that patients with schizophrenia suffer severe intellectual deficits during childhood and adolescence, while others imply that there is no basis for such severe deficits early in the development. Evidence for progressive deterioration in premorbid deficits has been presented, as well as studies showing stability of deficits. Some authors have provided evidence for a decline of intellectual ability from premorbid levels following the first psychotic episode, while others did not find evidence for such a decline. The focus of this chapter will be to review the literature pertaining to the presence of intellectual deficits during childhood and adolescence, and following the first psychotic episode in adult-onset schizophrenia in an effort to synthesize these disparate findings into a unified description of the course of intellectual functioning in schizophrenia.

Cognitive functioning after the onset of disease

A large body of evidence demonstrates that intellectual deviations from population norms are very common among chronic patients with schizophrenia. Between 75–85 per cent of all schizophrenia patients exhibit severe abnormal intellectual functioning (Kremen *et al.* 2000; Palmer *et al.* 1997; Weickert *et al.* 2000), scoring, an average of 19 IQ points below controls (Heinrichs and Zakzanis 1998). The deficit in general intellectual ability (IQ) is coupled with abnormalities in specific neuropsychological functions, particularly abnormal declarative memory, working memory, attention and executive functioning (Heinrichs and Zakzanis 1998; Palmer et al. 1997; Saykin et al. 1991).

Studies demonstrate that the deficits in IQ and in specific neuropsychological functions are already evident in patients after in the first psychotic episode. Saykin et al. (1994) studied 37 patients who were never exposed to neuroleptics medication. Patients showed a broad range of neuropsychological deficits, including in attention, abstraction, memory and learning. Patients performed 1 to 3 standard deviations (SD) below controls. Mohamed et al. (1999) studied 94 first episode patients of which the majority were neuroleptics naïve and demonstrated that as a group, patients were impaired on 29 out of the 30 neuropsychological measures assessed. Patients were performing between 1 to 2 standard deviations below controls on the majority of measures. Bilder et al. (2000) administered a comprehensive neuropsychological test battery to 94 first-episode patients after initial stabilization of psychosis. Patients were impaired on all 41 measures with the majority of deficits exceeding 1 SD. The magnitude of deficit in IQ was 1.7 SDs (equivalent to a 25 point difference). In a sample of 53 first episode patients, Bilder et al. (1991) demonstrated an average deficit of 24 IQ points.

Prospective longitudinal studies of schizophrenia patients following the first episode have suggested stability and even mild improvement over time. Censits et al. (1997) followed 30 first episode patients for 19 months. Patients remained 1 to 2 SDs below controls on all neuropsychological measures, with no significant change in performance over time. In another follow-up study, 35 first-episode or recent-onset schizophrenia patients were administered a comprehensive battery of neuropsychological tests during index hospitalization and at either 1 or 2 year follow-up examinations (Nopoulos et al. 1994). Neuropsychological deficits remained stable in most domains, with performance on tests of executive functions showing mild improvement over time.

Studies with longer duration of follow up show similar results. Gold et al. (1999) studied 54 first-episode or recent-onset schizophrenia patients and followed them for five years. They found a modest, 3-point improvement in IQ, especially in performance IQ. More specifically, 37 subjects improved their performance, 13 subjects performed worse, and four subjects showed no change. Change was also evident on specific neuropsychological measures; attention, memory and executive functions slightly improved, motor speed deteriorated. DeLisi et al. (1995) evaluated the longitudinal neuropsychological performance of 20 first episode patients at index hospitalization and at four year follow-up. The majority of the neuropsychological test scores did not change over time; improvement occurred in tests of concentration/speed, and overall global functioning. Hoff *et al.* (1999) studied language, executive, memory, processing speed, and sensory-perceptual functions in 42 patients with a first hospitalization for schizophrenia or schizophreniform disorder at approximate yearly intervals for the first 2–5 years of illness. Patients constantly scored 1 to 2 SDs below normal comparison subjects on neuropsychological test measures during the five-year course of the study. Patients exhibited some improvement on measures of language, executive functions and a mild decline in verbal memory.

Gender differences in cognitive functioning and the association with psychopathology

In their meta-analysis of neuropsychological performance in schizophrenia, Heinrichs and Zakzanis (1998) conclude that they found no significant relationships between IQ deficits and potential moderators including age, education, neuroleptic dose, sample gender composition, or age of illness onset. The correlations between neuropsychological functions and measures of psychopathology such as positive or negative symptoms are relatively modest (Saykin *et al.* 1994). In line with this observation, Mohamed *et al.* (1999) and Bilder *et al.* (2000) reported that worse neuropsychological performance was weakly correlated with severity of negative symptoms and neuroleptics dose. Higher correlations are observed between changes over time in neuropsychological functioning and change in psychopathology. Improvement in positive symptoms was associated with improvement in performance on measures of executive functions, memory and concentration/speed (Gold *et al.* 1999; Hoff *et al.* 1999). Gold *et al.* (1999) also reported that improvement in negative symptoms was a strong predictor for improvement in IQ. Censits *et al.* (1997), Hoff *et al.* (1999), and Bilder *et al.* (2000) explored sex differences in neuropsychological performance. No statistically significant gender differences in neuropsychological performance were evident in either study.

Taken together, these results suggest that schizophrenia patients exhibit severe and widespread neuropsychological deficits already at the first psychotic break. Specific neuropsychological deficits, such as in memory or executive functions, exist with a background generalized intellectual deficit. The deficits are largely constant over the first years following diagnosis, and improvement in the severity of symptomatology is associated with better cognitive functions.

Premorbid intellectual ability

Following Bleuler (1950) who described deterioration in school performance as a premorbid or prodromal sign in schizophrenia, a number of investigators have sought to determine whether lower IQ occurs as a precursor, or risk factor, for schizophrenia, or occurs only concomitantly with the overt expression of the illness.

The large majority of early studies of childhood and adolescence intellectual functioning of future schizophrenia patients were retrospective in nature, comparing the IQ scores of future schizophrenia patients with the IQ scores of their peers or schoolmates. For example, Albee et al. (1964) compared IQ scores of 122 second, 154 sixth and 103 eighth grade (ages 7, 12 and 14) future schizophrenia patients to all children in the same grade and school. These authors found significantly lower IQ scores in the future patients in all ages. The magnitude of deficits in future patients was between one half and two thirds of a standard deviation (8 to 10 IQ points). Offord and Cross (1971) studied 29 future patients through ninth grade and found them to be significantly impaired. The magnitude of impairment was 0.92 of a standard deviation (14 IQ points).

More recently, several epidemiological studies investigated the association between childhood and adolescence IQ and adult-onset schizophrenia. Epidemiological samples are representative of the population, and therefore protect against the ascertainment bias that often affects clinical samples. David et al. (1997) studied a population of 50,000 18-year-old Swedish male conscripts and found lower intellectual test scores in future schizophrenia patients. Davidson et al. (1999) reported similar results in a case-control study comparing 509 17-year-old Israeli male conscripts who were hospitalized one year or more after assessment and were compared to 9,215 never-hospitalized peers from the same school. The magnitude of deficit in this cohort was half a standard deviation (i.e., 8 IQ points) (Reichenberg et al. 2002). In contrast, Cannon et al. (1999) used a case-control design in a follow-up study of the Helsinki, Finland birth cohort, and found no significant differences in academic achievements between first to fourth grade (ages 7–11 years) between 400 future schizophrenia patients and 408 controls. However, future patients were less likely than controls to progress to high school. Isohanni et al. (1998) reported similar findings in the ninth grade (age 16) using the eleven thousand offspring in the North Finland birth cohort. Again, future patients were significantly more likely not to be in age-appropriate class. The lack of significant differences in academic achievements in the study by Ishoanni et al. may reflect the characteristics of the Finnish school system; future schizophrenia patients were not compared to age-matched controls but with younger individuals, thus masking true differences in intellectual performance. The findings from both studies may also suggest a progressive deterioration in intellectual performance as evident by age-appropriate class-level lagging and lack of progress to high school.

Only a few studies have examined the longitudinal course of cognitive deviance in future schizophrenia patients. Lane and Albee (1968) compared the IQ scores of 41 future schizophrenia patients to the performance of some 4,000 of their peers at both second and sixth grade (ages 7 and 12). Future patients were 13 points below controls at age 7, but only 11 points below controls at age 12. Results from two longitudinal prospective epidemiological studies suggest a similar pattern. Cannon *et al.* (2002) used data collected in the Dunedin Multidisciplinary Health and Development Study and followed up 1,000 children from the general population from birth to age 26. These authors found that the 36 future patients (defined as individuals with a schizophreniform disorder) performed more poorly than controls on standard IQ tests at each of five assessments between ages 3 and 11 years. The deficit in IQ was about 0.4 of a SD (i.e., 6 IQ points), with no evidence for progressive decline. In fact, group scores seemed to slightly improve over time. Cannon *et al.* (2000) found no significant change in IQ scores between ages 4 and 7 in the Philadelphia sample of the National Collaborative Perinatal Project (Borman *et al.* 1975). In both assessments, 72 future schizophrenia patients were significantly impaired in comparison to 7,941 controls with no psychiatric diagnosis. The magnitude of deficit did not seem to change over time. In contrast, Jones and colleagues (1994) studied schizophrenia among the 5,362 members of the National Survey of Health and Development birth-cohort in the UK to study the association between child development and risk for schizophrenia. Mean scores in all educational tests at ages 8, 11 and 15 years were consistently lower for 30 future schizophrenia patients than controls. This effect seemed to become stronger with age, as evident by the fact that these differences were consistently statistically significant only at age 15. The future patients showed deficits ranging between 4–7 IQ points.

The evidence of possible progressive decline in intellectual functioning during adolescence is supported by several additional studies of both clinical and epidemiological samples. Rabinowitz *et al.* (2002) in a retrospective study of 535 first episode schizophrenia patients documented progressive decline in intellectual functioning from childhood to age 18. Rabinowitz *et al.* (2000) studied time-related differences in intellectual functioning in schizophrenia using the cross-sectional Israeli conscripts cohort (Davidson *et al.* 1999). The authors reported that the severity of age 17 intellectual deficits in a test of non-verbal abstract reasoning in adult-onset schizophrenia patients was inversely related to the age of first hospitalization. Fuller *et al.* (2002) compared educational development test scores of 70 future schizophrenia patients from the fourth, eighth and eleventh grades (ages 8, 12 and 17) to state norms and found that test scores in the patients group dropped significantly between grades 8 and 11 (ages 13–16). Van Oel *et al.* (2002) retrospectively studied school performance beginning at age 6, in 49 twin pairs of whom at least one suffered from schizophrenia, and 43 healthy control twins. The authors found that the divergence in performance (towards underperformance), which distinguished twins from affected families from control twins, was evident starting at early adolescence. Kremen *et al.* (1998) followed up a community sample from early childhood and showed that a large decline in IQ scores between 4 and 7 years of age was associated with increased risk for psychotic symptoms in adulthood.

The evidence reviewed so far indicates that future schizophrenia patients exhibit abnormal intellectual functioning already at early childhood. The premorbid deficit seems to be larger when premorbid data are collected later in life (i.e., ages 17 or 18 vs. ages 4 to 11), suggesting a further reduction between childhood and the first onset of the psychotic symptoms. The deficit in IQ seems, however, to be of larger magnitude when assessed in first-episode patients in comparison to assessments of deficits at the premorbid stage. Thus, an additional decline might follow the onset of the disorder.

From premorbid to post-onset intellectual ability

To determine whether IQ deteriorates with the onset of schizophrenia, several studies compared premorbid and postmorbid IQ scores of schizophrenia patients. In an early study, Rappaport and Webb (1950) administered schizophrenia patients the same intelligence tests they had taken during high school. The patients, as a group, deteriorated by 34 points. Lubin *et al.* (1962) administered army intelligence tests to male schizophrenia patients and compared the scores to those obtained by the same patients at the time of induction. Patients deteriorated up to one-third of a SD on the different tests. Schwartzman and Douglas (1962) using a similar design demonstrated an average loss of 6 IQ points, with a mean interval of 10 years between premorbid and morbid tests of 50 schizophrenia patients. A matched sample of

30 normal controls gained the equivalent of 6 IQ points. The non-verbal subtests in the battery reflected greater deficit than the verbal tests. The conclusion drawn from these studies was that the onset of schizophrenia is characterized by a decline in intellectual abilities.

A study by Albee and colleagues (1963), however, challenged this conclusion. The authors compared premorbid childhood (second and sixth grade) IQ scores of 112 adult schizophrenia patients with IQ scores obtained during the psychosis. IQ scores were consistently about 10 points below normal, yet no significant difference was found between early premorbid IQ scores and scores during the psychosis. Russell *et al.* (1997) examined the childhood IQ scores of adult patients with schizophrenia who had attended a child psychiatry service, where measurement of intelligence was routine. Follow-up IQ scores of 34 of these patients were obtained an average of 19.4 years later. The mean child and adult IQ scores were more than one SD lower than those of the general population. There were, however, no significant differences between the child and adult IQ scores, suggesting that the impairment in intelligence observed already during childhood was stable over the follow-up period.

The results of Albee *et al.* (1963) and Russell *et al.* (1997) may, however, be due to a sampling bias since mainly low functioning individuals were studied, which may have influenced the outcome. The Albee *et al.* sample was drawn from inner city students, while the majority of patients in the Russell *et al.* study were drawn from a population of children who had received treatment at child psychiatry clinic due to psychiatric and learning problems, many of whom had an IQ of 80 or below already at first assessment. This study could thus be interpreted as assessing the stability of intellectual deficits in early-onset psychotic patients rather than the change from premorbid to postmorbid stage.

Rabinowitz *et al.* (2000) in the study of the Israeli male conscripts, found that the deficits in a measure of non-verbal abstract reasoning in individuals first hospitalized in the year prior to testing was twice the deficit observed in individuals first hospitalized after testing was conducted. Sheitman *et al.* (2000) compared premorbid IQ assessed during routine educational assessments and current IQ in 27 treatment-resistant schizophrenia patients. The patients declined from an average IQ score of 93 to an average score of 83. Caspi *et al.* (2003) administered army intelligence tests to 44 first episode psychotic patients after stabilization, and compared the scores to those obtained by the same individuals at the time of mandatory screening by the army. Changes in performance among patients were compared to changes in healthy control subjects matched for age at second assessment. There were no statistically significant changes between the first and the second assessments among the schizophrenia patients on any measure. However, a between-group comparison of changes showed that relative to the healthy comparisons, schizophrenia patients deteriorated on a measure of non-verbal abstract reasoning, and on a measure sensitive to mental speed and concentration.

Premorbid estimates of IQ have been used routinely as a means of comparing current intellectual deficits with intellectual potential before the onset of the illness. These premorbid estimates are based on the assumption that certain cognitive functions are insensitive to brain damage. A frequently used measure of premorbid intellectual ability is the ability to read and pronounce single words, an ability often acquired at an early age. Several studies have demonstrated the validity of using reading and pronunciation tests as estimates of premorbid intellectual ability in patients with schizophrenia (Kremen *et al.* 1996). Using such a measure of premorbid IQ, Gold (1998) reported an average 9-point difference between current post-morbid IQ score and premorbid performance in a sample of 103 schizophrenia patients (Gold, 1998). Bilder *et al.* (2000) observed an average 7-point difference between current post-morbid IQ score and premorbid performance in his sample of first episode patients. Goldberg *et al.* (1995) have demonstrated a 10 point IQ discrepancy between affected and unaffected twin pairs discordant for schizophrenia, suggesting that the genetic potential of the twin with schizophrenia would be ten points above their current IQ score. Similarly, in a study of individuals with genetic predisposition for schizophrenia ('high-risk'), those high-risk individuals who had experienced an increase in psychotic symptoms were found to exhibit a decline in IQ (Cosway *et al.* 2000). The magnitude of decline, as evident from the difference between estimated premorbid and current IQ scores, was of 10 points. A similar average magnitude of difference between estimated premorbid and current IQ scores was observed in another study of 117 consecutively admitted patients with chronic schizophrenia (Weickert *et al.* 2000). More specifically however, 51 per cent of these patients displayed an average general intellectual decline of 17 points from estimated premorbid levels; 24 per cent had low estimated premorbid intellect and low current intellectual levels (an average IQ of 80), and 25 per cent displayed average estimated premorbid intellectual levels and no IQ decline (average IQ of 100).

Caspi *et al.* (2003) and Weickert *et al.* (2000) found no statistically significant relationship between medication status and cognitive decline. Caspi *et al.* (2003) found no association between severity of psychotic symptoms or duration of untreated psychosis and cognitive change. Weickert *et al.* (2000) found no association between duration of illness or age of onset and cognitive decline.

Thus, the intellectual decline seems essentially independent of clinical symptoms or neuroleptics treatment.

Specificity of premorbid intellectual deficits

Studies of premorbid intellectual functioning in individuals who develop non-schizophrenic disorders show some variation in results. Mason (1956) compared scores on the Army General Classification Test between 368 future schizophrenia patients, 188 non-schizophrenia psychiatric patients and 290 army inductees with no mental disorders. Future schizophrenia patients scored significantly lower than controls, but the non-schizophrenic patients had no significant deficits. More recently, Reichenberg *et al.* (2002, 2005) showed premorbid deficits in IQ in males diagnosed with schizophrenia-spectrum disorders. The deficits were similar, yet milder, to those observed in male schizophrenia patients. Similar results were reported by David *et al.* (1997), who showed premorbid deficits in IQ in males diagnosed with other psychosis. The group of 'other psychosis' included patients with both affective and non-affective psychosis. Van Os *et al.* (1997) followed up 5,362 births in England for affective illness, and found lower childhood intellectual functioning in future patients. In contrast, Cannon *et al.* (2002) and Reichenberg *et al.* (2002) did not find evidence for premorbid intellectual deficits in non-psychotic affective disorders. It is plausible that some of the discrepancies are a result of inclusion of affective disorder patients both with and without psychotic symptoms, suggesting that psychosis, in general, is associated with deficits in premorbid IQ.

Gender differences in premorbid intellectual functioning

The existence of gender differences in cognitive impairments in schizophrenia has frequently been disputed (Haas and Castle 1997). The evidence reviewed above suggests no gender difference in neuropsychological performance in first-episode patients. Gender differences in premorbid intellectual functioning, however, have not been studied frequently. Although an early study (Offord 1974) suggested more severe premorbid IQ deficits among males, one large-scale clinical study and three epidemiological studies, however, demonstrated a different pattern. Bilder *et al.* (2000) in a large sample of first-episode schizophrenia patients reported significantly greater impairment in estimated premorbid IQ among female compared to male patients. Reichenberg *et al.* (2002) reported more severe intellectual deficits at age 17 in future female than male patients. Jones and Done (1997) and Weiser *et al.* (2000) reported similar findings.

Differential premorbid deficits

One of the more consistent findings in schizophrenia is the tendency of patients to show milder verbal than performance IQ deficits (Aylward *et al.* 1984; Heinrichs and Zakzanis 1998). Similar results were evident in some (Bilder *et al.* 1991, 2000), but not all (Gold *et al.* 1999) studies of first-episode patients. The findings in studies of premorbid functioning are also inconclusive. David *et al.* (1997) found more severe premorbid impairment in measures of verbal abilities. In contrast, Reichenberg *et al.* (2002) and Jones *et al.* (1994) found more severe premorbid deficits in measures of non-verbal intelligence. As described above, Caspi *et al.* (2003) found evidence for cognitive decline following the first psychotic episode on measures of non-verbal abstract reasoning and speed and concentration, but not on measures of verbal ability. In the follow-up study by Gold *et al.* (1999), improvement over time was especially evident for performance IQ. Taken as a whole, these results might suggest that verbal abilities are relatively spared by the disease process, whereas non-verbal abilities are more sensitive to the illness (Lezak 1995).

Summary and synthesis of the findings

The evidence reviewed in this chapter strongly supports the view that cognitive deficits are a major characteristic of schizophrenia patients and, in a subgroup of patients, are already evident many years before a clinical diagnosis of schizophrenia is assigned. It might be argued that the low intellectual functioning merely reflects the prodrome to the illness. However, we believe this is unlikely since the association between IQ and schizophrenia was evident even in individuals first admitted up to ten years after assessment (David *et al.* 1997; Davidson *et al.* 1999). The association between schizophrenia and intellectual abnormalities could be confounded by a third factor(s), causing both schizophrenia and low IQ. However, the studies reviewed controlled for a number of possible confounders such as social abnormalities, drug use, economic disadvantage, obstetric conditions and comorbid psychiatric diagnoses with no considerable attenuation of the association between low intellectual ability and schizophrenia (Cannon *et al.* 2002; David *et al.* 1997; Davidson *et al.* 1999; Heinrichs and Zakzanis 1998; Reichenberg *et al.* 2005).

The course and time of onset of the intellectual deficits through development is not yet clear. However, available data suggests that a deficit in childhood or adolescence intellectual ability (i.e., IQ <85) is evident in approximately one third of future patients (Davidson *et al.* 1999; Jones *et al.* 1994; Reichenberg *et al.* 2004; Weickert *et al.* 2000) and these individuals probably do not continue to deteriorate (Russell *et al.* 1997; Weickert *et al.* 2000). This group is probably also exhibiting widespread neuropsychological deficits (Weickert *et al.* 2000). An additional 25 per cent of patients show normal intellectual functioning both before and following the first psychotic episode, displaying only mild and specific neuropsychological deficits. The remaining majority of patients probably exhibit intellectual decline between childhood and the first onset of the disorder. The decline conceivably predates psychotic symptoms in some (Kremen *et al.* 1998), in some become manifest concurrently with the onset of psychotic symptoms the prodrome (Cosway *et al.* 2000), in some only appearing following the psychotic disorder, and in some is probably a combination of two or more of the above processes. This decline is probably at a magnitude of 10 IQ points or more. This group is likely to have a heterogeneous profile of specific neuropsychological deficits.

A decline is likely to occur during adolescence (Fuller *et al.* 2002), a time of robust structural and functional brain changes. Several studies have provided evidence for a process of 'pruning' in which excess or non-useful neural connections are terminated, leading to decrease over time in synaptic density (Huttenlocher and Dabholkar 1997), glucose metabolism (Chugani *et al.* 1987), and cortical gray matter volume (Giedd *et al.* 1999). A longitudinal study has shown that the decrease in cortical gray matter over ages 13–17 in normal children was four times greater in cases with childhood onset schizophrenia, suggesting over-pruning (Rapoport *et al.* 1999). Further studies are required in order to evaluate the validity of this assumption.

The specific neuropsychological deficits against a background of general intellectual impairment have been interpreted as an indication for a more fundamental, or 'core', cognitive deficit in schizophrenia (Heinrichs and Zakzanis 1998; Weickert and Goldberg 2000). Executive functions, working memory and attention have been suggested as the necessary and perhaps sufficient type of cognitive impairment in schizophrenia (Silver *et al.* 2003; Weickert and Goldberg 2000). Reichenberg *et al.* (2005) demonstrated that premorbid deficits in non-verbal abstract reasoning present an additional risk beyond the global premorbid intellectual deficit. Caspi *et al.* (2003) showed that intellectual decline was specific to measures of non-verbal reasoning and speed and concentration. Measures of reasoning strongly involve executive processes and working memory (Carpenter *et al.* 1990), suggesting that the proposed 'core' deficits are also more intimately related to the developmental trajectories of the disorder.

The deficits in general intellectual ability and in specific neuropsychological functions appear stable over the first few years since the onset of psychotic symptoms. There is even some evidence suggesting mild improvement over time. The long-term stability of neuropsychological impairment is still an open question. Some suggest that the neuropsychological impairment in schizophrenia remain stable (Censits *et al.* 1997; Heaton *et al.* 2001), yet there is some evidence suggesting that intellectual ability *continues* to deteriorate later in life, especially in institutionalized poor-outcome patients (Davidson *et al.* 1996; Friedman *et al.* 2001; Harvey *et al.* 1999). Future longitudinal studies are likely to address this question.

References

Albee, G., Lane, E. and Reuter, J. (1964). Childhood intelligence of future schizophrenics and neighborhood peers. *Journal of Psychology,* 58, 141–144.

Albee, G. W., Lane, E. A., Corcoran, C. and Werneke, A. (1963). Childhood and intercurrent intellectual performance of adult schizophrenics. *Journal of Consulting Psychology,* 27(4), 364–366.

Aylward, E., Walker, E. and Bettes, B. (1984). Intelligence in schizophrenia: meta-analysis of the research. *Schizophr Bull,* 10(3), 430–459.

Bilder, R. M., Goldman, R. S., Robinson, D., Reiter, G., Bell, L., Bates, J. A., Pappadopulos, E., Willson, D. F., Alvir, J. M., Woerner, M. G., Geisler, S., Kane, J. M. and Lieberman, J. A. (2000). Neuropsychology of first-episode schizophrenia: initial characterization and clinical correlates. *Am J Psychiatry,* 157(4), 549–559.

Bilder, R. M., Lipschutz-Broch, L., Reiter, G., Geisler, S., Mayerhoff, D. and Lieberman, J. A. (1991). Neuropsychological deficits in the early course of first episode schizophrenia. *Schizophr Res,* 5(3), 198–199.

Bleuler, E. (1950). *Dementia Praecox, or the Group of Schizophrenias (1911).* New York: International Universities Press.

Borman, S. H., Nichols, P. I. and Kennedy, W. A. (1975). *Preschool IQ: Prenatal and Early Developmental Correlates.* New York, NY: Halsted Press.

Cannon, M., Caspi, A., Moffitt, T. E., Harrington, H., Taylor, A., Murray, R. M. and Poulton, R. (2002). Evidence for early-childhood, pan-developmental impairment specific to schizophreniform disorder: results from a longitudinal birth cohort. *Arch Gen Psychiatry,* 59(5), 449–456.

Cannon, M., Jones, P., Huttunen, M. O., Tanskanen, A., Huttunen, T., Rabe-Hesketh, S. and Murray, R. M. (1999). School performance in Finnish children and later development of schizophrenia: a population-based longitudinal study. *Arch Gen Psychiatry,* 56(5), 457–463.

Carpenter, P. A., Just, M. A. and Shell, P. (1990). What one intelligence test measures: a theoretical account of the processing in the Raven Progressive Matrices Test. *Psychol Rev,* 97(3), 404–431.

Caspi, A., Reichenberg, A., Weiser, M., Rabinowitz, J., Kaplan, Z., Knobler, H., Davidson-Sagi, N. and Davidson, M. (2003). Cognitive performance in schizophrenia patients assessed before and following the first psychotic episode. *Schizophr Res,* 65(2–3), 87–94.

Censits, D. M., Ragland, J. D., Gur, R. C. and Gur, R. E. (1997). Neuropsychological evidence supporting a neurodevelopmental model of schizophrenia: a longitudinal study. *Schizophr Res,* 24(3), 289–298.

Chugani, H. T., Phelps, M. E. and Mazziotta, J. C. (1987). Positron emission tomography study of human brain functional development. *Ann Neurol,* 22(4), 487–497.

Cosway, R., Byrne, M., Clafferty, R., Hodges, A., Grant, E., Abukmeil, S. S., Lawrie, S. M., Miller, P. and Johnstone, E. C. (2000). Neuropsychological change in young people at high risk for schizophrenia: results from the first two neuropsychological assessments of the Edinburgh High Risk Study. *Psychol Med,* 30(5), 1111–1121.

David, A. S., Malmberg, A., Brandt, L., Allebeck, P. and Lewis, G. (1997). IQ and risk for schizophrenia: a population-based cohort study. *Psychol Med,* 27(6), 1311–1323.

Davidson, M., Harvey, P., Welsh, K. A., Powchik, P., Putnam, K. M. and Mohs, R. C. (1996). Cognitive functioning in late-life schizophrenia: a comparison of elderly schizophrenic patients and patients with Alzheimer's disease. *Am J Psychiatry,* 153(10), 1274–1279.

Davidson, M., Reichenberg, A., Rabinowitz, J., Weiser, M., Kaplan, Z. and Mark, M. (1999). Behavioral and intellectual markers for schizophrenia in apparently healthy male adolescents. *Am J Psychiatry,* 156(9), 1328–1335.

DeLisi, L. E., Tew, W., Xie, S., Hoff, A. L., Sakuma, M., Kushner, M., Lee, G., Shedlack, K., Smith, A. M. and Grimson, R. (1995). A prospective follow-up study of brain morphology and cognition in first-episode schizophrenic patients: preliminary findings. *Biol Psychiatry,* 38(6), 349–360.

Friedman, J. I., Harvey, P. D., Coleman, T., Moriarty, P. J., Bowie, C., Parrella, M., White, L., Adler, D. and Davis, K. L. (2001). Six-year follow-up study of cognitive and functional status across the lifespan in schizophrenia: a comparison with Alzheimer's disease and normal aging. *Am J Psychiatry,* 158(9), 1441–1448.

Fuller, R., Nopoulos, P., Arndt, S., O'Leary, D., Ho, B. C. and Andreasen, N. C. (2002). Longitudinal assessment of premorbid cognitive functioning in patients with schizophrenia through examination of standardized scholastic test performance. *Am J Psychiatry,* 159(7), 1183–1189.

Giedd, J. N., Blumenthal, J., Jeffries, N. O., Castellanos, F. X., Liu, H., Zijdenbos, A., Paus, T., Evans, A. C. and Rapoport, J. L. (1999). Brain development during childhood and adolescence: a longitudinal MRI study. *Nat Neurosci,* 2(10), 861–863.

Gold, J. M. (1998). Intellectual decline in schizophrenia patients (Letter). *American Journal of Psychiatry,* 155(7), 995–996.

Gold, S., Arndt, S., Nopoulos, P., O'Leary, D. S. and Andreasen, N. C. (1999). Longitudinal study of cognitive function in first-episode and recent-onset schizophrenia. *Am J Psychiatry,* 156(9), 1342–1348.

Goldberg, T. E., Torrey, E. F., Gold, J. M., Bigelow, L. B., Ragland, R. D., Taylor, E. and Weinberger, D. R. (1995). Genetic risk of neuropsychological impairment in schizophrenia: a study of monozygotic twins discordant and concordant for the disorder. *Schizophr Res,* 17(1), 77–84.

Haas, G. L. and Castle, D. J. (1997). Sex Differences in Schizophrenia. In M. S. Keshavan and R. M. Murray (eds) *Neurodevelopment and Adult Psychopathology,* pp. 155–177. Cambridge: Cambridge University Press.

Harvey, P. D., Silverman, J. M., Mohs, R. C., Parrella, M., White, L., Powchik, P., Davidson, M. and Davis, K. L. (1999). Cognitive decline in late-life schizophrenia: a longitudinal study of geriatric chronically hospitalized patients. *Biol Psychiatry,* 45(1), 32–40.

Heaton, R. K., Gladsjo, J. A., Palmer, B. W., Kuck, J., Marcotte, T. D. and Jeste, D. V. (2001). Stability and course of neuropsychological deficits in schizophrenia. *Arch Gen Psychiatry,* 58(1), 24–32.

Heinrichs, R. W. and Zakzanis, K. K. (1998). Neurocognitive deficit in schizophrenia: a quantitative review of the evidence. *Neuropsychology,* 12(3), 426–445.

Hoff, A. L., Sakuma, M., Wieneke, M., Horon, R., Kushner, M. and DeLisi, L. E. (1999). Longitudinal neuropsychological follow-up study of patients with first-episode schizophrenia. *Am J Psychiatry,* 156(9), 1336–1341.

Huttenlocher, P. R. and Dabholkar, A. S. (1997). Regional differences in synaptogenesis in human cerebral cortex. *J Comp Neurol,* 387(2), 167–178.

Isohanni, I., Jarvelin, M. R., Nieminen, P., Jones, P., Rantakallio, P., Jokelainen, J. and Isohanni, M. (1998). School performance as a predictor of psychiatric hospitalization in adult life.

A 28-year follow-up in the Northern Finland 1966 Birth Cohort. *Psychol Med,* 28(4), 967–974.

Jones, P., Rodgers, B., Murray, R. and Marmot, M. (1994). Child development risk factors for adult schizophrenia in the British 1946 birth cohort. *Lancet,* 344(8934), 1398–1402.

Jones, P. B. and Done, D. J. (1997). From birth to onset: a developmental perspective of schizophrenia in two national birth cohorts. In M. S. Keshavan and R. M. Murray (eds) *Neurodevelopment and Adult Psychopathology,* pp. 119–136. Cambridge: Cambridge University Press.

Kraepelin, E. (1919). *Dementia Praecox and Paraphrenia.* Edinburgh: E and S Livingstone.

Kremen, W. S., Buka, S. L., Seidman, L. J., Goldstein, J. M., Koren, D. and Tsuang, M. T. (1998). IQ decline during childhood and adult psychotic symptoms in a community sample: a 19-year longitudinal study. *Am J Psychiatry,* 155(5), 672–677.

Kremen, W. S., Seidman, L. J., Faraone, S. V., Toomey, R. and Tsuang, M. T. (2000). The paradox of normal neuropsychological function in schizophrenia. *J Abnorm Psychol,* 109(4), 743–752.

Kremen, W. S., Seidman, L.J., Faraone, S.V., Pepple, J.R., Lyons, M.J., Tsuang, M.T. (1996). The '3 Rs' and neuropsychological function in schizophrenia: An empirical test of the matching fallacy. *Neuropsychology,* 10, 22–31.

Lane, E. and Albee, G. (1968). On childhood intellectual decline of adult schizophrenics: A reassessment of an earlier study. *Journal of Abnormal and Social Psychology,* 73, 174–177.

Lezak, M. D. (1995). *Neuropsychological Assessment,* 3rd edn. New York, NY: Oxford University Press.

Lubin, A., Gieseking, C. F. and Williams, H. L. (1962). Direct measurement of cognitive deficit in schizophrenia. *Journal of Consulting Psychology,* 26(2), 139–143.

Mason, C. (1956). Pre-illness intelligence of mental hospital patients. *Journal of Consulting Psychology,* 20, 297–300.

Mohamed, S., Paulsen, J. S., O'Leary, D., Arndt, S. and Andreasen, N. (1999). Generalized cognitive deficits in schizophrenia: a study of first-episode patients. *Arch Gen Psychiatry,* 56(8), 749–754.

Nopoulos, P., Flashman, L., Flaum, M., Arndt, S. and Andreasen, N. (1994). Stability of cognitive 1functioning early in the course of schizophrenia. *Schizophr Res,* 14(1), 29–37.

Offord, D. R. (1974). School performance of adult schizophrenics, their siblings and age mates. *Br J Psychiatry,* 125, 12–19.

Offord, D. R. and Cross, L. A. (1971). Adult schizophrenia with scholastic failure or low IQ in childhood. A preliminary report. *Arch Gen Psychiatry,* 24(5), 431–436.

Palmer, B. W., Heaton, R. K., Paulsen, J. S., Kuck, J., Braff, D., Harris, M. J., Zisook, S. and Jeste, D. V. (1997). Is it possible to be schizophrenic yet neuropsychologically normal? *Neuropsychology,* 11(3), 437–446.

Rabinowitz, J., De Smedt, G., Harvey, P.D., Davidson, M. (2002). Relationship between premorbid functioning and symptom severity as assessed at first episode of psychosis. *American Journal of Psychiatry,* 159, 2021–2026.

Rabinowitz, J., Reichenberg, A., Weiser, M., Mark, M., Kaplan, Z. and Davidson, M. (2000). Cognitive and behavioural functioning in men with schizophrenia both before and shortly after first admission to hospital. Cross-sectional analysis. *Br J Psychiatry,* 177, 26–32.

Rapoport, J. L., Giedd, J. N., Blumenthal, J., Hamburger, S., Jeffries, N., Fernandez, T., Nicolson, R., Bedwell, J., Lenane, M., Zijdenbos, A., Paus, T. and Evans, A. (1999). Progressive cortical change during adolescence in childhood-onset schizophrenia. A longitudinal magnetic resonance imaging study. *Arch Gen Psychiatry,* 56(7), 649–654.

Rappaport, S. and Webb, W. (1950). An attempt to study intellectual deterioration by premorbid and psychotic testing. *Journal of Consulting Psychology,* 14, 95–98.

Reichenberg, A., Weiser, M., Caspi, A., Knobler, H. Y., Harvey, P. D., Rabinowitz, J. and Davidson, M. (2005). Premorbid intellectual functioning and risk of schizophrenia and spectrum disorders. *Journal of Clinical and Experimental Neuropsychology* (In Press).

Reichenberg, A., Weiser, M., Rabinowitz, J., Caspi, A., Schmeidler, J., Mark, M., Kaplan, Z. and Davidson, M. (2002). A population-based cohort study of premorbid intellectual, language, and behavioral functioning in patients with schizophrenia, schizoaffective disorder, and nonpsychotic bipolar disorder. *Am J Psychiatry*, 159(12), 2027–2035.

Russell, A. J., Munro, J. C., Jones, P. B., Hemsley, D. R. and Murray, R. M. (1997). Schizophrenia and the myth of intellectual decline. *Am J Psychiatry*, 154(5), 635–639.

Saykin, A. J., Gur, R. C., Gur, R. E., Mozley, P. D., Mozley, L. H., Resnick, S. M., Kester, D. B. and Stafiniak, P. (1991). Neuropsychological function in schizophrenia. Selective impairment in memory and learning. *Arch Gen Psychiatry*, 48(7), 618–624.

Saykin, A. J., Shtasel, D. L., Gur, R. E., Kester, D. B., Mozley, L. H., Stafiniak, P. and Gur, R. C. (1994). Neuropsychological deficits in neuroleptic naive patients with first-episode schizophrenia. *Arch Gen Psychiatry*, 51(2), 124–131.

Schwartzman, A. E. and Douglas, V. I. (1962). Intellectual loss in schizophrenia: Part I. *Canadian Journal of Psychology*, 16(1), 1–10.

Sheitman, B. B., Murray, M. G., Snyder, J. A., Silva, S., Goldman, R., Chakos, M., Volavka, J. and Lieberman, J. A. (2000). IQ scores of treatment-resistant schizophrenia patients before and after the onset of the illness. *Schizophr Res*, 46(2–3), 203–207.

Silver, H., Feldman, P., Bilker, W. and Gur, R. C. (2003). Working memory deficit as a core neuropsychological dysfunction in schizophrenia. *Am J Psychiatry*, 160(10), 1809–1816.

van Oel, C.J., Sitskoorn, M.M., Cremer, M.P. and Kahn, R.S. (2002). School performance as a premurbid marker for schizophrenia: a twin study. *Schizophrenia Bulletin*, 28(3), 401–414.

van Os, J., Jones, P., Lewis, G., Wadsworth, M. and Murray, R. (1997). Developmental precursors of affective illness in a general population birth cohort. *Arch Gen Psychiatry*, 54(7), 625–631.

Weickert, T. W. and Goldberg, T. E. (2000). The course of cognitive impairment in patients with schizophrenia. In T. Sharma and P. Harvey (eds) *Cognition in Schizophrenia*, pp. 3–15. New York, NY: Oxford University Press.

Weickert, T. W., Goldberg, T. E., Gold, J. M., Bigelow, L. B., Egan, M. F. and Weinberger, D. R. (2000). Cognitive impairments in patients with schizophrenia displaying preserved and compromised intellect. *Arch Gen Psychiatry*, 57(9), 907–913.

Weiser, M., Reichenberg, A., Rabinowitz, J., Kaplan, Z., Mark, M., Nahon, D. and Davidson, M. (2000). Gender differences in premorbid cognitive performance in a national cohort of schizophrenic patients. *Schizophr Res*, 45(3), 185–190.

Schizophrenia at the time of the first episode

Chapter 4

Early onset schizophrenia: cognitive and clinical characteristics

Sophia Frangou

Introduction

Schizophrenia commonly begins in young adulthood (Hafner *et al.* 1993). However, about 4 per cent of cases experience an unusually early onset of the disorder before 18 years of age (Cannon *et al.* 1999). Some of the studies reviewed here focused on patients with onset before the age of 12 (childhood-onset schizophrenia), others have examined adolescents (adolescent-onset schizophrenia) and some have included a mixture of children and adolescents. The boundary between childhood and adolescent onset schizophrenia reflects traditional divisions in the structure of psychiatric services rather than differences in presumed aetiology or pathophysiology. Therefore in this review we will use the term 'early-onset schizophrenia' (EOS) to describe both childhood and adolescent onset schizophrenia unless otherwise specified.

Several lines of evidence suggest that EOS is on a clinical and neurobiological continuum with adult onset schizophrenia but represents a more rare and severe form. Clinical studies have shown that EOS is associated with more severe clinical course (Werry *et al.* 1991; Asarnow *et al.* 1994; Maziade *et al.* 1996; Eggers and Bunk 1997), greater premorbid abnormalities (Watkins *et al.* 1988; Nicolson *et al.* 2000; Cannon *et al.* 2001; Vourdas *et al.* 2003) and increased severity of brain abnormalities (Thompson *et al.* 2001) and frequency of developmental deviance (Hollis 1995; Vourdas *et al.* 2003).

Clinical characteristics of EOS

The phenomenology of EOS

Kolvin *et al.* (1971) were the first to attempt to distinguish EOS from other psychotic and neurodevelopmental disorders of childhood. In their study the youngest child diagnosed as schizophrenic was 6.7 years old but most of their sample (about 80 per cent) developed the illness after the age of eight. Generally however, schizophrenia in very young children is rare but the incidence rises sharply between the ages of 12 and 14 (Galdos *et al.* 1993; Remschmidt *et al.* 1994; Hafner *et al.* 1995).

Few studies have examined the phenomenology of operationally defined EOS (Cantor *et al.* 1982; Green *et al.* 1992; Russell, 1994). However, such studies support continuity with the adult onset form. As in adult onset schizophrenia, auditory hallucinations and delusions are the most common psychotic features (Kolvin *et al.* 1971; Green *et al.* 1992; Russell, 1994). The presence of formal thought disorder is more variable across studies and depends on the sample and definition (Caplan *et al.* 2000).

Clinical and social outcome in EOS

The outcome of EOS patients both in terms of symptomatic recovery and psychosocial function appears to be poor, and possibly worse than that of the adult onset cases. In terms of clinical outcome, the rates of improvement reported after an average follow-up period of five years range between 3 per cent (Werry *et al.* 1991) and 56 per cent (Asarnow *et al.* 1994; Russell 1994). Studies with longer follow-up periods have consistently reported lower rates of improvement. Two studies followed up EOS patients for an average period of 16 years and reported that the majority of patients experienced continuous symptoms (Eggers 1978; Maziade *et al.* 1996); however full clinical remission was also noted in 5–20 per cent of EOS patients. The longest follow-up study, by Eggers and Bunk (1997), examined clinical outcome in a sample of 44 EOS patients over a period of 42 years. Half of the patients had continuous symptoms and 25 per cent were in partial remission. Premorbid function, mode and age of onset appear to be the best predictors of clinical outcome (Werry and McClellan 1992; Amminger *et al.* 1997; Eggers and Bunk 1997). Schmidt *et al.* (1995) compared both symptomatic and social outcome in EOS patients to that of adult onset schizophrenic patients. More than two-thirds of the 118 EOS cases in their sample had had at least one further schizophrenic episode during the 7-year follow-up period of the study and were in need of continuing psychiatric treatment. In the same study, EOS patients were more disadvantaged than adult onset cases in terms of social outcome. Greater impairment was noted for EOS patients particularly in the areas of self-care and social contacts.

Premorbid function in EOS

Developmental abnormalities

The severity of the clinical picture of EOS is also reflected in the degree of premorbid deficits observed. Relevant studies have reported wide-ranging abnormalities that include developmental delays, expressive and receptive language deficits, impaired gross motor functioning, learning and academic problems, and transient autistic-like symptoms (Watkins *et al.* 1988; Werry *et al.* 1991; Russell 1994; Alaghband-Rad *et al.* 1995). Although similar premorbid abnormalities have been observed in patients with adult-onset schizophrenia (Jones *et al.* 1994; Walker and Levine 1990) there are some quantitative differences between early- and adult-onset cases. Our group compared directly premorbid impairment in EOS and adult cases as part of the Maudsley Early Onset Schizophrenia Project (Vourdas *et al.* 2003). Consistent with other reports (Kolvin 1971; Watkins *et al.* 1988; Nicolson *et al.* 2000) we found that speech and language deficits were the most common developmental abnormalities in EOS. Such deficits were more frequent and severe the earlier the age of onset of schizophrenia, being most prevalent in childhood onset cases as also suggested by Hollis (1995). He studied a sample of 61 children and adolescent schizophrenics with a mean age of onset of 14.3 years from the Maudsley Children's Department, UK. He found that 23 per cent of them had speech and language impairments, which were greater in those patients who manifested schizophrenia before the age of 13.

There is less consistency with respect to motor abnormalities in EOS. The earliest study by Kolvin (1971) noted that only 3 per cent of developmental delays were due to delayed motor milestones. Watkins *et al.* (1988) found motor impairment in five out of the eight patients in their sample of schizophrenic children with onset before the age of 10. Motor deficits in this study included both delayed milestones and poor coordination. Hollis (1995) reported motor disturbance in 31 per cent of his sample. The abnormalities noted included restlessness, stereotyped movements, poor coordination and delayed milestones. Nicolson *et al.* (2000) found motor impairment in 57.1 per cent in their sample of childhood onset schizophrenia from the National Institute of Mental Health (NIMH), USA. Patients manifested delayed motor milestones as well as poor coordination and abnormal repetitive movements. In a previous analysis of a subgroup of this sample (Alaghband-Rad *et al.* 1995), the rate of motor impairment when restricted to delayed walking was 17 per cent and such developmental motor delays were more likely in those schizophrenic children that met either at least one (36 per cent) or all the criteria for infantile autism (13 per cent). In the Maudsley Early Onset Schizophrenia Study, there was a non-significant delay in motor milestones but more importantly about 3 per cent of the sample showed gross motor deficits as they had been unable to walk unsupported by the age of 2.

Abnormal neurological signs are another indicator of neurodevelopmental deviance. Increased rates of such abnormalities were reported even in the earliest studies of patients with childhood-onset schizophrenia (Kennard 1960; Gittelman and Birch 1967). Increased rates of neurologic abnormalities have also been found in adolescent-onset schizophrenia compared to healthy adolescents (Karp *et al.* 2001). Additionally, the number of neurologic signs decreased with age in the healthy controls but not in the EOS patients, which may be indicative of delay or absence of normal neurologic maturation during adolescence.

Premorbid adjustment

Poor premorbid function is one of the most consistent findings in schizophrenia. It has been reported in retrospective studies (Watt 1972; Watt and Lybensky 1976; Lewine *et al.* 1980; Baum and Walker 1995; Cannon *et al.* 1997; Malmberg *et al.* 1998), prospective birth cohort (Jones *et al.* 1994; Done *et al.* 1995; Olin and Mednick 1996; Mirsky *et al.* 1995) and high-risk studies (Aminger *et al.* 1999; Hans *et al.* 2000).

Premorbid adjustment deficits are also present in EOS patients. Kolvin (1971) found that 87 per cent of his subjects were premorbidly odd with 58 per cent having schizoid traits of being shy, withdrawn, timid and sensitive. Similarly, Asarnow and Ben-Meir (1988) and Watkins *et al.* (1988) demonstrated that poor premorbid social adaptation was particularly common in subjects with EOS. Hollis (1995) found that a premorbid history of social withdrawal was significantly more common in cases of EOS compared to non-psychotic patients. Two studies on treatment resistant EOS cases ascertained at the NIMH (Nicolson and Rapaport 1999; Alaghband-Rad *et al.* 1995) found that there had been concerns from parents and teachers about the social development and academic performance of more than half of their subjects.

In the Maudsley Early Onset Schizophrenia Study we found that 70.5 per cent of our EOS sample had at least one premorbid schizophrenia spectrum trait, most commonly social isolation (54 per cent) followed by having odd ideas or perceptions (41 per cent) (Vourdas *et al.* 2003). Problems in premorbid adjustment during childhood and adolescence were closely associated with developmental impairment in both genders (Vourdas *et al.* 2003). Premorbid function deteriorated further as EOS patients progressed to adolescence, particularly with respect to social isolation and poor scholastic performance. Premorbid adjustment was poorer in EOS compared to adult-onset cases both in our study and in other reports (Cannon-Spoor *et al.* 1982; Alaghband–Rad *et al.* 1995). Deficits in premorbid adjustment in childhood appear to have some degree of specificity to schizophrenia. Cannon *et al.* (2001) examined premorbid adjustment in childhood attendees of the child psychiatric services at our centre. Social withdrawal, abnormal suspiciousness and disturbed relationship with peers or adults other than family members were more common in those children who later developed schizophrenia rather than affective disorders. Furthermore, in the Maudsley Early Onset Schizophrenia Study we identified social isolation as well as strange beliefs and perceptions as being the most common premorbid schizoid/schizotypal characteristics of our sample of EOS cases. This is consistent with the observations of Poulton *et al.* (2000), from a prospective birth cohort study, who found that children reporting delusional beliefs and hallucinatory experiences at age 11 were sixteen times more likely than the rest of their cohort to be diagnosed with a schizophrenia spectrum disorders fifteen years later.

Cognitive function in EOS

Cognitive deficits are a consistent feature of schizophrenia and have been noted since the early descriptions of the disorder. In adult-onset schizophrenia, abnormalities have been reported in all aspects of cognition, with the largest effect size seen in general intellectual ability, verbal memory and executive function (Heinrichs and Zakzanis 1998). Several studies of adolescents with schizophrenia have confirmed the presence of cognitive deficits in this group. One of the earlier studies by Johnstone *et al.* (1989) found that such patients had poor language abilities and problems in long-term memory. More recent studies have extended this finding to include impairments in IQ, verbal memory and learning and executive function (Arsanow *et al.* 1994; Bedwell *et al.* 1999; Kumra *et al.* 2000; Kravariti *et al.* 2003a, b).

General intellectual ability

David *et al.* (1997) in a study of 18-year old male Swedish Army conscripts, found that intellectual functioning was a powerful predictor of future schizophrenia and this finding was replicated in a Israeli cohort of 16–17 year old males tested for eligibility for military service (Davidson *et al.* 1999). The proportion of cases falling within the highest IQ category in the study by Davidson *et al.* was six times higher than expected. This issue was further investigated by Isohanni *et al.* (1999) who showed that the distance from cognitive norm in either direction increases the odds for schizophrenia. It is unclear whether EOS patients are more impaired in measures of general intellectual ability than their adult-onset counterparts. This is mostly because studies of cognitive function of EOS patients have consistently excluded those with an IQ of less than 70. Even so, general intellectual ability in EOS has been repeatedly found to be in the low average range (Oie and Rund 1999; Oie *et al.* 1999; Rund *et al.* 1998, 1996; Kravariti *et al.* 2003a, b) and statistically lower than that of the healthy comparison subjects included in these studies.

Attention

EOS is probably associated with attentional impairment although the magnitude and consistency of this finding are variable. This contrasts with adult-onset schizophrenia where attentional dysfunction has been repeatedly found (Saykin *et al.* 1994; Bilder *et al.* 2000) even in first episode patients. The variability seen in EOS studies is probably related to the tests used to assess this cognitive domain and symptom severity at the time of testing. Kenny *et al.* (1997) found that although adolescents with EOS had widespread cognitive problems, abnormalities in divided attention were disproportionally large. Kumra *et al.* (2000) reporting from the NIMH study of EOS mentioned before found that both patients with schizophrenia as well as those with psychosis not otherwise specified shared a pattern of generalized cognitive deficits that included attention. In contrast, Oie *et al.* (1999) did not find any significant attentional impairment in schizophrenic adolescents when compared to matched healthy controls and patients with Attention Deficit Hyperactivity Disorder (ADHD).

These findings are in line with previous results from the same group that reported no evidence of disruption in vigilance or selective attention in EOS patients (Oie *et al.* 1998a, b; Rundt *et al.* 1998). Similarly, EOS patients participating in the Maudsley Early Onset Schizophrenia Study did not show deficits in attention and concentration (Kravariti *et al.* 2003a, b).

Executive function

Executive function encompasses a broad range of cognitive processes including planning, abstraction, cognitive set-shifting, motivation and self-regulation. A wide range of tests is used to examine this cognitive domain. Examination of executive function in EOS is so far quite limited because the number of available studies is small and have concentrated on few aspects of executive function. Kenny *et al.* (1997) found that compared with normal subjects, adolescents with schizophrenia demonstrated generalized cognitive impairment on measures of attention, memory, and executive function with the largest effect sizes seen in working memory.

Oie *et al.* (1999) in their sample of adolescent schizophrenics found deficits in abstraction and cognitive set shifting. Their results are similar to those reported by the NIMH group (Kumra *et al.* 2000). In the Maudsley Early Onset Schizophrenia Study executive function was assessed using the Tower of London Test to measure planning and problem-solving, the Executive Golf task to measure spatial working memory, the Trail Making Test, Part A and B, to examine sequencing and mental flexibility and a modified version of Baddeley's Working Memory Task to investigate dual task performance (Kravariti *et al.* 2003b). In the Tower of London Test patients showed deficits in planning accuracy and speed of visual motor processing. In contrast to adult-onset schizophrenics, they showed reduced subsequent planning time (a measure of time spent planning and thinking about the next problem-solving move), which may suggest greater impulsivity. Deficits were also observed in the spatial working memory task. Examination of the pattern of patients' performance in this task suggested that the observed deficit could be accounted for mostly by patients' inability to generate an efficient strategy, and less so by difficulties in maintaining information in working memory. Patients performed poorly on sequencing and set shifting as measured by the Trails Making task. Here their observed deficit could not be attributed to reduced motor speed/reaction time, as no deficit could be detected in this variable.

Memory

In adult-onset cases the median effect size for memory impairment is about 0.74 and shows significant evidence of variability (Heinrichs and Zakzanis 1998).

There are only a few studies on memory function in EOS with contradictory results. Oie and Rund (1999) assessed verbal and visual memory in EOS using the California Verbal Learning Test and Kimura Recurring Figures respectively. They found that visual memory impairment was greater than two standard deviations in adolescents with schizophrenia compared to controls. In the Maudsley Early Onset Schizophrenia Study memory was tested using the Wechsler Memory Scale-Revised (WMS-R) (Kravariti *et al.* 2003a). In the Maudsley Early Onset Schizophrenia Study deficits in visual memory were small, in the region of 0.2 standard deviations from the control mean. The most pronounced memory deficit in our sample was in the verbal memory subscale. Furthermore, patients' score in the composite General memory Scale of the WMS-R was disproportionally lower than their Full Scale IQ score. The difference was 10 points and is amongst the largest reported in the schizophrenia literature. Further studies on memory function in EOS are needed to clarify the nature and degree of impairment in this cognitive domain.

Concluding remarks

The studies reviewed here provide consistent evidence that early- and adult-onset schizophrenia are on the same continuum. Clinical and cognitive data suggest increased severity in EOS cases on multiple levels. The study of EOS is therefore more likely to yield useful insights into the complex relationships between brain development and the pathophysiology of schizophrenia.

References

Alaghband-Rad J, McKenna K, Gordon CT *et al.* (1995). Childhood-onset schizophrenia: the severity of premorbid course. *Journal of the American Academy of Child and Adolescent Psychiatry*, 34, 1273–1283.

Amminger GP, Resch F, Mutschlechner R, Friedrich MH, Ernst E (1997). Premorbid adjustment and remission of positive symptoms in first-episode psychosis. *European Child and Adolescent Psychiatry*, 6, 212–218.

Amminger GP, Pape S, Rock D, *et al.* (1999). Relationship between childhood behavioral disturbance and later schizophrenia in the New York High-Risk Project. *American Journal of Psychiatry*, 156, 525–530.

Asarnow RF, Asamen J, Granholm E, Sherman T, Watkins JM, Williams ME (1994a). Cognitive/neuropsychological studies of children with a schizophrenic disorder. *Schizophrenia Bulletin*, 20, 647–669.

Asarnow JR, Tompson MC, Goldstein MJ (1994b). Childhood onset schizophrenia: a follow-up study. *Schizophrenia Bulletin*, 20, 599–617.

Asarnow JR, Ben-Meir S (1988). Children with schizophrenia spectrum and depressive disorders: a comparative study of premorbid adjustment, onset pattern and severity of impairment. *Journal of Child Psychology and Psychiatry*, 29, 477–488.

Baum KM, Walker EF (1995). Childhood behavioral precursors of adult symptom dimensions in schizophrenia. *Schizophrenia Research*, 16, 111–120.

Bedwell JS, Keller B, Smith AK, Hamburger S, Kumra S, Rapoport JL (1999). Why does postpsychotic IQ decline in childhood-onset schizophrenia? *American Journal of Psychiatry*, 156, 1996–1997.

Bilder RM, Goldman RS, Robinson D *et al.* (2000). Neuropsychology of first-episode schizophrenia: initial characterization and clinical correlates. *American Journal of Psychiatry*, 157, 549–559.

Cannon M, Jones P, Gilvarry C, *et al.* (1997). Premorbid social functioning in schizophrenia and bipolar disorder: similarities and differences. *American Journal of Psychiatry*, 154, 1544–1550.

Cannon M, Jones P, Huttunen MO *et al.* (1999). School performance in Finnish children and later development of schizophrenia: a population-based longitudinal study. *Archives of General Psychiatry*, 56, 457–463.

Cannon M, Walsh E, Hollis C *et al.* (2001). Predictors of later schizophrenia and affective psychosis among attendees at a child psychiatry department. *British Journal of Psychiatry*, 178, 420–426.

Cannon-Spoor HE, Potkin SG, Wyatt RJ (1982). Measurement of premorbid adjustment in chronic schizophrenia. *Schizophrenia Bulletin*, 8, 470–484.

Cantor S, Evans J, Pearce J, Pezzot-Pearce T (1982). Childhood schizophrenia: present but not accounted for. *American Journal of Psychiatry*, 139, 758–762.

Caplan R, Guthrie D, Tang B, Komo S, Asarnow RF (2000). Thought disorder in childhood schizophrenia: replication and update of concept. *Journal of the American Academy of Child and Adolescent Psychiatry*, 39, 771–778.

David AS, Malmberg A, Brandt L, Allebeck P, Lewis G (1997). IQ and risk for schizophrenia: a population-based cohort study. *Psychological Medicine*, 27, 1311–1323.

Davidson M, Reichenberg A, Rabinowitz J et al. (1999). Behavioral and intellectual markers for schizophrenia in apparently healthy male adolescents. *American Journal of Psychiatry*, 156, 1328–1335.

Done DJ, Crow TJ, Johnstone EC, Sacker A (1994). Childhood antecedents of schizophrenia and affective illness: social adjustment at ages 7 and 11. *BMJ*, 309, 699–703.

Eggers C (1978). Course and prognosis of childhood schizophrenia. *Journal of Autism and Childhood Schizophrenia*, 8, 21–36.

Eggers C, Bunk D (1997). The long-term course of childhood-onset schizophrenia: a 42-year follow up. *Schizophrenia Bulletin*, 23, 105–117.

Galdos PM, van Os JJ, Murray RM (1993). Puberty and the onset of psychosis. *Schizophrenia Research*, 10, 7–14.

Gittelman M, Birch HG (1967). Childhood schizophrenia. Intellect, neurologic status, perinatal risk, prognosis, and family pathology. *Archives of General Psychiatry*, 17, 16–25.

Green WH, Padron-Gayol M, Hardesty AS, Bassiri M (1992). Schizophrenia with childhood onset: a phenomenological study of 38 cases. *Journal of the American Academy of Child and Adolescent Psychiatry*, 31, 968–976.

Hafner H, Maurer K, Loffler W, Riecher-Rossler A (1993). The influence of age and sex on the onset and early course of schizophrenia. *British Journal of Psychiatry*, 162, 80–86.

Hans SL, Marcus J, Nuechterlein KH, Asarnow RF, Styr B, Auerbach JG (1999). Neurobehavioral deficits at adolescence in children at risk for schizophrenia: The Jerusalem Infant Development Study. *Archives of General Psychiatry*, 56, 741–748.

Hans SL, Auerbach JG, Asarnow JR, Styr B, Marcus J (2000). Social adjustment of adolescents at risk for schizophrenia: the Jerusalem Infant Development Study. *Journal of the American Academy of Child and Adolescent Psychiatry*, 39, 1406–1414.

Heinrichs RW, Zakzanis KK (1998). Neurocognitive deficit in schizophrenia: a quantitative review of the evidence. *Neuropsychology*, 12, 426–445.

Hollis C (1995). Child and adolescent (juvenile onset) schizophrenia. A case control study of premorbid developmental impairments. *British Journal of Psychiatry*, 166, 489–495.

Johnstone EC, Owens DG, Bydder GM, Colter N, Crow TJ, Frith CD (1989). The spectrum of structural brain changes in schizophrenia: age of onset as a predictor of cognitive and clinical impairments and their cerebral correlates. *Psychological Medicine*, 19, 91–103.

Jones P, Rodgers B, Murray R, Marmot M (1994). Child development risk factors for adult schizophrenia in the British 1946 birth cohort. *Lancet*, 19 (344), 1398–1402.

Isohanni I, Jarvelin MR, Jones P, Jokelainen J, Isohanni M (1999). Can excellent school performance be a precursor of schizophrenia? A 28-year follow-up in the Northern Finland 1966 birth cohort. *Acta Psychiatrica Scandinavica*, 100, 17–26.

Karp BI, Garvey M, Jacobsen LK et al. (2001). Abnormal neurologic maturation in adolescents with early-onset schizophrenia. *American Journal of Psychiatry*, 158, 118–122.

Kennard MA (1960). Value of equivocal signs in neurologic diagnosis. *Neurology*, 10, 753–764.

Kenny JT, Friedman L, Findling RL, Swales TP, Strauss ME, Jesberger JA, Schulz SC (1997). Cognitive impairment in adolescents with schizophrenia. *American Journal of Psychiatry*, 154, 1613–1615.

Kravariti E, Morris RG, Rabe-Hesketh S, Murray RM, Frangou S (2003a). The Maudsley early onset schizophrenia study: cognitive function in adolescents with recent onset schizophrenia. *Schizophrenia Research*, 61, 137–148.

Kravariti E, Morris RG, Rabe-Hesketh S, Murray RM, Frangou S (2003b). The Maudsley early-onset schizophrenia study: cognitive function in adolescent-onset schizophrenia. *Schizophrenia Research*, 65, 95–103.

Kumra S, Wiggs E, Bedwell J *et al.* (2000). Neuropsychological deficits in pediatric patients with childhood-onset schizophrenia and psychotic disorder not otherwise specified. *Schizophrenia Research*, 42, 135–144.

Kolvin C, Ounsted M, Humphrey M, McNay A (1971). The phenomenology of childhood psychoses. *British Journal of Psychiatry*, 118, 385–395.

Lewine RR, Watt NF, Prentky RA, Fryer JH (1980). Childhood social competence in functionally disordered psychiatric patients and in normals. *Journal of Abnormal Psychology*, 89,132–138.

Malmberg A, Lewis G, David A, Allebeck P (1998). Premorbid adjustment and personality in people with schizophrenia. *British Journal of Psychiatry*, 172, 308–313.

Maziade M, Gingras N, Rodrigue C *et al.* (1996). Long-term stability of diagnosis and symptom dimensions in a systematic sample of patients with onset of schizophrenia in childhood and early adolescence. I: nosology, sex and age of onset. *British Journal of Psychiatry*, 169, 361–370.

Mirsky AF, Kugelmass S, Ingraham LJ, Frenkel E, Nathan M (1995). Overview and summary: twenty-five year follow-up of high-risk children. *Schizophrenia Bulletin*, 21, 227–239.

Nicolson R, Rapoport JL (1999). Childhood-onset schizophrenia: rare but worth studying. *Biological Psychiatry*, 46, 1418–1428.

Nicolson R, Lenane M, Singaracharlu S *et al.* (2000). Premorbid speech and language impairments in childhood-onset schizophrenia: association with risk factors. *American Journal of Psychiatry*, 157, 794–800.

Oie M, Rund BR, Sundet K (1998a). Covert visual attention in patients with early-onset schizophrenia. *Schizophrenia Research*, 34, 195–205.

Oie M, Rund BR, Sundet K, Bryhn G (1998b). Auditory laterality and selective attention: normal performance in patients with early-onset schizophrenia. *Schizophrenia Bulletin*, 24, 643–652.

Oie M, Rund, BR (1999). Neuropsychological deficits in adolescent-onset schizophrenia compared with attention deficit hyperactivity disorder. *American Journal of Psychiatry*, 156, 1216–1222.

Oie M, Sundet K, Rund BR (1999). Contrasts in memory functions between adolescents with schizophrenia or ADHD. *Neuropsychologia*, 37, 1351–1358.

Olin SC, Mednick SA (1996). Risk factors of psychosis: identifying vulnerable populations premorbidly. *Schizophrenia Bulletin*, 22, 223–240.

Poulton R, Caspi A, Moffitt TE, Cannon M, Murray R, Harrington H (2000). Children's self-reported psychotic symptoms and adult schizophreniform disorder: a 15-year longitudinal study. *Archives of General Psychiatry*, 57, 1053–1058.

Remschmidt HE, Schulz E, Martin M, Warnke A, Trott GE (1994). Childhood-onset schizophrenia: history of the concept and recent studies. *Schizophrenia Bulletin*, 20, 727–745.

Rund BR, Oie M, Sundet K (1996). Backward-masking deficit in adolescents with schizophrenic disorders or attention deficit hyperactivity disorder. *American Journal of Psychiatry*, 153, 1154–1157.

Rund BR, Zeiner P, Sundet K, Oie M, Bryhn G (1998). No vigilance deficit found in young schizophrenic or ADHD subjects. *Scandinavian Journal of Psychology*, 39, 101–107.

Russell AT (1994). The clinical presentation of childhood-onset schizophrenia. *Schizophrenia Bulletin,* 20, 631–646.

Saykin AJ, Shtasel DL, Gur RE *et al.* (1994). Neuropsychological deficits in neuroleptic naive patients with first-episode schizophrenia. *Archives of General Psychiatry,* 51, 124–131.

Schmidt M, Blanz B, Dippe A, Koppe T, Lay B (1995). Course of patients diagnosed as having schizophrenia during first episode occurring under age 18 years. *European Archives of Psychiatry and Clinical Neurosciences,* 245, 93–100.

Thompson PM, Vidal C, Giedd JN *et al.* (2001). Mapping adolescent brain change reveals dynamic wave of accelerated gray matter loss in very early-onset schizophrenia. *Proceedings of the National Academy of Science USA,* 98, 11650–11655.

Vourdas A, Pipe R, Corrigall R, Frangou S (2003). Increased developmental deviance and premorbid dysfunction in early onset schizophrenia. *Schizophrenia Research,* 62, 13–22.

Walker E, Lewine RJ (1990). Prediction of adult-onset schizophrenia from childhood home movies of the patients. *American Journal of Psychiatry,* 147, 1052–1056.

Watkins JM, Asarnow RF, Tanguay PE (1988). Symptom development in childhood onset schizophrenia. *Journal of Child Psychology and Psychiatry,* 29, 865–878.

Watt NF (1972). Longitudinal changes in the social behavior of children hospitalized for schizophrenia as adults. *Journal of Nervous and Mental Disorders,* 155, 42–54.

Watt NF, Lubensky AW (1976). Childhood roots of schizophrenia. *Journal of Consult Clinical Psychology,* 44, 363–375.

Werry JS, McClellan JM, Chard L (1991). Childhood and adolescent schizophrenic, bipolar, and schizoaffective disorders: a clinical and outcome study. *Journal of the American Academy of Child and Adolescent Psychiatry,* 30, 457–465.

Werry JS, McClellan JM (1992). Predicting outcome in child and adolescent (early onset) schizophrenia and bipolar disorder. *Journal of the American Academy of Child and Adolescent Psychiatry,* 31, 147–150.

Chapter 5

Brain imaging studies in childhood-onset schizophrenia

Nitin Gogtay and Judith L. Rapoport

Introduction

Converging evidence indicates that serious childhood psychiatric disorders reflect subtle abnormalities of brain development. Clinical and neuropsychological studies indicate abnormal brain function in child psychiatric populations (Goodman 1994) and childhood psychiatric disorders are strongly associated with neurological and neurodevelopmental disorders (Rutter et al. 1970). With the advent of non-invasive brain MRI methodology, imaging data can now be safely acquired for pediatric populations. Interpretation of these data is substantiated by preclinical studies on the organization and function of neural circuits in the developing brain, and the molecular mediators of these changes.

As both computerized axial tomography (CAT) and positron emission tomography (PET) scanning in children utilize ionizing radiation, these techniques have rarely been feasible or desirable for pediatric patients. Magnetic resonance imaging (MRI) and magnetic resonance spectroscopy (MRS) on the other hand are non invasive, relatively simple, and allow reliable, automated quantitative measurements of multiple brain regions to gather both normative and disease-specific cross-sectional and longitudinal data in children (Collins *et al.* 1999; Giedd *et al.* 1996, 1999a; Thompson *et al.* 2000, 2001). These techniques have made brain imaging a key part of child psychiatric research (Gogate *et al.* 2001), including the study of childhood-onset psychoses.

Childhood-Onset Schizophrenia (COS), defined as onset of psychotic symptoms before the 13th birthday, is a rare and severe form of the illness, which is continuous with its adult counterpart and has been under study at the NIMH since 1990 (Nicolson and Rapoport 1999). These cases resemble chronic poor outcome adult cases but are less contaminated by substance abuse, and/or prolonged institutionalization. As is true for many medical disorders, early onset populations are more severely affected and may have unique and/or more salient pathophysiology and familial/genetic risk factors (Childs and Scriver 1986).

Thus the availability of pediatric COS subjects and their age-matched norms enable us to study brain development during teenage years and may expand the understanding of the disease.

In this chapter we review structural brain-imaging studies of schizophrenia in childhood and adolescence. In addition to supporting the continuity with later onset disorder, these studies present evidence for a striking disease-specific progressive brain change seen during adolescence for COS.

Childhood-onset schizophrenia

History and background

Childhood-onset schizophrenia has been recognized since the early twentieth century (Kraepelin 1919) and children can be diagnosed with unmodified DSM criteria. Such cases are rare and many patients with affective or other atypical psychoses are often misdiagnosed as COS (Werry 1992; McKenna *et al.* 1994; Gordon *et al.* 1994). COS resembles poor outcome adult cases with respect to the frequency of insidious onset and poor premorbid functioning. The early developmental abnormalities in social, motor, and language domains in COS are particularly severe compared to that for the later onset patients (Alaghband-Rad *et al.* 1995; Green *et al.* 1992; Hollis 1995). Additionally, although not observed in the studies of early development of adult-onset schizophrenia (Done *et al.* 1994; Walker and Lewine 1990; Jones *et al.* 1994), transient autistic symptoms such as hand flapping and echolalia occur in toddler years for a substantial minority of the children (Alaghband-Rad *et al.* 1995; Green *et al.* 1992; Russell *et al.* 1989) most probably reflecting a more compromised early brain development.

NIMH COS cohort

Since 1990, children with early onset psychosis have been recruited nationally for diagnostic screening for COS at the NIMH. Diagnosis of COS is confirmed after an extensive evaluation, which includes in patient observation during a three-week drug washout period. To date, 74 patients have participated in the study, including 43 boys and 31 girls with a mean age of 14.06 + 2.67 years and mean age of onset of psychosis at 10.07 + 1.9 years. Once the diagnosis is confirmed, a structural brain MRI scan is obtained with prospective re-scanned at two-year intervals.

Automated brain MRI analyses

A typical MR image consists of approximately 8 million 1mm^3 voxels or volume elements, each of which is assigned a certain number based upon the magnetic characteristics of the tissue within the voxel. In image analysis each of the voxels is classified as gray matter, white matter, or cerebrospinal fluid, and the tissue types are then classified based on voxel intensity and using artificial neural networks. This classification is then combined with a probabilistic brain atlas to determine the structure or region to which the classified voxel belongs (Collins *et al.* 1999) to measure total and regional gray and white matter volumes in an automated manner (Figure 5.1) (Giedd *et al.* 1996).

It is then possible to assess brain volumetric changes over a period of time using longitudinal rescans. Although automated measures carry a distinct advantage of unbiased measurements of brain volume, many smaller structures such as the globus pallidus, hippocampus, amygdala and thalamus still need to be measured using hand tracing by human experts (Giedd *et al.* 1996).

Studies in childhood-onset schizophrenia

Reports on structural brain abnormalities in childhood-onset schizophrenia are scarce. One early computerized axial tomography (CT) scan study of 15 adolescents (mean age = 16 + 1.5) with schizophrenia or schizophreniform

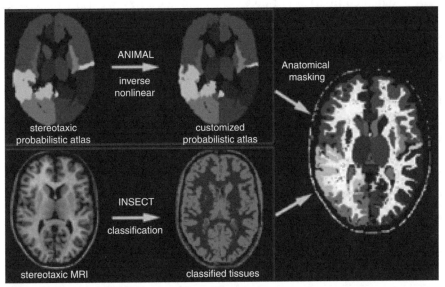

Figure 5.1 INSECT (Intensity Normalized Stereotaxic Environment for Classification of Tissue) is an automated program for classifying each voxel of a brain MR image into gray matter, white matter, or cerebrospinal fluid based on the intensity of the voxel. ANIMAL (Automatic Nonlinear Image Matching and Anatomical Labeling) is also an automated approach that labels a voxel's location in space based on prior anatomic knowledge. The Montreal Neurological Institute (MNI) program is unique in that it combines the two techniques. This allows for an automated voxel-intensity and anatomically informed classification of the brain tissue (Collins *et al.* 1999).

disorder demonstrated larger ventricular volume in the schizophrenic group, with higher ventricular brain ratio associated with poor treatment response, as had been described for adult patients (Schulz *et al.* 1983). A more recent CT study of 19 children with very early onset schizophrenia (mean age = 11.3 + 2.3) also showed ventricular enlargement (Badura *et al.* 2001).

The bulk of brain MRI studies of childhood schizophrenia come from the NIMH sample, with more recent contributions from other groups (Matsumoto *et al.* 2001a, b; Sowell *et al.* 2000; James *et al.* 2002). All the automated MRI analyses on this population come from the NIMH sample.

Cross-sectional studies

Most studies show children with schizophrenia to have: increased lateral ventricular volume, decreased total brain volume, decreased gray matter volume, and increased basal ganglia volume (the last most probably secondary to medication effect (Frazier *et al.* 1996; Rapoport *et al.* 1997, 1999; Kumra *et al.* 2000; Sowell *et al.* 2000)). There is less agreement with respect to reduced volume of temporal lobe structures (Jacobsen *et al.* 1996; Matsumoto *et al.* 2001a, b), which in these studies were measured manually.

An updated comparison of 60 COS (mean age 14.27 + 2.41) with 110 age (mean age 14.18 + 2.44) and sex matched healthy volunteers has now extended our previous observations. As seen in Table 5.1, the decreased brain volume in COS is due to a robust (10 per cent) decrease in cortical gray matter, while the

Table 5.1 Anatomic brain MRI measures at (initial scan) for COS and age and sex matched community controls

Brain region	COS patients mean ($\pm$ SD)	Healthy controls mean ($\pm$ SD)	ANOVA		ANCOVA	
Automated measures	(N = 60)	(N = 110)	F	p	F	p
Total cerebral volume	1078.62 (117.96)	1108.05 (116.31)	2.46	0.119	–	–
Total gray matter	687.31 (77.49)	718.05 (76.29)	6.24	0.0135	10.36	0.002
Total white matter	391.31 (50.70)	390.00 (49.50)	0.03	0.870	10.36	0.002[+]
Frontal gray matter	211.91 (25.46)	222.60 (23.03)	7.76	0.006	10.61	0.001
Temporal gray matter	178.08 (20.410)	183.89 (18.83)	3.49	0.064	1.05	0.306
Parietal gray matter	111.92 (13.77)	119.65 (13.52)	12.53	0.0005	17.66	0.00004
Occipital gray matter	61.42 (9.39)	65.55 (10.55)	6.41	0.0123	4.13	0.0436
Lateral ventricles	16.44 (8.42)	11.84 (6.17)	16.54	0.00007[+]	22.97	0.000004[+]

[+]COS > NV.

The mean age for COS was 14.27 (SD = 2.41) and for community controls 14.18 (SD = 2.44) (p = 0.814).
ANOVA and ANCOVA: Analysis of variance and covariance (covariate = total cerebral volume)

uncorrected total white matter volume does not differ significantly between the COS and healthy groups. Of note is the strikingly reduced parietal gray matter volume, which may be characteristic of early onset schizophrenia as discussed below.

Recently, a study with 9 COS subjects and 11 normal children (mean age 11 years), using statistical parametric mapping of gray and white matters and CSF, also found increased ventricular volume and decreased temporal and frontal gray matter volumes (Sowell et al. 2000). Although this small study did not show parietal gray matter reduction, the ventricular enlargement in this study was predominantly posterior, suggesting that posterior brain regions may be selectively affected in the earlier illness.

Prospective brain imaging studies in COS

Prospective brain MRI rescan measures for the NIMH COS sample show striking progressive abnormalities (Figure 5.2). Increasing ventricular volume and decreasing total cortical, frontal, temporal, and parietal gray matter volumes were seen across two, four and six years after their initial scan, and regional gray-white segmentation shows that the progressive loss is seen for gray matter only (Jacobsen et al. 1998; Rapoport et al. 1997, 1999; Giedd et al. 1999b).

More recent studies of adult onset schizophrenia (AOS), using comparable methodology, have found significant but more subtle progressive gray matter

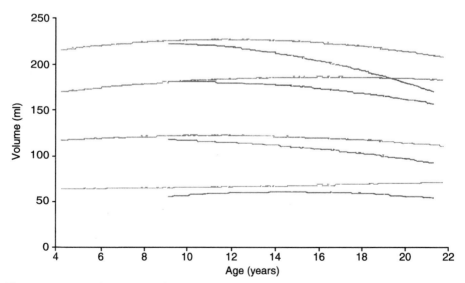

Figure 5.2 Regional gray matter loss in COS compared to age- and sex-matched controls (Giedd et al. 1999b; Rapoport et al. 1999).

loss (Gogate *et al.* 2001). Similar to that seen for COS, progressive ventricular expansion and cortical gray matter loss, mostly in the frontal and temporal region, is also seen in the AOS patients, although parietal gray matter loss appears more specific to COS (Mathalon *et al.* 2001; DeLisi 1999a, b; Gur *et al.* 1998; Lieberman *et al.* 2001). The NIMH COS study showed no significant total temporal lobe differences on initial scan (Table 5.1).

The striking changes seen for COS must occur only during a limited period, since age of onset is not significantly related to cortical gray matter volume in adult patients (Lim *et al.* 1996; Marsh *et al.* 1997), and the degree of cortical loss seen in COS would not be sustainable over time without dementia. Thus adolescence may provide a time-limited window in which the progressive brain changes in schizophrenia are most easily observed. The greater severity of these patients may be a confounding factor, as seen by the effect size comparisons of longitudinal MRI studies, which show that the brain changes seen for COS during adolescence are more pronounced than those seen for the adult patients (Gogate *et al.* 2001). More recent longitudinal analysis of our quantitative brain imaging data for a larger group of 36 COS patients with one or more scans, suggests that the rate of gray matter loss slows as these COS patients reach age 20 (Sporn *et al.* 2003). We continue to follow these patients and anticipate continued slowing of change with age.

Diagnostic specificity of brain abnormalities in childhood-onset schizophrenia

The progressive gray matter loss in COS is confounded by the effects of illness severity and the probably related lower cognitive level of the COS subjects. To address these confounds of chronic stress of illness, cognitive level, and medication exposure, we compared the brain developmental changes for COS to a group of age, sex, IQ and treatment matched non-schizophrenic patients who had been referred for the COS study but were diagnosed as 'Psychosis not otherwise specified' (NOS). These subjects had only transient psychotic symptoms together without formal thought disorder, marked behavioral dyscontrol, and were given a provisional label of 'multi-dimensionally impaired (MDI)'(Kumra *et al.* 1998; McKenna *et al.* 1994). At follow-up, none became schizophrenic but most continued to have behavioral and affective problems necessitating residential or special school placement and long term medication management (Nicolson *et al.* 2001).

A prospective brain MRI comparison study of patients with childhood-onset schizophrenia (n = 23, mean age = 13.9 + 2.5) and pediatric patients with 'atypical psychosis' (n = 19; mean age = 13.3 + 3) was carried out to test the hypothesis that cortical gray matter loss would occur for COS, but not for the adolescents with atypical psychoses (Gogtay *et al.* 2004). The atypical psychosis group was matched with the COS group with respect to age, sex, IQ, premorbid functioning, medication treatment and hospitalization. Both groups were also compared with age and sex matched healthy controls (n = 38, mean age = 13.2 + 3). The mean follow-up period was 2.5 + 0.8 years. The COS group had significantly greater total and regional gray matter loss than did the 'atypical psychosis' or healthy control groups (ANOVA post hoc *p* values from 0.002 to 0.02) as seen in Figure 5.3. The atypical psychosis and control groups did not differ significantly from each other.

Thus the progressive cortical loss, at least as measured with this relatively crude parcellation, appears specific to schizophrenia. This finding is in agreement with the recent reports of Pantelis *et al.* (2003) in which high-risk unmedicated late adolescent subjects who progressed to affective illness did not show progressive brain tissue loss, while the ones progressing to first episode did.

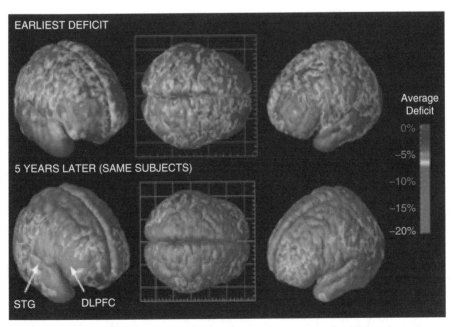

Figure 5.3 Progressive and region-specific loss of cortical gray matter in childhood-onset schizophrenia compared with age- and sex-matched community controls. STG – superior temporal gyrus; DLPFC – dorsolateral prefrontal cortex. Loss of gray matter shown as deficit per year (Thompson *et al.* 2001).

Clinical correlates of gray matter loss

A larger patient sample has enabled examination of clinical correlates of the gray matter loss. Poor premorbid functioning and baseline clinical severity as measured by the Brief Psychiatric Rating Scale (BPRS) were associated with a faster rate of gray matter reduction (standardized coefficient $= 0.34$, $r^2 = 0.12$, $p < 0.05$; and standardized coefficient $= 0.31$, $r^2 = 0.09$, $p < 0.05$ respectively) (Sporn *et al.* 2003). There was no significant relationship between the rate of cortical gray loss and sex, ethnicity, familial schizotypy, age of onset, duration of illness, full scale IQ, or information and comprehension subscale raw scores.

Unexpectedly however, when treatment and outcome measures were separately examined in relation to gray matter loss, percentage improvement on the BPRS scale was associated with a steeper slope for of gray matter reduction, i.e. more improvement was associated with greater loss (standardized coefficient $= 0.47$, $r^2 = 0.22$, $p < 0.01$) (Sporn *et al.* unpublished data). No treatment variable, including medication type, total or per weight dose, or clinical rating scale scores at follow-up, was associated with the rate of gray matter reduction, and there was no significant correlation between gray matter loss and cognitive test performance. With pooled analyses including baseline, follow-up, and clinical change scores, the clinical improvement measures showed the strongest correlation with rate of gray matter loss (Sporn *et al.* submitted).

Dynamic mapping of structural brain changes

Longitudinal re-scans of the NIMH COS adolescent sample were analyzed using a cortical pattern matching method developed at the UCLA Neuroimaging Laboratory (Thompson *et al.* 2001). Three scans per subject obtained at approximately two-year intervals were quantified, using a program in which three-dimensional distribution of gray matter in the brain is first computed and then mathematically compared from one scan to the next. The method utilized a computational tensor matching strategy that aligns corresponding landmarks on the cortical surface, across time, and across subjects, with greater spatial detail than previously obtainable (Thompson *et al.* 2000). This mapping of region specific brain cortical development across time and between subject groups has far greater resolution, and thus allows detection of dynamic changes in regional gray matter using time one, time two, and time three subtractions.

Subtraction maps of the youngest COS and controls show that the parietal gray matter volume loss occurs initially, with frontal and temporal gray matter changes appearing later across the adolescent years, providing support,

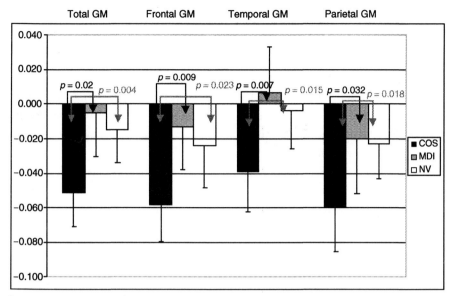

Figure 5.4 Comparison of percent change in total and regional gray matter volumes between COS (n = 19), MDI (n = 23) and NV (normal volunteers; N = 38) across a two and a half year period. *P* values are obtained with one-way ANOVA with Tukey HSD post hoc test. Error bars indicate standard deviation. MDI and NV do not differ significantly for any measure (all *p* >0.6). GM – gray matter (Gogtay *et al.* 2004).

with more established quantitative methods, for the back to front 'wave' of progressive gray matter loss in COS.

In order to relate this cortical wave of gray matter loss in COS to the pattern seen in normal development, we have recently analyzed 66 prospective scans from 20 healthy children from ages 4 to 18 (three or more scans each). Preliminary analysis of normal cortical development in this group does not show any back to front pattern (Gogtay *et al.* unpublished data).

Sibling studies of COS

A recent comparison of 15 healthy full siblings of COS (mean age = 19.14, SD = 5.99) and 32 age and sex matched community controls shows that the COS siblings have smaller parietal gray matter volumes (F(dF) = 5.69 (1,44), *p* = 0.02, Gogtay *et al.* 2003). This finding was more prominent for the younger (age 18 and below; n = 8) siblings, while the older sibling group (n = 7) showed a trend for total and frontal gray matter volume reduction. These preliminary findings in healthy siblings, if substantiated suggest that a back to front pattern (parieto-frontal) of gray matter loss may be a familial trait marker. An extended prospective study of sibling brain development in COS is currently underway at the NIMH.

Other imaging studies

There has only been one PET study of COS. Cerebral glucose metabolism was examined in 16 adolescent subjects from the NIMH childhood-onset schizophrenia sample and 26 healthy adolescents matched for age, sex, and handedness using positron emission tomography (PET) and ^{18}F-fluorodeoxyglucose (FDG) (Jacobsen and Rapoport 1998). Subjects performed an auditory continuous performance task (CPT) during FDG uptake. Childhood-onset schizophrenics made less correct and more incorrect identification on the CPT than did healthy subjects. PET findings indicated only mild hypofrontality, in spite of their poorer performance. Intriguingly, abnormally increased cerebellar metabolism was the most striking finding.

Few functional MR imaging studies have been conducted for childhood-onset schizophrenia, in part because functional imaging demands a level of cooperation or cognitive ability too difficult for the very ill participants. Because radiation is not a problem with this technique, Thomas and colleagues have conducted a proton magnetic resonance spectroscopy study of 10 children with schizophrenia and 12 healthy children (Thomas *et al.* 1998). They found that the ratio of N-acetylaspartate to creatine was significantly lower in the frontal lobes of schizophrenic children. Although the role of N-acetylaspartate has not been firmly established, it is thought to be a marker of neuronal density or neuronal volume (Renshaw *et al.* 1995).

Conclusions and future directions

The mechanism of these striking and progressive brain changes in schizophrenia remains unknown. The gray matter loss is consistent with the 'reduced neuropil' hypothesis for schizophrenia (Glantz and Lewis 2000; Harrison 1999; Selemon and Goldman-Rakic 1999) and also with the models of subtle, progressive and widespread disruption and decreasing connectivity of multiple cortical regions (McGlashan and Hoffman 2000; Woods 1998). One neurodevelopmental hypothesis of schizophrenia proposes an early (and fixed) lesion in the pre or perinatal period resulting in a disturbed late maturational response (Weinberger 1987). Animal models of schizophrenia supporting this hypothesis show that developmentally specific early lesions can disrupt the later maturing regions such as the frontal–limbic circuitry, and that such effects could be the interaction of genetic (variability and vulnerability) and environmental factors (Lipska and Weinberger 1995; Lipska *et al.* 2002).

Our data in part support a modification of this model, as our COS patients show both a more pronounced evidence of early brain impairment as indicated by more impaired development in the first years of life (Alaghband-Rad *et al.* 1995), as well as striking later progression (Nicolson *et al.* 2000).

We consider that the basis for this progression is similar to that proposed by Woods (1998), which considers schizophrenia as a progressive neurodevelopmental disorder that may reflect the action of genes showing greater expression in adolescence.

It is thus possible that the neurodevelopmental genes will have multiple roles across different time periods and that etiological agents causing abnormalities in early development will have related but different effects at later stages depending upon gene-environment interaction.

The progressive brain changes could also represent a plastic response of the brain to the illness, an argument also supported by our recent data. The decrease in regional and total gray matter shows a significant relationship with measures of clinical improvement across this period (Sporn *et al.* submitted). This could thus be a plastic response that may be 'restitutive' in nature. Clearly, brain plasticity cannot represent the only basis for these changes, as the healthy siblings of the probands also show some cortical gray matter changes on initial scan (Gogtay *et al.* 2003). These formulations however are not exclusionary. It may be that early clinical improvement is simply a byproduct of elimination of malfunctioning synapses. It is intriguing that the COS slopes seem to diverge from normal around age 10, the mean age of onset of psychosis for this group. This study cannot address the question of whether the gray matter loss 'triggers' the illness. However, the recent study of Pantelis *et al.* where pre-schizophrenic subjects showed gray matter loss while the ones developing into affective illness did not, suggests that this may be the case (Pantelis *et al.* 2003).

The search for mechanisms producing these progressive changes and their clinical correlations are important future research targets. Establishing patterns of cortical development in normal children is a critical part of these efforts. Similarly, imaging COS probands and their well siblings may address the issue of progressive loss as a trait marker. Finally, complementary studies using other modalities such as MRS and using higher strength machines will be important for understanding the pathophysiology of this devastating childhood illness.

References

Alaghband-Rad, J., McKenna, K., Gordon, C.T., Albus, K.E., Hamburger, S.D., Rumsey, J.M., Frazier, J.A., Lenane, M.C. and Rapoport, J.L. (1995) Childhood-onset schizophrenia: the severity of premorbid course. *J Am Acad Child Adolesc Psychiatry* 34 (10), 1273–1283.

Badura, F., Trott, G.E., Mehler-Wex, C., Scheuerpflug, P., Hofmann, E., Warmuth-Metz, M., Nadjmi, M., Solymosi, L. and Warnke, A. (2001) A study of cranial computertomograms in very early and early onset schizophrenia. *J Neural Transm* 108 (11), 1335–1344.

Childs, B. and Scriver, C.R. (1986) Age at onset and causes of disease. *Perspect Biol Med* 29 (3 Pt 1), 437–460.

Collins, D.L., Zijdenbos, A.P., Baare, W.F.C. and Evans, A.C. (1999) ANIMAL + INSECT: Improved cortical structure segmentation. In *Proceedings of the Annual Conference on Information Processing in Medical Imaging (IPMI)*, pp. 210–223. Visegrad, Hungary: Springer.

DeLisi, L.E. (1999a) Regional brain volume change over the life-time course of schizophrenia. *J Psychiatr Res* 33 (6), 535–541.

DeLisi, L.E. (1999b) Defining the course of brain structural change and plasticity in schizophrenia. *Psychiatry Res* 92 (1), 1–9.

Done, D.J., Crow, T.J., Johnstone, E.C. and Sacker, A. (1994) Childhood antecedents of schizophrenia and affective illness: social adjustment at ages 7 and 11. *BMJ* 309 (6956), 699–703.

Frazier, J.A., Giedd, J.N., Hamburger, S.D., Albus, K.E., Kaysen, D., Vaituzis, A.C., Rajapakse, J.C., Lenane, M.C., McKenna, K., Jacobsen, L.K., Gordon, C.T., Breier, A. and Rapoport, J.L. (1996) Brain anatomic magnetic resonance imaging in childhood-onset schizophrenia. *Arch Gen Psychiatry* 53 (7), 617–624.

Giedd, J.N., Blumenthal, J., Jeffries, N.O., Castellanos, F.X., Liu, H., Zijdenbos, A., Paus, T., Evans, A.C. and Rapoport, J.L. (1999a) Brain development during childhood and adolescence: a longitudinal MRI study [letter]. *Nat Neurosci* 2, 861–863.

Giedd, J.N., Jeffries, N.O., Blumenthal, J., Castellanos, F.X., Vaituzis, A.C., Fernandez, T., Hamburger, S.D., Liu, H., Nelson, J., Bedwell, J., Tran, L., Lenane, M., Nicolson, R. and Rapoport, J.L. (1999b) Childhood-onset schizophrenia: progressive brain changes during adolescence [see comments]. *Biol Psychiatry* 46 (7), 892–898.

Giedd, J.N., Snell, J.W., Lange, N., Rajapakse, J.C., Casey, B.J., Kozuch, P.L., Vaituzis, A.C., Vauss, Y.C., Hamburger, S.D., Kaysen, D. and Rapoport, J.L. (1996) Quantitative magnetic resonance imaging of human brain development: ages 4–18. *Cereb Cortex* 6 (4), 551–560.

Glantz, L.A. and Lewis, D.A. (2000) Decreased dendritic spine density on prefrontal cortical pyramidal neurons in schizophrenia [see comments]. *Arch Gen Psychiatry* 57 (1), 65–73.

Gogate, N., Giedd, J., Janson, K. and Rapoport, J.L. (2001) Brain imaging in normal and abnormal brain development: new perspectives for child psychiatry. *Clinical Neuroscience Research* 1, 283–290.

Gogtay, N., Sporn, A., Clasen, L.S., Greenstein, D., Giedd, J.N., Lenane, M., Gochman, P.A., and Rapoport, J.L. (2003) Structural brain MRI abnormalities in healthy siblings of patients with childhood-onset schizophrenia. *Am J Psychiatry* 160, 569–571.

Godtay, N., Sporn, A., Clasen, L.S., *et al.* (2004) Comparison of progressive cortical gray matter loss in childhood-onset schizophrenia with that in childhood-onset atypical psychoses. *Arch Gen Psychiatry* 61(1): 17–22.

Goodman, R. (1994) Brain disorders. In M. Rutter, E. Taylor, and L. Hersov, *Child and Adolescent Psychiatry: Modern Approaches*, 3rd edn, pp. 172–190. London: Blackwell.

Gordon, C.T., Frazier, J.A., McKenna, K., Giedd, J., Zametkin, A., Zahn, T., Hommer, D., Hong, W., Kaysen, D., Albus, K.E. *et al.* (1994) Childhood-onset schizophrenia: an NIMH study in progress. *Schizophr Bull* 20 (4), 697–712.

Green, W.H., Padron-Gayol, M., Hardesty, A.S. and Bassiri, M. (1992) Schizophrenia with childhood onset: a phenomenological study of 38 cases. *J Am Acad Child Adolesc Psychiatry* 31 (5), 968–976.

Gur, R.E., Cowell, P., Turetsky, B.I., Gallacher, F., Cannon, T., Bilker, W. and Gur, R.C. (1998) A follow-up magnetic resonance imaging study of schizophrenia. Relationship of neuroanatomical changes to clinical and neurobehavioral measures. *Arch Gen Psychiatry* 55 (2), 145–152.

Harrison, P.J. (1999) The neuropathology of schizophrenia. A critical review of the data and their interpretation. *Brain* 122 (Pt 4), 593–624.

Hollis, C. (1995) Child and adolescent (juvenile onset) schizophrenia. A case control study of premorbid developmental impairments. *Br J Psychiatry* 166 (4), 489–495.

Jacobsen, L.K., Giedd, J.N., Castellanos, F.X., Vaituzis, A.C., Hamburger, S.D., Kumra, S., Lenane, M.C. and Rapoport, J.L. (1998) Progressive reduction of temporal lobe structures in childhood-onset schizophrenia. *Am J Psychiatry* 155 (5), 678–685.

Jacobsen, L.K., Giedd, J.N., Vaituzis, A.C., Hamburger, S.D., Rajapakse, J.C., Frazier, J.A., Kaysen, D., Lenane, M.C., McKenna, K., Gordon, C.T. and Rapoport, J.L. (1996) Temporal lobe morphology in childhood-onset schizophrenia [published erratum appears in Am J Psychiatry 1996 June; 153 (6), 851]. *Am J Psychiatry* 153 (3), 355–361.

Jacobsen, L.K. and Rapoport, J.L. (1998) Research update: childhood-onset schizophrenia: implications of clinical and neurobiological research. *J Child Psychol Psychiatry* 39 (1), 101–113.

James, A.C., Javaloyes, A., James, S. and Smith, D.M. (2002) Evidence for non-progressive changes in adolescent-onset schizophrenia: follow-up magnetic resonance imaging study. *Br J Psychiatry* 180, 339–344.

Jones, P., Rodgers, B., Murray, R. and Marmot, M. (1994) Child development risk factors for adult schizophrenia in the British 1946 birth cohort. *Lancet* 344 (8934), 1398–1402.

Kraepelin, E. (1919) 1919 edn, Huntington, NY: Robert E. Krieger.

Kumra, S., Giedd, J.N., Vaituzis, A.C., Jacobsen, L.K., McKenna, K., Bedwell, J., Hamburger, S., Nelson, J.E., Lenane, M. and Rapoport, J.L. (2000) Childhood-onset psychotic disorders: magnetic resonance imaging of volumetric differences in brain structure. *Am J Psychiatry* 157 (9), 1467–1474.

Kumra, S., Jacobsen, L.K., Lenane, M., Zahn, T.P., Wiggs, E., Alaghband-Rad, J., Castellanos, F.X., Frazier, J.A., McKenna, K., Gordon, C.T., Smith, A., Hamburger, S. and Rapoport, J.L. (1998) 'Multidimensionally impaired disorder': is it a variant of very early-onset schizophrenia? [see comments]. *J Am Acad Child Adolesc Psychiatry* 37 (1), 91–99.

Lieberman, J., Chakos, M., Wu, H., Alvir, J., Hoffman, E., Robinson, D. and Bilder, R. (2001) Longitudinal study of brain morphology in first episode schizophrenia. *Biol Psychiatry* 49, 487–499.

Lim, K.O., Harris, D., Beal, M., Hoff, A.L., Minn, K., Csernansky, J.G., Faustman, W.O., Marsh, L., Sullivan, E.V. and Pfefferbaum, A. (1996) Gray matter deficits in young onset schizophrenia are independent of age of onset. *Biol Psychiatry* 40, 4–13.

Lipska, B.K., Halim, N.D., Segal, P.N. and Weinberger, D.R. (2002) Effects of reversible inactivation of the neonatal ventral hippocampus on behavior in the adult rat. *J Neurosci* 22, 2835–2842.

Lipska, B.K. and Weinberger, D.R. (1995) Genetic variation in vulnerability to the behavioral effects of neonatal hippocampal damage in rats. *Proc Natl Acad Sci USA* 92 (19), 8906–8910.

Marsh, L., Harris, D., Lim, K.O., Beal, M., Hoff, A.L., Minn, K., Csernansky, J.G., DeMent, S., Faustman, W.O., Sullivan, E.V. and Pfefferbaum, A. (1997) Structural magnetic resonance imaging abnormalities in men with severe chronic schizophrenia and an early age at clinical onset. *Arch Gen Psychiatry* 54, 1104–1112.

Mathalon, D.H., Sullivan, E.V., Lim, K.O. and Pfefferbaum, A. (2001) Progressive brain volume changes and the clinical course of schizophrenia in men: a longitudinal magnetic resonance imaging study. *Arch Gen Psychiatry* 58, 148–157.

Matsumoto, H., Simmons, A., Williams, S., Hadjulis, M., Pipe, R., Murray, R. and Frangou, S. (2001a) Superior temporal gyrus abnormalities in early-onset schizophrenia: similarities and differences with adult-onset schizophrenia. *Am J Psychiatry* 158 (8), 1299–1304.

Matsumoto, H., Simmons, A., Williams, S., Pipe, R., Murray, R. and Frangou, S. (2001b) Structural magnetic imaging of the hippocampus in early onset schizophrenia. *Biol Psychiatry* 49 (10), 824–831.

McGlashan, T.H. and Hoffman, R.E. (2000) Schizophrenia as a disorder of developmentally reduced synaptic connectivity. *Arch Gen Psychiatry* 57 (7), 637–648.

McKenna, K., Gordon, C.T., Lenane, M., Kaysen, D., Fahey, K. and Rapoport, J.L. (1994) Looking for childhood-onset schizophrenia: the first 71 cases screened [see comments]. *J Am Acad Child Adolesc Psychiatry* 33 (5), 636–644.

Nicolson, R., Lenane, M., Brookner, F., Gochman, P., Kumra, S., Spechler, L., Giedd, J.N., Thaker, G.K., Wudarsky, M. and Rapoport, J.L. (2001) Children and adolescents with psychotic disorder not otherwise specified: A two to eight year follow-up. *Comprehensive Psychiatry* 42 (4), 319–325.

Nicolson, R., Lenane, M., Singaracharlu, S., Malaspina, D., Giedd, J.N., Hamburger, S.D., Gochman, P., Bedwell, J., Thaker, G.K., Fernandez, T., Wudarsky, M., Hommer, D.W. and Rapoport, J.L. (2000) Premorbid speech and language impairments in childhood-onset schizophrenia: association with risk factors. *Am J Psychiatry* 157 (5), 794–800.

Nicolson, R. and Rapoport, J.L. (1999) Childhood-onset schizophrenia: rare but worth studying. *Biol Psychiatry* 46 (10), 1418–1428.

Pantelis, C., Velakoulis, D., McGorry, P.D., Wood, S.J., Suckling, J., Phillips, L.J., Yung, A.R., Bullmore, E.T., Brewer, W., Soulsby, B., Desmond, P. and McGuire, P.K. (2003) Neuroanatomical abnormalities before and after onset of psychosis: a cross-sectional and longitudinal MRI comparison. *Lancet* 361, 281–285.

Rapoport, J.L., Giedd, J., Kumra, S., Jacobsen, L., Smith, A., Lee, P., Nelson, J. and Hamburger, S. (1997) Childhood-onset schizophrenia. Progressive ventricular change during adolescence [see comments]. *Arch Gen Psychiatry* 54 (10), 897–903.

Rapoport, J.L., Giedd, J.N., Blumenthal, J., Hamburger, S., Jeffries, N., Fernandez, T., Nicolson, R., Bedwell, J., Lenane, M., Zijdenbos, A., Paus, T. and Evans, A. (1999) Progressive cortical change during adolescence in childhood-onset schizophrenia. A longitudinal magnetic resonance imaging study. *Arch Gen Psychiatry* 56 (7), 649–654.

Renshaw, P.F., Yurgelun-Todd, D.A., Tohen, M., Gruber, S. and Cohen, B.M. (1995) Temporal lobe proton magnetic resonance spectroscopy of patients with first-episode psychosis. *Am J Psychiatry* 152 (3), 444–446.

Russell, A.T., Bott, L. and Sammons, C. (1989) The phenomenology of schizophrenia occurring in childhood. *J Am Acad Child Adolesc Psychiatry* 28 (3), 399–407.

Rutter, M., Graham, P. and Yule, W. (1970) A neuropsychiatric study in childhood. In: Clinics in Developmental Medicine, 35/36. S.I.M.P. Heinemann, London:

Schulz, S.C., Koller, M.M., Kishore, P.R., Hamer, R.M., Gehl, J.J. and Friedel, R.O. (1983) Ventricular enlargement in teenage patients with schizophrenia spectrum disorder. *Am J Psychiatry* 140 (12), 1592–1595.

Selemon, L.D. and Goldman-Rakic, P.S. (1999) The reduced neuropil hypothesis: a circuit based model of schizophrenia [see comments]. *Biol Psychiatry* 45 (1), 17–25.

Sowell, E.R., Levitt, J., Thompson, P.M., Holmes, C.J., Blanton, R.E., Kornsand, D.S., Caplan, R., McCracken, J., Asarnow, R. and Toga, A.W. (2000) Brain abnormalities in early-onset schizophrenia spectrum disorder observed with statistical parametric mapping of structural magnetic resonance images. *Am J Psychiatry* 157 (9), 1475–1484.

Sporn, A.L., Addington, A.M., Gogtay, N., *et al.* (2004). Pervasive developmental disorder and childhood-onset schizophrenia: comorbid disorder or a phenotypic variant of a very early onset illness? *Biol Psychiatry* 55(10): 989–94.

Sporn, A.L., Greenstein, D.K., Gogtay, N., *et al.* (2003). Progressive Brain Volume Loss During Adolescence in Childhood-Onset Schizophrenia. *Am J Psychiatry* 160(12): 2181–2189.

Thomas, M.A., Ke, Y., Levitt, J., Caplan, R., Curran, J., Asarnow, R. and McCracken, J. (1998) Preliminary study of frontal lobe 1H MR spectroscopy in childhood-onset schizophrenia. *J Magn Reson Imaging* 8 (4), 841–846.

Thompson, P.M., Giedd, J.N., Woods, R.P., MacDonald, D., Evans, A.C. and Toga, A.W. (2000) Growth patterns in the developing brain detected by using continuum mechanical tensor maps. *Nature* 404, 190–193.

Thompson, P.M., Vidal, C., Giedd, J.N., Gochman, P., Blumenthal, J., Nicolson, R., Toga, A.W. and Rapoport, J.L. (2001) From the cover: mapping adolescent brain change reveals dynamic wave of accelerated gray matter loss in very early-onset schizophrenia. *PNAS* 98 (20), 11650–11655.

Walker, E. and Lewine, R.J. (1990) Prediction of adult-onset schizophrenia from childhood home movies of the patients. *Am J Psychiatry* 147, 1052–1056.

Weinberger, D.R. (1987) Implications of normal brain development for the pathogenesis of schizophrenia. *Arch Gen Psychiatry* 44 (7), 660–669.

Werry, J.S. (1992) Child and adolescent (early onset) schizophrenia: a review in light of DSM-III-R. *J Autism Dev Disord* 22 (4), 601–624.

Woods, B.T. (1998) Is schizophrenia a progressive neurodevelopmental disorder? Toward a unitary pathogenetic mechanism [see comments]. *Am J Psychiatry* 155 (12), 1661–1670.

Chapter 6

Neurocognitive deficits and first-episode schizophrenia: characterization and course

Irene M. Bratti and Robert M. Bilder

Introduction

It is now widely acknowledged that neurocognitive deficits are an important aspect of the schizophrenia syndrome. Clinicians increasingly recognize the pervasive impact these deficits may have on daily functioning, and there is a new optimism that neurocognitive deficits may be at least partially ameliorated by novel psychopharmacological and non-pharmacological treatments. This chapter aims to describe the overall pattern of neurocognitive deficit at the time of the first episode of psychotic illness, characterize the pre- and post-illness course of deficits, and summarize current knowledge about the relations of these deficits to a range of other clinical characteristics.

The perspective gained from the study of first-episode patients is unique in several respects. Perhaps most important is the degree to which results may generalize to a large population of individuals who develop schizophrenia. Early neurocognitive studies focused on chronic samples, which were potentially biased to over-represent individuals with suboptimal course of illness and/or lack of additional resources that might have prevented their long-term institutional care. Studies of genetic high-risk samples are of enormous value but necessarily under-represent a large group of individuals where familial illness is not apparent. More recent studies of prodromal syndromes offer their own unique insights, but substantial proportions of the participants in these studies will never develop schizophrenia, and conversely, such samples fail to include individuals who develop schizophrenia without experiencing pronounced prodromal symptoms. At the first episode, there is a unique opportunity to observe the characteristics of illness early in the process, often without artifacts of extensive treatment, and to document the longitudinal course as it unfolds. As we highlight below, it may further be possible to gain insights about developmental course using follow-back methods. Thus we believe that observations of first episode samples open an important window on both the antecedents and post-onset course of neurocognitive deficits in schizophrenia.

Generalized neurocognitive deficit

Dating back to the historic work of Spearman, a distinction has been made between general and more specific cognitive abilities (Spearman 1927). It is interesting to note that most current approaches to neurocognitive assessment reflect a blend of assessment methods with origins that are distinguished

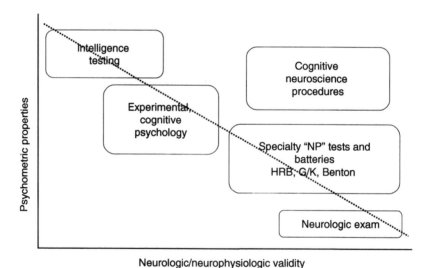

Fig. 6.1 Psychometric properties vs neurologic/neurophysiologic validity of neurocognitive assessment procedures.

Neurocognitive assessment procedures widely used in schizophrenia research developed from historical roots that involve a tradeoff between psychometric properties and neurologic/ neurophysiologic validity. On the one hand are procedures derived from the intelligence-testing tradition, which have strong psychometric properties enabling inferences about individual differences, but these were developed with virtually complete agnosticism to underlying brain functions. On the other hand are procedures developed from clinical neurology, which aim to detect pathognomonic signs of dysfunction in specific brain regions, but are poor at characterizing individual differences, since all individuals except those affected perform perfectly. Many additional neuropsychological and experimental or cognitive test procedures have been developed that involve some compromise along these dimensions. In theory, cognitive neuroscience research aims to satisfy both aims, and develop novel procedures that offer psychometric precision in the measurement of neural system functions.

by their roots in psychometric or neurological traditions. On the one hand, there is a psychometric tradition, with its origins in the development of IQ testing during the late nineteenth and early twentieth century. This tradition emphasized strong statistical and psychometric measurement principles, and refinement of measures has long been guided by empirical analyses of underlying factor structure (including Spearman's division of intelligence into general and specific abilities). This work has continued to influence modern thinking, with influential contributions including the work of Jensen and colleagues (Jensen 1998, 2000), and the work that has extended the Horn-Cattell theoretical distinction between crystallized and fluid intelligences (e.g., Woodcock-Johnson) (McArdle *et al.* 2002; Woodcock 1993). While measures deriving from the psychometric tradition typically have strong psychometric properties, most measures were developed without explicit consideration of relations to brain function. Behavioral, experimental and more recently cognitive psychology have in parallel generated a diversity of procedures, which have largely shared with intelligence testing a solid attention to refined measurement principles, along with an agnosticism about relations to brain function.

A parallel but largely independent neurological tradition spawned a diversity of procedures for assessing dysfunction in specific brain systems. The neurological exam offers an extreme example of these procedures, which are typically designed to elicit pathognomonic signs of specific localized brain disturbances. These methods are strong in their capacity to identify focal central nervous system lesions, but would horrify a psychometrician interested in assessing variability in broader groups of individuals, most of whom do not have such specific lesions. Classic neuropsychological examination procedures are largely derived from the neurologic tradition, but efforts have been made to increase their sensitivity to variation across ability levels. Despite these efforts, some widely used neuropsychological procedures have very poor psychometric properties except in samples suffering from specific disorders (e.g., procedures from the Boston Diagnostic Aphasia Exam are well suited to examining variation in aphasics but ceiling effects are often apparent in non-aphasic samples). It should further be recognized that many neuropsychological procedures that are widely used (e.g., Wisconsin Card Sorting Test) have origins in the Gestalt tradition of the 1930s and were refined after the Second World War to study patients with penetrating missile wounds to the head. More recent developments in neuropsychological testing have attempted to preserve knowledge about the sensitivity and specificity to dysfunction in dissociable brain systems, along with attention to psychometric principles. The ultimate (perhaps aspirational) goal in the study of both healthy cognition and pathological states are procedures that incorporate both our expanded knowledge of cognitive neuroscience, and which have psychometric properties enabling their application across individuals with wide variation in ability.

Application of tests derived from this diversity of historic threads has converged to indicate that people with the diagnosis of schizophrenia show a substantial generalized deficit, even at the time of the first episode. Two widely used indices of generalized neurocognitive performance have been applied in first-episode schizophrenia research–general measures of intelligence quotient, or IQ, and composite scores or profiles derived from batteries comprising multiple neuropsychological tests. While both can provide a measure of an individual's overall cognitive functioning, they usually have clear distinctions. Neuropsychological batteries typically focus on assessment of multiple fluid cognitive abilities, such as measures of memory, executive function and attention, that are very sensitive to brain dysfunction. IQ tests, on the other hand, usually have a greater emphasis on assessment of crystallized intellectual abilities (general knowledge, vocabulary) that are less sensitive to brain dysfunction. Indeed some of these IQ measures may be useful in estimating premorbid ability in individuals who have suffered brain damage. The IQ tests tend to have a stronger representation of verbal functioning and notably tend to exclude measures of memory. This is important as learning and memory functions are among those measures most consistently associated with deficits in schizophrenia. For these reasons, the magnitude of deficit documented in studies using IQ may be smaller than the magnitude of deficit observed on a composite neurocognitive battery, due to the inclusion in the neurocognitive battery of more measures sensitive to the deficits of schizophrenia. At the same time, it should be recognized that in some small number of studies, the magnitude of IQ deficit may appear large relative to other more specific cognitive deficits, primarily because the IQ test has stronger psychometric measurement properties.

Multiple studies have now reported IQ test scores in patients with first-episode schizophrenia (FES), and results consistently reveal a 10–25 point deficit in Full Scale IQ (FSIQ) for patients with FES compared to controls matched on other demographic parameters or population norms (Bilder *et al.* 2000; Russell *et al.* 1997; Aylward *et al.* 1984). This difference amounts to approximately a 0.7–1.7 standard deviation (SD) below the average population IQ. In Heinrichs and Zakzanis's meta-analysis of patients with both first-episode and chronic schizophrenia, the effect size for the WAIS-R IQ was 1.24 (Heinrichs and Zakzanis 1998).

Sampling issues must also be considered carefully in interpretation of IQ test scores. For example, a study by Townsend *et al.* using the WAIS III found very modest deficits (Townsend *et al.* 2001) of approximately 5 points compared to population norms, but the study did not include a control group, rendering the results difficult to interpret. Without a control group it is difficult to know what the sample's predicted performance should have been. Similarly, it is critical in evaluating any study with a control group to determine on precisely what variables the control group was matched to the patients. For instance, studies have shown that even for patients whose FSIQ is in normal range, it is often lower than expected given the FSIQ of the patients' siblings and first-degree relatives (Aylward *et al.* 1984; Gilvarry *et al.* 2000). Egan *et al.* demonstrated that patients with schizophrenia (N = 120) had FSIQs 15 points lower than their unaffected siblings (N = 189), though the study did not use an FES population (Egan *et al.* 2001). Similarly, using the NART scores as an estimate of premorbid IQ, Gilvarry *et al.* found an IQ difference of approximately 11.33 points between non-FES patients with schizophrenia and their siblings (Gilvarry *et al.* 2000). Given that 15 IQ points equals 1 SD, these patients demonstrated IQ deficits of close to 1 SD compared to their siblings. Furthermore, there is evidence that first-degree relatives themselves show deficits that are typically intermediate between those observed in patients and healthy individuals who do not have a similar family history of schizophrenia (see below for more complete discussion). Discrepancies observed in studies with family controls thus will systematically underestimate the actual deficit of the patients with respect to an unselected healthy population.

Many newer studies have evaluated patients with FES using general neuropsychological batteries. Most of these studies have concluded that there is a large generalized deficit across diverse neurocognitive domains that is approximately 1–2 SD below controls (Bilder *et al.* 2000; Mohamed *et al.* 1999; Hoff *et al.* 1998; Censits *et al.* 1997; Saykin *et al.* 1994). This was also reported in a large meta-analysis that included some first- and early-episode patients, but was comprised mainly of individuals with chronic schizophrenia (Heinrichs and Zakzanis 1998) with deficits ranging from 0.46 to 1.41 SD below population norms.

It appears that on measures of general neurocognitive function, by an individual's first episode of psychosis he or she is already performing approximately 1 to 2 standard deviations below comparable groups of healthy individuals appropriately matched on demographic variables. While this overall range of deficit may appear broad, it should be noted that estimates of effect size obtained from different studies may vary widely based on the reliability of the test scores used (the more reliable, the greater the sensitivity to deficit) and the nature of the comparison group. Furthermore, given that multiple studies have demonstrated at least a 1 SD deficit on IQ testing, we may conclude that the general deficit on neuropsychological batteries is over 1 SD, as neuropsychological measures tend to be more sensitive to the deficits of schizophrenia, leading to overall lower scores than IQ tests.

Specific neurocognitive deficits

Regarding the specific patterns of neuropsychological deficit, heterogeneity in construct definition makes it difficult to determine specific constructs that may be differentially impaired in FES. For instance, while some studies classified the Stroop word-color test under attention (Censits et al. 1997), others classified it under executive function (Hoff et al. 1999; Townsend et al. 2001; Riley et al. 2000), or speed of processing (Saykin et al. 1994; Mohamed et al. 1999). Though patients with FES do show specific cognitive deficits, the magnitude of the specific deficit pattern pales in comparison to the statistical size and likely clinical significance of the generalized deficit (Bilder et al. 2000). For example, Bilder and colleagues (Bilder et al. 2000) found a generalized deficit of approximately 1.5 SD in their first episode sample, and the deviations of individual functional domains from this generalized deficit amounted to only about 0.5 SD.

One of the most widely available (but not the most informative) sources of cognitive pattern information comes from the widely administered IQ tests. A consistent finding in samples of patients with both FE and chronic schizophrenia is a discrepancy between Verbal and Performance IQ. For example, using the WAIS-R, FES patients' verbal IQ was better than their performance IQ by about 8 points (Bilder et al. 2000). No other consistent deficit patterns have been identified on the WAIS (Bilder et al. 2000; Aylward et al. 1984). This V-P split can be considered a reflection of the discrepancy between crystallized and fluid intellectual abilities (as noted above), or more specifically a reflection of impairments in speeded processing, attention, abstraction, and novel problem-solving skills relative to basic language skills.

On more comprehensive neurocognitive batteries, Bilder et al. found that measures of memory and executive function were both more severely impaired than the generalized deficit of 1.5 SD below healthy volunteer levels (Bilder et al. 2000). Other studies have found that tasks of executive function (Riley et al. 2000; Mohamed et al. 1999; Censits et al. 1997), memory tasks (Riley et al. 2000; Addington et al. 2003; Mohamed et al. 1999; Censits et al. 1997; Saykin et al. 1994), attentional tasks (Addington et al. 2003; Mohamed et al. 1999;

Censits *et al.* 1997; Saykin *et al.* 1994), and speed-of-cognitive processing tasks (Townsend *et al.* 2001; Mohamed *et al.* 1999; Saykin *et al.* 1994) are significantly worse than other functional domains. These studies all converge to suggest that memory, executive, and attentional dysfunctions comprise areas of relative impairment in schizophrenia, and that these relative deficits are clearly apparent by the time of the first episode.

Multiple studies have demonstrated that verbal memory is specifically impaired in first-episode patients (Addington *et al.* 2003; Saykin *et al.* 1994; Hoff *et al.* 1999; Censits *et al.* 1997; Bilder *et al.* 2000). Censits *et al.* found that verbal memory performance was over 2 SD below controls (Censits *et al.* 1997). Hoff *et al.* reported that verbal memory was the only neuropsychological score to show decline over time in a longitudinal study (Hoff *et al.* 1999). Saykin *et al.* found that verbal memory and learning tasks accounted for approximately 46 per cent of the variance between the performance of FES patients and control subjects and that after accounting for verbal memory and learning, all other neurocognitive measures accounted for less than 5 per cent of variance (Saykin *et al.* 1994). Verbal memory was also highly impaired in a meta-analysis of samples of patients with both FE and chronic schizophrenia at 1.4 SD below population norms (Heinrichs and Zakzanis 1998). In a review of the literature, Green found that delayed verbal memory was associated with all three reviewed measures of functional outcome—community functioning, social problem solving, and specific skill acquisition (Green 1996) (see below for more details). Other studies did not find that FES patients had worse performance on verbal memory (Riley *et al.* 2000; Townsend *et al.* 2001). Their results, however, may be somewhat compromised by multiple comparisons with an uncorrected p value, a small sample size, and controls matched only on age (Riley *et al.* 2000), or no control group (Townsend *et al.* 2000).

Since there are typically moderate to strong correlations among different neurocognitive domains, the question arises whether there is a core deficit that may underlie both the generalized deficit and some or all of the specific deficits. For example, one could imagine that a fundamental deficit in attention might limit learning/memory functions. In their study, Bilder *et al.* (2000) examined the difference between patients with higher and lower levels of global neurocognitive ability. Patients with higher general ability scales had relatively poor memory function, while patients with low general ability had both relative memory and executive deficits (Bilder *et al.* 2000). These results suggested that memory deficits might be most sensitive to the neurocognitive deficit in schizophrenia, while additional executive deficits might contribute to more severe overall cognitive disability. Other studies have also found that those FES subjects who did poorly on tests of executive function also did more poorly than other subjects on all other cognitive tests (Addington *et al.* 2003). Hoff *et al.* found in a longitudinal study that patients who went into remission tended to show greater improvements in executive tasks than other FES patients and control subjects (Hoff *et al.* 1999). Bilder *et al.* also found that when memory deficits were controlled for using regression techniques, the only other significant contribution to distinguishing patient performance from control performance were motor skills like speed and dexterity (Bilder *et al.* 2000). These findings converge to suggest that some features of learning/memory performance are particularly sensitive to the more general cognitive deficits of schizophrenia. Further deficits in executive and motor function may explain additional variation in overall cognitive ability, and distinguishes those patients with the greatest degree of impairment.

Relative neurocognitive strengths – language

Language remains a complicated neurocognitive area to study as it involves different aspects of cognition. These includes fairly crystallized measures such as vocabulary, as well as more fluid measures often considered dependent on executive functions, such as verbal fluency and measures of verbal abstraction ability (which are frequently found to be impaired). There are also different potential deficits in speech production vs. speech comprehension. Some studies show a relative sparing of vocabulary (Townsend *et al.* 2001). This finding is in keeping with the relatively better performance of schizophrenic patients on verbal IQ measures vs. performance IQ. In their meta-analysis, Heinrichs and Zakzanis found that vocabulary was moderately spared (SD = 0.69) (Heinrichs and Zakzanis 1998). Bilder *et al.* found that language tasks were relatively spared, with an average deficit of approximately 1.0 SD below baseline vs. an overall average of 1.5 SD below other neuropsychological measures (Bilder *et al.* 2000). In their cross-sectional study, Saykin *et al.* found language sparing in patients with chronic schizophrenia, but not in FES patients (Saykin *et al.* 1994); however, the individuals in their FES sample were still psychotic at the time of testing. Their language measures also included verbal abstraction tests, which are likely more affected by current psychotic symptoms than more crystallized abilities such as vocabulary. Regarding premorbid deficits, in a retrospective analysis of academic performance before the onset of symptoms, Ang and Tan demonstrated that language performance remained stable and did not differ from matched controls, even as other skills, such as mathematics, deteriorated in the period between ages 12 and 16 (Ang and Tan 2004).

Summary of specific neurocognitive strengths and deficits

In summary, at first episode people with schizophrenia demonstrate specific areas of cognitive deficit, over and above the 1–2 SD general deficit. Tests of memory, executive function, attention, and speed of processing are specifically impaired. Verbal memory is selectively impaired at approximately 2 SD below the general deficit (Bilder *et al.* 2000; Saykin *et al.* 1994). In a number of studies, executive functioning was impaired in those with overall poorer cognitive functioning, and spared in those with less overall cognitive disability. Language, especially more crystallized measures such as vocabulary, appeared to be relatively spared.

Course of neuropsychological deficits

Premorbid/prodromal course

It is apparent that by the first episode of psychosis, people with schizophrenia already have significant cognitive impairments compared to their healthy peers and siblings. Are these deficits present from birth or do they appear at some identifiable period in development? Several studies have assessed premorbid or prodromal cognitive functioning in individuals who later developed schizophrenia. Regarding IQ, Davidson *et al.* reviewed data from a large cohort of Israeli adolescent males assessed for the national draft board who later developed schizophrenia (N = 509) vs. healthy individuals (N = 9215). They found that poor adolescent intellectual functioning was a strong predictor of later development of schizophrenia. Furthermore, there was a linear relationship between lower intellectual functioning and risk of schizophrenia (Davidson *et al.* 1999). David *et al.* also concluded in a population-based cohort study that low IQ is itself a predictor of risk of schizophrenia (David *et al.* 1997). Others have also found a correlation between low premorbid IQ and schizophrenia risk (Jones *et al.* 1994). Kremen *et al.* conducted a prospective general population study, in which they concluded that a larger than expected decline in IQ from ages four to seven was a predictor of later progression to psychosis. It appeared that the key predictive factor was IQ decline, because subjects with low age four IQs and similarly low age seven IQs did not have an elevated risk for psychosis. Though a low age seven IQ also predicted psychotic symptoms, a large IQ decline was more predictive of later psychosis than either age seven IQ alone, or parents' socioeconomic status (Kremen *et al.* 1998).

Using standardized scholastic tests, Fuller *et al.* demonstrated that while students who later developed schizophrenia (n = 70) were below the

50th percentile for state student performance at all grade levels, this difference was non-significant at the fourth and eighth grade. However by the eleventh grade the premorbid students were significantly below the 50th percentile: four of six measures (reading, language, sources of information, and the composite score) were below the premorbid group's previous fourth grade performance by eleventh grade. The effect sizes for the difference from 50th percentile in reading, language, sources of information, and composite score ranged from 0.32–0.41 in premorbid individuals. The vocabulary and mathematics scores were not significantly below the 50th percentile by the eleventh grade. Language scores showed a linear decline from the fourth grade, while the other measures showed improvement between fourth and eighth grade, only to drop by grade 11 (Fuller *et al.* 2002). For the majority of the measures, therefore, a significant cognitive impairment became evident somewhere between the ages of 13 and 16. This scholastic decline was not correlated with severity of later positive, negative, or disorganized symptoms. There was also little correlation between performance on a later neurocognitive battery administered after the onset of schizophrenia. The authors posit that perhaps scholastic testing is measuring different cognitive dimensions than the later neuropsychological battery. Though this study is one of the few to examine actual and not calculated premorbid test performance, the results are compared to the 50th percentile population norm, rather than a matched control group. It thus remains unclear what magnitude of deficit these individuals may have had with respect to expectations that would be based on their individual family and sociocultural backgrounds. Despite this caveat, the Fuller *et al.* findings concur with those of Kremen, that decline in cognitive function prior to the overt onset of schizophrenia may be a characteristic of individuals who will go on to develop schizophrenia.

In another follow-back study, where prospectively acquired data were mined from academic records, individuals who would later go on to develop schizophrenia were compared to a group of healthy people recruited from the same community (Bilder *et al.* 1995; Reiter *et al.* 1995). Comparison of academic achievement scores (math, reading) revealed a significant deficit (effect size ~ 1 SD) for the to-become-patient group detectable as early as the first grade. These individuals did not show further relative decline in performance, but showed a stable deficit of similar magnitude on these achievement tests into the high school years. In contrast, analysis of the actual grades earned in their courses showed a subtle decline in the years from the seventh through the eleventh grade (approximately ages 13–17), suggesting a possible adolescent decline in cognitive ability. These findings are consistent with several ideas

1) that a decline in cognitive ability may presage the onset of schizophrenia, 2) that there are some substantial deficits that can be detected very early, and 3) that additional deterioration may occur in the premorbid period. Notably, the test scores and grades included in this study were all obtained prior to the time when family members noticed any behavioral changes in the to-be-patients, suggesting that the cognitive decline may precede other prodromal features of schizophrenia.

Ang and Tan also used standardized academic performance tests to evaluate premorbid function and change in function between two groups of tests administered at ages 12 and 16. The study group was comprised of 30 people who later developed first-episode schizophrenia around age 20, and 30 healthy volunteers matched on age, gender, socioeconomic status, and performance on the first standardized tests. The authors concluded that mathematics scores declined significantly between the two testing periods, but that language scores did not (see above). FES patients were noted to be showing declines in cognitive performance as measured by academic tests up to four years before the onset of significant symptoms (Ang and Tan 2004). Mathematic skills are more fluid than the relatively crystallized language skills, and thus may be more sensitive to cognitive decline.

Cannon *et al.* did not find academic impairment in children aged 7–11 who went on to develop schizophrenia, schizoaffective disorder, and schizophreniform disorder, compared to age-matched healthy individuals in a case-control population study. They compared the grades of approximately 400 children who went on to develop a schizophrenia-spectrum disorder, to 408 healthy individuals, on three factors derived from school subjects—academic, sports and handicraft—and a behavioral factor. The children who went on to develop a schizophrenia-spectrum disorder showed significant impairment compared to healthy individuals only on the sports and handicrafts factor, possibly suggesting subtle motor deficits in vulnerable children. However, despite performing as well as healthy individuals, the pre-schizophrenic children were significantly less likely to go on to high school (Cannon *et al.* 1999). There are several reasons why in this study pre-schizophrenic children might not have shown academic impairment or decline. First, during the early school years grades are often based less on objective scholastic performance than during later years, and this study does not include results from standardized testing that may be a more valid measure of early cognition than school grades. Furthermore, the studies by Fuller *et al.*, Bilder *et al.*, and Ang and Tan suggest that there is a significant cognitive decline between the ages of 12 and 17, which would not be observed in the time-course of this study. It should be noted that despite similar academic performances, the children who later developed schizophrenia were less likely to proceed to high school, suggesting a subtle cognitive or social impairment not captured by the fairly crude measure of school grades.

The evidence from follow-back studies indicates that as early as age 6 or 7, people who go on to develop schizophrenia are showing academic impairments and lower IQ scores. The data also suggest further cognitive decline, as evidenced by deterioration in academic performance and IQ. There was a significant IQ decline between ages four and seven in Kremen *et al*'s study. Fuller *et al.*, Bilder *et al.* and Ang and Tan all suggested an academic decline between ages 12 and 17. Significantly, these declines in cognitive performance occurred several years before the onset of any prodromal symptoms.

Change in cognitive function accompanying psychosis onset and after the first episode

Earlier in the chapter we examined the magnitude and quality of the general cognitive deficit, and the pattern of specific deficits, as they appear at the first break in schizophrenia. Less is known, however, about the longitudinal course of cognitive function from the premorbid or prodromal period to the period after the first break. Several cross-sectional studies have attempted to address this question. One popular method for retrospective estimation of change in IQ based on cross-sectional testing is to compare scores on current IQ tests with scores on measures used to estimate premorbid IQ, such as the National Adult Reading Test (NART). The NART, modifications of the NART, and similar measures (such as the more recently developed Wechsler Test of Adult Reading) rely on the premise that certain reading skills, especially the reading of phonetically irregular words, along with measures of general knowledge or vocabulary, correlate strongly with FSIQ in healthy populations, and are insensitive to deterioration. Several studies using the NART administered after patients became ill have been interpreted as suggesting a cognitive decline compared to the WAIS FSIQ or other neurocognitive measures administered during the same testing period (Addington *et al.* 2003; Townsend *et al.* 2002; Gilvarry *et al.* 2000). However, the NART has been demonstrated to be a poor measure of premorbid IQ at the high and low extremes of the IQ scale. In the case of people with schizophrenia, the correlation with IQ scores may be lower and the estimation error would be biased to overestimate the premorbid FSIQ (by as much as 15 points) in schizophrenia patients (Russell *et al.* 2000). Further complicating matters is the fact that studies using the NART or similar premorbid estimates to contrast with current IQ scores make a fundamental assumption that the pathologic process in schizophrenia does not have a substantial impact on the acquisition of basic reading skills or other crystallized intellectual abilities; this assumption may well be wrong. Indeed, the deficit observed on these premorbid indices with respect to expectations based on population norms offer support for the idea that people who will go on to develop schizophrenia have pre-onset pathology that interferes with their acquisition of these skills, and thus the validity of conclusions drawn from studies using NART or similar measures must be interpreted cautiously.

There is an ever-increasing number of prospectively acquired longitudinal data documenting the course of cognitive dysfunction following the onset of schizophrenia. Russell *et al.* reported on 34 subjects who had been IQ tested during childhood as part of a child psychiatry assessment. Over 19 years later, the FSIQ of these schizophrenic subjects had gone down 1.9 points, from 84.1 during childhood to 82.2 as chronically ill schizophrenic inpatients (Russell *et al.* 1997). However, the use of different tests across time points, small sample size, lack of control group, and sampling bias (these subjects were recruited from a childhood psychiatric clinic) make generalization of these results difficult. Using a similar approach to determine the amount of decline in intellectual ability that may accompany onset of schizophrenia, Bilder and colleagues examined the discrepancies between premorbid Scholastic Aptitude Test (SAT) scores and current (post-onset, after clinical stabilization of the first episode) IQ scores. The relationship between earlier (age 16 to 18) SAT scores and current (age ~25) IQ was based on correlations observed in a healthy comparison group from the same community. While the healthy individuals had no decline in scores (by definition), the people with schizophrenia showed a 7 point decline (approximately $\frac{1}{2}$ SD) relative to the IQ predicted from their SAT score (Bilder 1; Reiter 1). This magnitude of decline may over-estimate the magnitude of intellectual deterioration accompanying the first episode, since the sample included only the college bound subgroup of people with schizophrenia. This subgroup includes those individuals with the highest levels of premorbid ability among those who go on to develop schizophrenia, and presumably they are at greater risk of intellectual decline compared to those who had poorer premorbid function. Overall, it seems likely that there is a change in intellectual ability accompanying the first episode of illness, but that this may be subtle and is likely less than $\frac{1}{2}$ SD in magnitude. In a comprehensive meta-analysis on intelligence and schizophrenia assessing studies before 1984, the authors conclude that there is no consistent finding of IQ decline during the course of the illness (Aylward *et al.* 1994).

Regarding the course of deficits as documented by more comprehensive neuropsychological batteries, a cross-sectional study by Saykin *et al.* found that FES patients performed approximately 0.5 SD better on a neurocognitive battery than patients with chronic schizophrenia, but the pattern of deficits remained the same (Saykin *et al.* 1994). However, the FES patients and the chronically ill patients were not matched, and most likely represented different population samples. Other studies demonstrate that patients with chronic schizophrenia perform approximately 0.3 to 1.0 SD worse than FES patients on general neuropsychological batteries (Bilder *et al.* 1992; Hoff *et al.* 1998), though this data is derived from cross-sectional studies and also may be subject to selection biases.

Concerning longitudinal data, in a four to five year follow-up study with 42 people, Hoff *et al.* found that FES patients did not show deterioration on a neuropsychological battery, other than a mild decline in verbal memory scores. The individuals with schizophrenia showed a mild improvement in testing over the years on all measures–except verbal memory and sensory-perceptual tasks–secondary to practice effects, but no more than the healthy volunteers did. The overall deficit for patients with schizophrenia was thus maintained at 1–2 SD below healthy volunteers (Hoff *et al.* 1999). Censits *et al.* found no decline in neurocognitive measures over 19 months in either FES patients (N = 30), previously treated, patients with chronic schizophrenia (N = 30), or healthy individuals (N = 38), despite an overall large neurocognitive deficit of over 1 SD in patients (see above). Gold *et al.* found that after five years, most neurocognitive scores remained the same for 54 first-episode patients. However, several scores improved, including measures of visual attention, verbal memory, and executive function (Gold *et al.* 1999). Goldman *et al.* found no deterioration and only slight improvement in neurocognitive scores following their first episode sample over the first three years of treatment (Goldman, 1996).

While most studies find almost no areas of deterioration, Stirling *et al.*, in a 10 year follow-up study, found that there was a significant decline in FES performance on three of nine neurocognitive measures–object assembly, picture completion, and memory for design. The other six measures studied, however, including the WCST, verbal fluency tests and verbal memory tests, did not deteriorate or showed mild but non-significant improvement (Stirling *et al.* 2003).

A fascinating series of studies in older patients has suggested that people with schizophrenia may be vulnerable to more substantial deterioration (Harvey *et al.* 1999). Since this topic is covered fully in another chapter, it will not be discussed further here.

The longitudinal data suggest that after the onset of schizophrenia, there is at most a subtle decline in cognitive function of no more than 0.5 SD. Many studies demonstrate no decline or some improvement at follow-up. However, the follow-up periods of the available studies may not be long enough to draw a definitive conclusion about possible cognitive decline after first-episode.

Neurocognitive deficits and relationship to first-degree relatives

In the last several years, there has been an increasing interest in determining patterns of neurocognitive deficits in first-degree relatives of people with schizophrenia, in the hope of identifying various cognitive endophenotypes of the disorder. The concept of the endophenotype has been evolving in schizophrenia, as research into the genetic underpinnings of the disorder has been unsuccessful in identifying consistent candidate genes. The difficulty lies in the presumed complex inheritance of this polygenic disease. The endophenotype can be defined as a component characteristic of a disorder, which can be identified and measured, and which has a simpler inheritance pattern than the full phenotype of the illness. Endophenotypes can be of various natures, including biochemical, neuroanatomical, or neuropsychological. Gottesman and Gould identified five necessary features for endophenotypes to be useful in psychiatry research: 1) the endophenotype is associated with illness in the population, 2) it is hereditable, 3) it is state-independent and does not vary with illness course, 4) within families, illness and endophenotype co-segregate, and 5) the endophenotype found in affected family members is found in non-affected family members more frequently than in the general population (Gottesman and Gould 2003).

Because people with schizophrenia show a profound general neuropsychological impairment even at first presentation, it can be difficult to identify candidate cognitive endophenotypes in patients, especially as other severe axis I disorder patients (such as bipolar disorder patients) can show similarly significant cognitive deficits. However, if specific cognitive impairments can be demonstrated in first-degree relatives, especially if those impairments are not found in the relatives of those with other axis I disorders, they may identify cognitive endophenotypes, more common in affected families than in the general population as a whole, and in the population of families with other axis I disorders in particular.

Studies have demonstrated that first-degree relatives show impairments in measures of IQ (Zalla *et al.* 2004; Egan *et al.* 2001; Kremen *et al.* 1998), verbal memory (Egan *et al.* 2001; Kremen *et al.* 1998; Goldberg *et al.* 1995), visual memory (Kremen *et al.* 1998; Goldberg *et al.* 1995), attention (Egan *et al.* 2001; Laurent *et al.* 1999; Asarnow *et al.* 2002), executive function (Egan *et al.* 2001; Goldberg *et al.* 1995; Zalla *et al.* 2004; Laurent *et al.* 1999; Asarnow *et al.* 2002), language (Egan *et al.* 2001; Laurent *et al.* 1999), and psychomotor speed (Goldberg *et al.* 1995).

However, other studies fail to find impairments in some measurements of IQ (Gilvarry *et al.* 2000), executive function (Zalla *et al.* 2004; Laurent *et al.* 1999), attention, and visual memory (Laurent *et al.* 1999).

Studies have also compared the relatives of people with schizophrenia to relatives of people with other axis I disorders, such as bipolar disorder (Zalla *et al.* 2004; Kremen *et al.* 1998; Gilvarry *et al.* 2000) and ADHD (Asarnow *et al.* 2002). Some have found that the relatives of people with schizophrenia perform poorly compared to relatives of people with other axis I disorders (Kremen *et al.* 1998; Asarnow *et al.* 2002); others have not (Gilvarry *et al.* 2000; Zalla *et al.* 2004).

Another important reason to identify possible cognitive deficits in relatives of people with schizophrenia is related to the difficulty in appropriately matching schizophrenic patients to control subjects. Frequently, the measures used to match patients and controls are affected by the illness itself, such as educational level and IQ. This may underestimate the expected ability of the patient group, leading to falsely elevated scores for the individuals with schizophrenia on non-affected or more crystallized measures (like language, see above). This same concern can be considered for the first-degree relatives of schizophrenic subjects (Kremen *et al.* 1995). Kremen *et al.* examined this issue by comparing first-degree relatives to control subjects on measures of the WRAT-R reading, spelling, and arithmetic subtests, as well as on full scale IQ. They concluded that relatives have an attenuated level of deficit compared to schizophrenic subjects, but that the concern regarding appropriate matching measures for relatives and controls still applied. They suggested that a better matching strategy was to equate patients, or relatives, and control subjects on more crystallized tests, such as the WRAT-R reading scores, or the NART. Goldberg *et al.* compared sets of monozygotic twins discordant (N = 20 pairs), and concordant (N = 8 pairs) for schizophrenia, to 7 normal monozygotic twin sets. They concluded that the discordant non-affected siblings trended towards worse performance on measures of verbal and visual memory, WCST and other tests of executive function, and tests requiring information processing speed of response. However, the authors note that the differences were only of trend significance and that the performance of the unaffected twins was generally at the low end of the average range, suggesting attenuated, rather than impaired, performance. The authors also note that the affected twins did significantly worse than their unaffected siblings on measures of FSIQ, memory, attention, WCST, and information processing response speed, and that even affected twins who performed in the normal range on several variables were still performing significantly lower than their unaffected twin (Goldberg *et al.* 1995).

It is worth noting again that there is enormous diversity in the tests used to evaluate the neuropsychological performance of first-degree relatives, and, much like the studies of FES samples, different tests may be included under the same cognitive categories in different studies.

That aside, it appears that the first-degree relatives of people with schizophrenia have a similar pattern of deficits to those of first-episode schizophrenia subjects, including impairment in measures of verbal memory, visual memory, attention, speed of processing, and executive function. Similarly to the evidence available for first-episode schizophrenia, the data for verbal memory and, to a lesser extent, visual memory and attention, appears to be the most robust. The impairments on measures of executive function are inconsistent, and may, as they appear to do in the first-episode population, vary with level of general cognitive function (i.e., those who are most impaired may be those who also have impairments in executive function). Furthermore, the performance of unaffected relatives generally seems to lie between the performances of their relative with schizophrenia, and that of normal control subjects (Cannon *et al.* 1994; Goldberg *et al.* 1995; Kremen *et al.* 1998), suggesting that their performance is attenuated, rather than impaired, by the genetic inheritance of the disease.

Neurocognitive deficits and relationship to symptoms

Regarding the relationship between cognitive deficits and clinical symptoms, the data remains to some degree contradictory. At this time, the evidence appears strongest for the relationship between cognition and negative symptoms. Several studies have concluded that affective flattening and other negative symptoms are related to an overall larger global deficit (Addington *et al.* 2003; Bilder *et al.* 2000; Censits *et al.* 1997), and poorer attention and memory scores after episode stabilization (Bilder *et al.* 2000; Censits *et al.* 1997). Gold *et al.* found verbal and full scale IQ scores correlated with negative symptoms at baseline, and that improvement in negative symptoms over the five year follow-up period accounted for 10 per cent of the improvement in verbal IQ (Gold *et al.* 1999). However, other studies have found only weak (Mohamed *et al.* 1999) or no relationship (Hoff *et al.* 1999) of cognitive deficit patterns and negative symptoms. Stirling *et al.* in a 10 year follow-up study of first-episode patients found that while baseline neurocognitive performance had almost no relationship to severity of negative symptoms at 10 years, there was a strong relationship between neurocognitive scores at the follow-up period and negative symptoms (Stirling *et al.* 2003).

Regarding positive symptoms and cognition, Hoff *et al.* found that positive symptom improvement over time was associated with improvements in executive function, spatial memory, concentration speed-of-processing tasks, and global cognitive measures (Hoff *et al.* 1999). Censits *et al.* concluded that bizarre ideation was strongly correlated with language functioning (Censits *et al.* 1997). Gold *et al.* found improvement in the Trail Making B score was the only neurocognitive measure related to improvement in positive symptoms, and that there was no relationship between baseline neurocognitive functioning and positive symptom score (Gold *et al.* 1999). In the study described above, Stirling *et al.* found that neither baseline nor follow-up neurocognitive scores had a significant relationship to positive symptoms at 10 years (Stirling *et al.* 2003). Similarly, Mohamed *et al.* found no relationship between scores on a neurocognitive battery and positive symptoms (Mohamed *et al.* 1999).

In regard to disorganized symptoms and cognition, little data is available. Mohamed *et al.* and Gold *et al.* found no relationship between neuropsychological performance and disorganized symptoms (Mohamed *et al.* 1999; Gold *et al.* 1999). In a study of chronically ill people with schizophrenia, Bilder *et al.* found that language, memory, and global deficits correlated with the disorganized symptom cluster, which includes alogia, attentional impairment, formal thought disorder, and bizarre behavior (Bilder *et al.* 1985). In their FES sample, Bilder *et al.* found significant correlations between alogia and memory, executive, attentional, visuospatial, and global deficits, and between attentional impairment and executive deficits. However, thought disorder and bizarre behavior were not significantly associated with any neurocognitive measure (Bilder *et al.* 2000).

Neurocognitive deficits and relationship to outcome

There is a limited amount of data available at this time regarding neuropsychological deficits in first episode schizophrenia and the relationship to functional outcome. Bilder *et al.* found that neuropsychological deficits accounted for approximately 5–25 per cent of the variance in ratings of first episode course and social/vocational outcome after two years (Bilder *et al.* 2000).

Verdoux *et al.* found that verbal and visual memory deficits were a predictor of worse clinical outcome at one year. They found no relationship of WCST performance to any sort of outcome measure, and they found no significant association between any cognitive performance and social outcome (Verdoux *et al.* 2003).

Stirling *et al.* followed 49 first-episode patients for an average of over 10 years. They compared performance on a limited neurocognitive battery at baseline to neurocognitive performance at follow-up, as well as both neurocognitive scores to outcome measures including measures of work performance, social competence, and GAF scores. Regarding the relationship of neurocognitive performance to outcome, the authors conclude that baseline cognitive scores bear no significant relationship to outcome variables 10 years later. Outcome at follow-up, however, was significantly associated with most neurocognitive measures, including a general composite of the neurocognitive performance. The best predictors of poor outcome were scores on the WCST and WAIS picture arrangement subscale (Stirling *et al.* 2003).

Addington and Addington evaluated the relationship between neuro-cognitive test performance and social functioning in FES patients at baseline (Addington and Addington 1999), and again 2.5 years later (Addington and Addington 2000). At baseline, data on 80 individuals demonstrated no relationship between neurocognitive performance and current social functioning, though visuospatial and verbal ability, verbal memory, cognitive flexibility, and vigilance tests were associated with measures of social problem-solving. Poor performance on cognitive flexibility tests was also associated with lower quality of life scores; 2.5 years later, 65 of the original patients were reassessed for symptoms, quality of life, social functioning, and problem-solving. Neurocognitive testing was not repeated. Again, the authors concluded that there were no associations between neurocognitive functioning at baseline and community functioning 2.5 years later. However, the relationship between cognition—especially vigilance—verbal ability and verbal memory, and social problem solving remained intact at follow-up. The relationship between cognitive flexibility and social problem-solving weakened at follow-up. Negative symptoms confounded the relationship between both social functioning, where it weakened the association with cognition, and with quality of life. When the authors controlled for negative symptoms were controlled for, there was no significant relationship between cognitive measures and quality of life scores.

In a review that included first-episode and chronically ill individuals, Green identified three areas of functional outcome–community functioning, social problem-solving, and specific skill acquisition. He noted that delayed verbal memory deficits were significantly associated with difficulties in all three measures. Vigilance (a measure of attention) was related to the acquisition of specific social skills, and in two of four studies it was also related to social problem-solving. Card sorting (a measure of executive function) was related to community functioning, inconsistently related to skill acquisition, and not related to social problem-solving (Green 1996). In a year 2000 review update and meta-analysis Green *et al.* reanalyzed 37 studies that included both chronically ill patients and recently ill patients. The results of their meta-analysis demonstrated that secondary verbal memory, immediate verbal memory, executive functions as measured by the WCST (or similar tests), and vigilance are all significantly related to functional outcome, both in terms of social skill acquisition and problem-solving, and actual community outcome and activities of daily living. The effect sizes ranged form small medium (card sorting and vigilance), to medium (secondary verbal memory), to medium large (immediate verbal memory) (Green *et al.* 2000).

The data on the effect of the neurocognitive deficit at first episode on functional outcome is still fairly sparse, however some tentative conclusions can be reached. So far, the ability to predict long-term outcome at baseline testing remains modest, though there are fairly strong correlations between outcome measures and neuropsychological performance at the same testing period. The strongest relationships, after general level of cognitive functioning, are between verbal memory performance and functional outcome, with somewhat less consistent relationships between attention and executive function, and outcome.

Summary and conclusion

At the time of the first episode of schizophrenia, there is a generalized cognitive deficit that ranges from 1 to 2 standard deviations below that of healthy comparison groups. FES patients show relatively better performance on certain measures of verbal and crystallized cognitive function and greater impairment on neuropsychological measures that are more sensitive to brain dysfunction. There are selective areas of increased impairment, including verbal and visual memory, attention, executive function, and speed of processing. Verbal memory impairments are the most robust and the most profound, even in individuals with overall better cognitive function. Executive functioning appears to be selectively impaired, at least in a subgroup of patients who have overall poorer cognitive functioning. Cognitive impairments in people with schizophrenia are documented as early as age six or seven, which is usually the first time that they receive any formal psychological tests, and the underlying pathology is almost certainly present in some form at birth. However there appears to be a period of further decline between the ages of 12 and 17, even before overt prodromal signs of the illness are observed by family members. After the first episode of psychosis has stabilized clinically, there is no convincing evidence of further neurocognitive decline, though the follow-up periods in the longitudinal studies to date may not be long enough to draw definitive conclusions, and there is evidence of decline in later life. The first-degree relatives of people with schizophrenia also show subtle cognitive deficits. The pattern of deficit is similar in patients and their relatives, with the performance of first-degree relatives falling between that of their ill family member and matched controls. There is limited data on cognitive performance and its relationship to clinical symptoms. The available evidence is weak, though the strongest relationship is between cognitive performance and negative symptoms. There is also a paucity of data on the relationship between cognitive deficits and functional outcome, though the strongest predictors of outcome appear to be the same areas that are most impaired, including verbal memory, executive functioning, and attention. This is an area of strong research interest and new information is rapidly accumulating to determine more precisely the relations of neurocognitive deficits to specific real-world outcomes.

Neurocognitive assessment methods yield information useful in understanding both higher-level functional outcomes, and more basic functional neural systems. In this chapter, we have attempted to provide a general description of the magnitude, pattern and longitudinal course of these deficits and their relations to some key clinical parameters. Elsewhere we have commented on the implications this evidence has for understanding the likely neurodevelopmental pathology that underlies vulnerability to the schizophrenia syndrome (Lencz *et al.* 2001a, 2001b). These issues are also addressed by other contributions in this book. It is hoped that increased interdisciplinary attention to all aspects of schizophrenia, from genes to jobs will help dissect the multiplicity of pathological processes that contribute to the disability associated with this syndrome and its effective treatments.

The neurocognitive deficits observed in first episode schizophrenia are an obvious burden to the patients who directly suffer these limitations, their caregivers who must provide supportive roles for which they may often be under-prepared, and a society that has so far failed to allocate adequate resources for their care. Despite decades of experience with psychopharmacological agents that help treat some symptoms of this syndrome, the neurocognitive deficits have proven particularly refractory to treatment. There is some promise in the development of new treatments that specifically target cognitive dysfunction, and it is hoped that this challenge will be addressed by large-scale efforts on the part of academia, government and industry. New approaches at providing cognitive rehabilitation services to people early in the course of schizophrenia may also have promise. Until these efforts bear fruit, it is crucial that we strive to increase clinical awareness of neurocognitive deficits and the likely profound impact these deficits have on a wide range of other functions and quality of life.

References

Addington, J. and Addington, D. (1999). Neurocognitive and social functioning in schizophrenia. *Schizophr. Bull.* 25(1): 173–82.

Addington, J. and Addington, D. (2000). Neurocognitive and social functioning in schizophrenia: a 2.5 year follow-up study. *Schizophr. Res.* 44(1): 47–56.

Addington, J., Brooks, B. L., and Addington, D. (2003). Cognitive functioning in first episode psychosis: initial presentation. *Schizophr. Res.* 62(1–2): 59–64.

Ang, Y. G. and Tan, H. Y. (2004). Academic deterioration prior to first episode schizophrenia in young Singaporean males. *Psychiatry Res.* 121(3): 303–07.

Asarnow, R. F. *et al.* (2002). Neurocognitive impairments in nonpsychotic parents of children with schizophrenia and attention-deficit/hyperactivity disorder: the University of California, Los Angeles Family Study. *Arch. Gen. Psychiatry* 59(11): 1053–60.

Aylward, E., Walker, E. and Bettes, B. (1984). Intelligence in schizophrenia: meta-analysis of the research. *Schizophr. Bull.* 10(3): 430–59.

Bilder, R. M. *et al.* (2000). Neuropsychology of first-episode schizophrenia: initial characterization and clinical correlates. *Am. J. Psychiatry* 157(4): 549–59.

Bilder, R. M. *et al.* (1992). Intellectual deficits in first-episode schizophrenia: evidence for progressive deterioration. *Schizophr. Bull.* 18(3): 437–48.

Bilder, R. M. *et al.* (1985). Symptomatic and neuropsychological components of defect states. *Schizophr. Bull.* 11(3): 409–19.

Bilder, R. M., Reiter, G., Bernstein, K. and Lieberman, J. A. (1995). Deterioration of cognitive function accompanies the onset of schizophrenia: from premorbid SAT to postmorbid FSIQ. *Journal of the International Neuropsychological Society* 157, 1.

Cannon, M. *et al.* (1999). School performance in Finnish children and later development of schizophrenia: a population-based longitudinal study. *Arch. Gen. Psychiatry* 56(5): 457–63.

Cannon, T. D. *et al.* (1994). Neuropsychological functioning in siblings discordant for schizophrenia and healthy volunteers. *Arch. Gen. Psychiatry* 51(8): 651–61.

Censits, D. M. *et al.* (1997). Neuropsychological evidence supporting a neurodevelopmental model of schizophrenia: a longitudinal study. *Schizophr. Res.* 24(3): 289–98.

David, A. S. *et al.* (1997). IQ and risk for schizophrenia: a population-based cohort study. *Psychol. Med.* 27(6): 1311–23.

Davidson, M. *et al.* (1999). Behavioral and intellectual markers for schizophrenia in apparently healthy male adolescents. *Am. J .Psychiatry* 156(9): 1328–35.

Egan, M. F. *et al.* (2000). Relative risk of attention deficits in siblings of patients with schizophrenia. *Am. J. Psychiatry* 157(8): 1309–16.

Egan, M. F. *et al.* (2001). Relative risk for cognitive impairments in siblings of patients with schizophrenia. *Biol. Psychiatry* 50(2): 98–107.

Fuller, R. *et al.* (2002). Longitudinal assessment of premorbid cognitive functioning in patients with schizophrenia through examination of standardized scholastic test performance. *Am. J. Psychiatry* 159(7): 1183–89.

Gilvarry, C. *et al.* (2000). Premorbid IQ in patients with functional psychosis and their first-degree relatives. *Schizophr. Res.* 41(3): 417–29.

Gold, S. *et al.* (1999). Longitudinal study of cognitive function in first-episode and recent-onset schizophrenia. *Am. J. Psychiatry* 156(9): 1342–48.

Goldberg, T. E. *et al.* (1995). Genetic risk of neuropsychological impairment in schizophrenia: a study of monozygotic twins discordant and concordant for the disorder. *Schizophr. Res.* 17(1): 77–84.

Goldman, R. S., Bilder, R. M., Walder, D., Bates, J., Lieberman, J. (1996). Longitudinal Neuropsychological change in first-episode schizophrenia. *Biological Psychiatry* 39, 520.

Gottesman, I. I. and Gould, T. D. (2003). The endophenotype concept in psychiatry: etymology and strategic intentions. *Am. J. Psychiatry* 160(4): 636–45.

Green, M. F. (1996). What are the functional consequences of neurocognitive deficits in schizophrenia? *Am. J. Psychiatry* 153(3): 321–30.

Green, M. F. *et al.* (2000). Neurocognitive deficits and functional outcome in schizophrenia: are we measuring the right stuff? *Schizophr. Bull.* 26(1): 119–36.

Harvey, P. D. *et al.* (1999). Cognitive decline in late-life schizophrenia: a longitudinal study of geriatric chronically hospitalized patients. *Biol. Psychiatry* 45(1): 32–40.

Heinrichs, R. W. and Zakzanis, K. K. (1998). Neurocognitive deficit in schizophrenia: a quantitative review of the evidence. *Neuropsychology.* 12(3): 426–45.

Hoff, A. L. *et al.* (1999). Longitudinal neuropsychological follow-up study of patients with first-episode schizophrenia. *Am. J. Psychiatry* 156(9): 1336–41.

Hoff, A. L. *et al.* (1998). Sex differences in neuropsychological functioning of first-episode and chronically ill schizophrenic patients. *Am. J. Psychiatry* 155(10): 1437–39.

Jensen, A. R. (1998). Jensen on Jensenism. *Intelligence* 26(3): 181–208.

Jensen, A. R. (2000). Intelligence: A new look – Special review. *Personality and Individual Differences* 28(1): 191–94.

Jones, P. *et al.* (1994). Child development risk factors for adult schizophrenia in the British 1946 birth cohort. *Lancet* 344(8934): 1398–402.

Kremen, W. S. *et al.* (1998). IQ decline during childhood and adult psychotic symptoms in a community sample: a 19-year longitudinal study. *Am. J. Psychiatry* 155(5): 672–77.

Kremen, W. S. *et al.* (1998). Neuropsychological risk indicators for schizophrenia: a preliminary study of female relatives of schizophrenic and bipolar probands. *Psychiatry Res.* 79(3): 227–40.

Kremen, W. S. *et al.* (1995). The 3 Rs and neuropsychological function in schizophrenia: a test of the matching fallacy in biological relatives. *Psychiatry Res.* 56(2): 135–43.

Laurent, A. *et al.* (1999). Neuropsychological functioning among non-psychotic siblings and parents of schizophrenic patients. *Psychiatry Res.* 87(2–3): 147–57.

Lencz, T., Bilder, R. M. and Cornblatt, B. (2001a). The timing of neurodevelopmental abnormality in schizophrenia: An integrative review of the neuroimaging literature. *CNS Spectrums* 6(3): 233–55.

Lencz, T., Cornblatt, B. and Bilder, R. M. (2001b). Neurodevelopmental models of schizophrenia: Pathophysiologic synthesis and directions for intervention research. *Psychopharmacology Bulletin* 35(1): 95–125.

McArdle, J. J. *et al.* (2002). Comparative longitudinal structural analyses of the growth and decline of multiple intellectual abilities over the life span. *Dev. Psychol.* 38(1): 115–42.

Mohamed, S. *et al.* (1999). Generalized cognitive deficits in schizophrenia: a study of first-episode patients. *Arch. Gen. Psychiatry* 56(8): 749–54.

Reiter, G., Bilder, R. M., Freyeisen, P., Bell, L. and Lieberman, J. A. (1995). Premorbid achievement in first episode schizophrenia. *Journal of the International Neuropsychological Society* 157, 1.

Riley, E. M. *et al.* (2000). Neuropsychological functioning in first-episode psychosis–evidence of specific deficits. *Schizophr. Res.* 43(1): 47–55.

Russell, A. J. *et al.* (2000). The National Adult Reading Test as a measure of premorbid IQ in schizophrenia. *Br. J. Clin. Psychol.* 39(Pt 3): 297–305.

Russell, A. J. *et al.* (1997). Schizophrenia and the myth of intellectual decline. *Am. J. Psychiatry* 154(5): 635–39.

Saykin, A. J. *et al.* (1994). Neuropsychological deficits in neuroleptic naive patients with first-episode schizophrenia. *Arch. Gen. Psychiatry* 51(2): 124–31.

Spearman, C. (1927). *The Abilities of Man, Their Nature and Measurement*. New York: The Macmillan Company.

Stirling, J. *et al.* (2003). Neurocognitive function and outcome in first-episode schizophrenia: a 10-year follow-up of an epidemiological cohort. *Schizophr. Res.* 65(2–3): 75–86.

Townsend, L. A., Malla, A. K. and Norman, R. M. (2001). Cognitive functioning in stabilized first-episode psychosis patients. *Psychiatry Res.* 104(2): 119–31.

Townsend, L. A. *et al.* (2002). Changes in cognitive functioning following comprehensive treatment for first episode patients with schizophrenia spectrum disorders. *Psychiatry Res.* 113(1–2): 69–81.

Verdoux, H. *et al.* (2002). Social and clinical consequences of cognitive deficits in early psychosis: a two-year follow-up study of first-admitted patients. *Schizophr. Res.* 56(1–2): 149–59.

Woodcock, R. W. (1993). An information-processing view of Gf-Gc theory. *Journal of Psychoeducational Assessment Monograph Series*: Advances in Psychoeducational Assessment. Woodcock-Johnson Psychoeducational Battery - Revised. Brandon, VT: Clinical Psychology Publishing (pp. 80–102).

Zalla, T. *et al.* (2004). Executive dysfunctions as potential markers of familial vulnerability to bipolar disorder and schizophrenia. *Psychiatry Res.* 121(3): 207–17.

Chapter 7

Structural and functional brain abnormalities in first-episode schizophrenia

Tonmoy Sharma and Veena Kumari

Introduction

Abundant evidence implicates abnormalities in almost all cortical and subcortical regions at least to some degree in schizophrenia. Understanding features of brain abnormalities in the first-episode (FE) psychosis is important for furthering our knowledge of the brain basis of schizophrenia. The FE is a crucial stage in the course of the disorder; it represents a transition from a premorbid to a morbid state and provides a valuable starting point for prospective and longitudinal studies. Characterization of brain abnormalities in FE psychosis allows not only exclusion of confounding effects of chronicity, medication and institutionalization but also, when compared to the abnormalities seen in the later chronic course, to establish which abnormalities are already present at the onset, which might show a progressive decline or change in association with antipsychotic treatment, and which might not be present during the FE but emerge during the chronic course of the disorder; those present at the onset are more likely to be of developmental origin, whereas those emerging later in the course are perhaps more likely to be of degenerative nature.

Recent technical advances in neuroimaging have offered much insight into brain abnormalities in schizophrenia. In particular, magnetic resonance imaging (MRI) has provided information on structural abnormalities, magnetic resonance spectroscopy (MRS) on neurochemical abnormalities while positron emission tomography (PET) and functional MRI (fMRI) have enabled us to characterize functional abnormalities in the brains of living schizophrenia patients. Most of the brain abnormalities noted at the illness onset appear to have cognitive and clinical significance. Some abnormalities, especially functional, may be amenable to successful treatment of symptoms.

Structural brain abnormalities: Nature and significance

Recent advances in MRI have led to a surge in studies of brain alterations in schizophrenia over the last two decades (McCarley *et al.* 1999; Wright *et al.* 2000; Shenton *et al.* 2001). A review of structural MRI studies (Shenton *et al.* 2001) has revealed alterations in cavum septi pellucidi (92 per cent of all studies which measured this structure), lateral ventricles (80 per cent), amygloid/hippocampal complex (74 per cent), third ventricles (73 per cent), basal ganglia (68 per cent), superior temporal gyrus (STG, 67 per cent; 100 per cent for grey matter), corpus callosum (63 per cent), temporal lobe (61 per cent), planum temporale (60 per cent), frontal lobe (60 per cent), parietal lobe (60 per cent), occipital lobe (44 per cent), thalamus (42 per cent), cerebellum (31 per cent), and whole brain volume (22 per cent) in schizophrenia patients. Some inconsistency in the replicability of alterations is likely to be due to the stage of the illness at which the measurements were taken, in addition to other factors such as gender which also influence the nature and degree of the abnormality observed (Shenton *et al.* 2001). Another review (Wright *et al.* 2000), focusing specifically on studies which allowed the magnitude of observed deficits to be estimated, has revealed 26 per cent proportionately larger lateral ventricles (based on 30 studies), 2 per cent reduction in the whole brain volume (31 studies), 2 per cent reduction in the temporal lobe volume (25 studies), and 6 per cent reduction in the hippocampus (24 studies) in patients with schizophrenia (also not taking the stage of the illness into account) compared to healthy controls.

Studies of brain structure in FE psychosis have revealed smaller whole brain volume, cortical grey matter, temporal lobe grey matter and thalamic volumes (Fannon *et al.* 2000, Ettinger *et al.* 2002), and enlarged lateral and third ventricles (Fannon *et al.* 2000), in FE patients compared to healthy controls. In a subgroup of minimally medicated male patients from this sample, Sumich *et al.* (2002) found that the hippocampus and planum temporale were smaller relative to healthy controls, with the reduction strongest in the left hippocampus. The lateral temporal lobe decrement in volume has been replicated in other samples (Kim *et al.* 2003). Smaller amygdale in neuroleptic-naïve FE patients has also been reported (Joyal *et al.* 2003). These findings with region of interest measurement have been replicated and analysed further by other techniques (Narr *et al.* 2004). Analysis of the shape change using surface-based mesh modelling revealed reductions in the left hemisphere and in anterior and midbody CA1 and CA2 hippocampal regions. Some of the abnormalities seen in FE seem to be specific for schizophrenia. Hirayasu *et al.* (1998)

found that FE schizophrenia patients had smaller grey matter volume in the posterior STG compared to FE patients and healthy controls and a significant left smaller than right asymmetry. Reduction on the prefrontal cortex has been controversial, with reports of volume decrement in FE schizophrenia patients in some studies (Hirayasu *et al.* 2001; Crespo-Facorro *et al.* 2000) but not in others (Molina *et al.* 2004). It is possible that the abnormality on the prefrontal cortex is more functional than structural or may become more evident as chronicity develops. Studies also suggest that at illness onset the caudate nucleus volume is smaller or comparable to healthy controls but may show enlargement with antipsychotic treatment, particularly with typical antipsychotics (Chakos *et al.* 1994, 1995; Gur *et al.* 1998; Corson *et al.* 1999; Gunduz *et al.* 2002).

In a controversial paper that goes against accepted wisdom from the early interventionists in schizophrenia, who have postulated that prolonged untreated psychosis may have serious effects such as poor response to neuroleptic medications, poor clinical outcomes, and direct neurotoxicity, Ho *et al.* (2003a) examined a large sample of patients (N = 156) with DSM-IV schizophrenia, schizophreniform disorder, or schizoaffective disorder who were evaluated during their first episode of psychosis. They measured total brain tissue, grey and white matter, CSF, and measures of brain surface anatomy. The mean duration of untreated initial psychosis in this sample was 74.3 weeks. Correlations between neurocognitive functioning, brain volumetric measurements, and surface anatomy measurements with duration of untreated initial psychosis did not reach statistical significance. The absence of strong correlations suggests that untreated initial psychosis has little, if any, direct toxic neural effects.

In general, most data indicate that brain abnormalities are present early on in the course of schizophrenia. The next section will consider the evidence for the ongoing changes subsequent to the first psychotic episode.

Longitudinal studies of brain morphology during early schizophrenia

The question of whether morphological changes in schizophrenia are of developmental origin or are progressive remains unsettled and can be resolved only with longitudinal follow-up studies of FE patients. Deciding whether schizophrenia is a progressive illness has implications for early intervention.

There is growing evidence that, at least in some patients, there is continued alteration of brain structures over time. However, it is unclear whether this is an atrophic process or neurodevelopmental failure, given the failure of neuropathological studies to show degenerative change (Weinberger *et al.* 2002). DeLisi and colleagues (1997a, 1998) followed-up 50 FE patients and 20 healthy controls over an average of 4.5 years. Greater enlargement of lateral ventricles and reduction of hemispheric volume was observed over time in the patients compared with controls. They also observed differences in the rates of brain change in left and right hemispheres, right cerebellum, C4 of corpus callosum, and left lateral ventricle between patients and controls, whereas the temporal lobe, hippocampus and caudate nucleus did not show significant brain change over time in either group. In addition, they found that patients receiving continuous medication showed less change in axial ventricular volume bilaterally and in right hippocampus, and a similar trend in temporal lobe. These findings suggest a general progressive change during the first five years following onset of psychosis, with a sparing of the medial temporal lobe and caudate nucleus. In a recent follow-up study of 26 of these patients and 10 controls at a 10 year follow-up after their first evaluation DeLisi *et al.* (2004) reported significantly greater ventricular enlargement during the second five years in the patient cohort compared with controls. The rate of ventricular change during the first five years was significantly correlated with age at first hospitalization, and ventricular enlargement in years 5–10 was correlated with the amount of time spent in hospital. There was however no relationship linking ventricular enlargement to poorer outcome.

Gharaibeh and colleagues (2000) studied change in the midline brain shape over 3–5 years following illness onset. A rapid change was observed in the patients but not in healthy controls. Kasai *et al.* (2003) observed a reduction in STG volume over time in FE patients, this change being specific to the left posterior STG. They compared FE patients with schizophrenia and affective disorder (13 with schizophrenia and 15 with affective psychosis, 13 of whom had a manic psychosis) and 22 healthy control subjects. Follow-up scans occurred, on average, 1.5 years after the initial scan. Patients with first-episode schizophrenia showed significant decreases in grey matter volume over time in the left Heschl gyrus (6.9 per cent) and left planum temporale (7.2 per cent) compared with patients with first-episode affective psychosis or control subjects. This study showed that in schizophrenia, but not in affective psychosis, progressive structural changes in brain volume are seen. Ho *et al.* (2003b) studied a well-characterized sample of 73 recent-onset schizophrenic patients and 23 controls, and followed them for three years. They found accelerated enlargement in cortical sulcal cerebrospinal fluid spaces early in the course of the illness. Patients, but not controls, showed progressive reduction in frontal lobe white matter volume and a reciprocal increase in frontal lobe cerebrospinal fluid volume.

Some studies, however, have not been able to demonstrate such decrement over time. Lieberman *et al.* (2001) followed-up FE patients and healthy controls at 12 months after the first episode. Although the patients had larger lateral and third ventricles compared to healthy controls at each time-point, there did not seem to be a significant decrement in cortical and hippocampal volumes over time. The study by Kasai *et al.* (2003) also failed to find change in the amygdaloid-hippocampal complex in FE patients over the course of 1.5 years.

The findings from these studies suggest that a continuous active abnormal process occurs after the first episode. Some inconsistency in results is likely to be due to the use of different scanning protocols and methods for measuring brain volumes, in addition to the confounding variables such as gender, medication and illness outcome. It is also worth noting that although some studies did not observe greater changes in brain volumes of schizophrenia patients during the first 10 years of the illness, compared to the changes seen in controls, no study has observed effects in the opposite direction (i.e. greater change in controls) suggesting that some structures may show progressive alterations during the early course. It is possible that disruptions in neurodevelopment or neural plasticity may act alone or in combination to bring about these progressive brain deficits in schizophrenia.

Cognitive correlates of MRI-detected brain alterations

As noted by Bratti and Bilder in the preceding chapter, FE patients show generalized cognitive deficit ranging from 1–2 standard deviation below that of healthy controls, with more severe and selective impairments on measures of verbal and visual memory, attention, executive function, and speed of processing. It has been thought since the time of Kraepelin (1919) and Beuler (1911) that cognitive deficits are expression of underlying brain pathology. A recent review (Antonova *et al.* 2004) confirms that at least some cognitive deficits seen in this disorder are indeed associated with the degree of structural brain alterations. In particular, consistent relationships have been noted between (i) whole brain volume and general intelligence, (ii) archicortical, but not paleocortical, prefrontal cortex and executive functions, and (iii) temporal lobe, hippocampus and parahippocampal gyrus and performance speed and accuracy, memory and executive function, verbal endowment and abstraction, respectively (Antonova *et al.* 2004).

Currently only a small number of studies are available that focus on the relationship of structural brain alterations to cognitive deficits in FE patients, but they appear to present a similar picture to that noted for chronic schizophrenia. Specifically, larger grey matter volume is found to be associated with higher (premorbid) IQ in FE patients (Zipursky et al. 1998). Larger anterior cingulate volume is found to predict (better) executive functioning more strongly than performance on tests of language, attention, memory, visuospatial function and general IQ (Szeszko et al. 2000). Along similar lines, progressive decreases in frontal lobe grey and white matter volumes have been found to be related to poorer executive functioning over a period of three years since the illness onset (Ho et al. 2003b). Positive associations have been noted between parahippocampal volume and logical memory and verbal IQ in FE patients (De Lisi et al. 1991; Hoff et al. 1992). Hippocampus volume (bilaterally) is found to be associated with learning (De Lisi et al. 1991). Reduced volume of the anterior hippocampal formation has been found to be associated with lower scores on measures of executive and motor functions (Bilder et al. 1995); given that these domains are generally thought to be sensitive to the integrity of frontal lobe systems, this observation has been taken to suggest that neurodevelopmental faults affecting the morphology of the anterior hippocampal formation may be evident later on in life as deficient fronto-limbic control. A later study from the same group (Szeszko et al. 2002) also reported that larger anterior hippocampus predicts better executive functioning and motor function (more strongly than memory language) but, in this instance, only in male FE patients (i.e. absent in female patients). There is weak evidence (i.e. not surviving for multiple correlations) for a relationship between anomalous cerebral asymmetry and impaired language processing in FE patients (Delisi et al. 1997b). Volume reduction in the cerebral cortex, including the precentral, superior and middle temporal, and lingual gyri has been found to predict deficits in signs of sensory integration in FE patients (Dazzan et al. 2004). Finally, there are data indicating that some structure–function associations noted in healthy controls might be absent in FE patients, for example, the positive association of cerebellum to certain cognitive functions (Szeszko et al. 2003a; Ettinger et al. 2004), while others not emerging significantly in controls may be found in FE patients, for example, positive relationship of grey matter density of the left thalamic nucleus, left angular, and supramarginal gyrus, and left inferior frontal and post-central gyri to performance on a sustained attention task (Salgado-Pineda et al. 2003).

Overall, current evidence indicates that brain alterations are present at the onset of symptoms and relate meaningfully to cognitive impairments commonly seen in this disorder. More recent, though limited at present, data also indicate that reductions in certain brain regions, for example in the frontal lobe, are associated with worsening of relevant cognitive functions (Ho *et al.* 2003b). More longitudinal data are required to compare the rate of changes in these two modes of illness expression during the course of the disorder.

Clinical significance of MRI-detected brain alterations

Several theorists implicate dysfunctions in brain structures reported to be aberrant in FE patients in formation and/or maintenance of symptoms of schizophrenia. Disruption of cortico-cerebellar-thalamo-cortical circuitry, which has a role in coordination of both motor and cognitive processes (Middleton and Strick 1994; Schmahmann 1996; Schmahmann and Sherman 1997), has been proposed as an essential feature of schizophrenia (Andreasen *et al.* 1998, 1999). Prefronto-temprolimbic structural and functional connectivity (Weinberger and Lipska, 1995) and prefronto-temprolimbic interactions with ventral striatum (Buchsbaum 1990; Grace 1991; Gray 1995, 1998; O'Donnell and Grace 1998) are proposed as the basis for symptomatology and/or cognitive disturbances in schizophrenia. Malfunctioning of the neuronal projections of the prefrontal cortex to thalamus via striatum, which play an important role in initiation of mental activity, has been considered the basis of negative syndrome (review, Semkovska *et al.* 2001) while faulty dopaminergic pathways have been implicated in formation of positive symptoms (Gray 1995, 1998).

There have been a number of studies investigating the relationship of brain morphology to the type and magnitude of symptom levels in the FE. Buttressing the suggestion of an association between frontal lobe dysfunction and negative symptoms, progressive decreases in frontal lobe white matter volume and enlargement in frontal lobe cerebrospinal fluid volume over a course of three years after the onset are found to be associated with greater negative symptom severity (Ho *et al.* 2003b). Among male FE patients, greater reversal in a composite measure of cerebellar asymmetry (i.e., torque) is found to correlate with increased negative symptoms before the initiation of antipsychotic medication (Szeszko *et al.* 2003b).

A high prevalence of abnormal (larger) cavum septi pellucidi in schizophrenia has been considered to reflect neurodevelopmental abnormalities in midline structures of the brain. Very recently, larger cavum septi pellucidi has been found to be associated with more severe thinking disturbance and smaller left parahippocampal gyrus grey matter volumes (Kasai *et al.* 2004); the latter observation was specific to schizophrenia and not seen in patients with affective psychoses. FE patients with paranoid psychosis are found to have smaller left amygdala volumes than the patients with nonparanoid psychosis (Sumich *et al.* 2002). The volume of the left anterior STG is reported to correlate inversely with psychotic symptoms (Kim *et al.* 2003). A positive but weak relationship (i.e. did not survive correction for multiple comparisons) of right posterior STG to negative symptoms was also noted in this study (Kim *et al.* 2003); this observation needs to be replicated before being taken seriously.

While some studies demonstrate a straightforward relationship between structural alterations (i.e. reductions and enlargements associated with the disorder) and severity of symptoms, others apparently reveal counterintuitive associations. For example, larger volumes of the parahippocampal gyrus (Prasad *et al.* 2004a) and entorhinal cortex (Prasad *et al.* 2004b) is found to be associated with presence of delusions/delusional disorder in FE drug-naïve patients though, on average, these structures are smaller in patients compared to healthy controls. These observations have been explained (Prasad *et al.* 2004a, b) exploiting previous data showing that the parahippocampal gyrus and entorhinal cortex play an important role in memory functions and delusional subjects recall more threatening propositions, fewer specific memories to positive cues, and more categorical memories than healthy and non-delusional subjects. An over-inclusive retrieval style, specific recall of threatening events, and errors in checking such memories against external reality could account for the formation of delusions in patients with relatively larger entorhinal cortex. A smaller entorhinal cortex in non-delusional patients, on the other hand, may prevent them from retrieving such memories efficiently, hence less likelihood of forming delusions while showing other characteristics of the illness (Prasad *et al.* 2004a, b). Furthermore, there are also data showing no relationship of reductions in the cortical grey matter, temporal lobe grey matter, and whole brain volume as well as significant enlargement of the lateral and third ventricles to positive or negative symptoms (Fannon *et al.* 2000). Another study from the same research group did not detect any relationship between thalamic volume reductions and positive or negative symptoms (Ettinger *et al.* 2001).

In addition to symptom formation and/or maintenance, structural brain abnormalities may also be predictive of other clinical aspects of the illness. For example, insight into the illness, which is considered an aspect of the illness that is vital for treatment compliance, has been found to be specifically and positively related to right dorsolateral prefrontal cortex volume in FE patients (Shad *et al.* 2004). Responsiveness to medication may also be predicted by morphological impairment prior to treatment initiation. Studies of chronic patients indicate that the structural integrity of the dorsolateral prefrontal cortex and temporal regions predicts responsiveness to clozapine in chronic schizophrenia (Konicki *et al.* 2001; Molina *et al.* 2003). There are no published studies addressing this issue directly in FE patients. Relatively greater ventricular enlargement over time (12 months to 3 years since the onset) has been reported be associated with poor outcome patients in follow-up studies of FE patients (Lieberman *et al.* 2001; Ho *et al.* 2003b) although not consistently so (DeLisi *et al.* 1998, 2004). The finding of progressive ventricular enlargement in patients with poor outcome schizophrenia is taken as empirical support for the hypothesis that persistent positive and negative symptoms result in progressive brain changes in the form of ventricular enlargement, possibly due to neurodegeneration (Lieberman *et al.* 2001). Greater cerebral asymmetry has been found to be associated with full recovery and adequate social/vocational functioning in FE patients over a two-year period in one study (Robinson *et al.* 2004). Decreases in cerebral grey matter volume over one year are found to correlate with two-year outcomes, and, independently of that, with higher cumulative dosage of antipsychotic medication in FE patients (Cahn *et al.* 2002).

It seems reasonable to suggest that the relationships between alterations in individual brain structures and symptoms of schizophrenia are subtle and more complex than the observed relationships of structural brain alterations to neurocognitive functions. This is perhaps due to relatively greater temporal stability of structural alterations and cognitive deficits than symptoms (Hughes *et al.* 2003). The evidence, although limited at present, can be taken to suggest that structural alterations present at the illness onset and during the early course of schizophrenia could potentially inform about the outcome of this disorder.

Neurochemical abnormalities: nature, course and significance

MRS studies allow the investigation of the developmental biochemistry of the living brain and, in recent years, have provided evidence of neuronal dysfunction in schizophrenia. The neurochemical abnormality most intensively studied with MRS in schizophrenia concerns the levels of N-Acetylaspartate (NAA) in various regions of the brain. NAA is found in high concentrations in the central nervous system, almost exclusively in neurons, and believed to be a marker of both neuronal loss and cellular dysfunction.

Studies have, in general, shown reductions of frontal and temporal NAA in medicated and chronic schizophrenia patients (review, Rowland *et al.* 2001).

NAA/creatine ratios are also found to be reduced for the frontal (Cecil *et al.* 1999) and the temporal lobe in antipsychotic-naive FE patients compared to healthy controls (Renshaw *et al.* 1995; Cecil *et al.* 1999); these observations suggest lower neuronal viability and are consistent with findings of reduced volume in both frontal and temporal regions in schizophrenia. One study, however, noted comparable NAA/choline rations in the left medial temporal and left dorsolateral prefrontal regions in first-episode patients and healthy controls (Wood *et al.* 2003). Reduced NAA concentrations in schizophrenia might reflect pathological states related to glutamatergic changes (Bertolino and Weinberger 1999; Rubin *et al.* 1995). Animal studies, for example, demonstrating that NAA concentrations in the frontal cortex are reduced in adult male rats subjected to perinatal stress (Poland *et al.* 1999) or neonatal hippocampal damage (Bertolino *et al.* 2002), suggest frontal NAA brain deficits in schizophrenia to be of developmental origin.

There is evidence of reduced NAA concentration in the anterior cingulate in chronic schizophrenia (Deicken *et al.* 1997) even in absence of volume loss (Deicken *et al.* 1999), and of increase in NAA in this region with atypical, but not typical, antipsychotic treatment (Braus *et al.* 2001, 2002a). The NAA/creatine ratio in frontal lobe of chronic schizophrenia, however, has been reported to remain unchanged after antipsychotic treatment (Pae *et al.* 2004) or even to reduce within the first year of antipsychotic treatment (Bustillo *et al.* 2002). Some inconsistency in results is likely to be due to a different region of interest in the frontal cortex in these studies. Studies of FE patients investigating antipsychotic influences with clearly defined regions of interest would be valuable.

Reduced NAA concentrations in the frontal lobe are found to be associated with frontal lobe-based neuropsychological dysfunctions in schizophrenia patients (Deicken *et al.* 1997; Bertolino *et al.* 2003). There is also evidence for a significant negative relationship of frontal NAA concentration to severity of symptoms, particularly positive symptoms and general psychopathology in chronic schizophrenia (Sigmundsson *et al.* 2003). In an FE sample, thalamic NAA has been found to correlate negatively with duration of prodromal symptoms, and choline in anterior cingulate and thalamus to correlate positively with duration of untreated psychosis (Theberge *et al.* 2004). It has been suggested that the neuronal damage, detectable via lower NAA, may be occurring before the onset of psychosis while the association of increased choline with longer duration of untreated psychosis could indicate that psychosis-related membrane alterations precede the appearance of NAA reductions (Theberge *et al.* 2004). Few reliable data are currently available specifically focusing on the relationship of neurochemical abnormalities to cognitive and clinical outcomes in FE samples, with most studies utilizing relatively small samples with limited power to examine such relationships.

Hippocampal NAA reduction in schizophrenia is considered an established finding (review, Deicken *et al.* 2000). Hippocampal NAA/creatine plus phosphocreatine appears to be selectively affected early in the course of illness and may improve with antipsychotic treatment in FE patients (Fannon *et al.* 2003). Very recently, relevant interesting data have emerged from animal studies, in particular those which show that compared with socially housed rats, isolation rearing results in disrupted prepulse inhibition of the startle response (which is reversible with antipsychotic medication; review Geyer *et al.* 2001) and reduced NAA in the temporal cortex (Harte *et al.* 2004). These data suggest that temporal lobe NAA reduction also may be of developmental origin and relevant to neurodevelopmental hypothesis of schizophrenia. Investigations of neurochemical abnormalities noted (but less consistently) in some other regions such as basal ganglia in chronic/medicated schizophrenia patients (review, Deicken *et al.* 2000) are yet to be confirmed in neuroleptic-naïve FE samples.

Some models of schizophrenia have emphasized glutamate dysfunction in schizophrenia (Javitt and Zukin 1991; Olney and Farber 1995; Carlsson *et al.* 1999) and the availability of relevant tools has allowed these models to be tested with *in vivo* measures of glutamate metabolism specially in FE, antipsychotic-naïve patients. Supporting these models, there is recent evidence that the level of glutamine is significantly higher in the left anterior cingulate cortex and thalamus of the patients with schizophrenia than in the healthy controls (Theberge *et al.* 2002).

Antipsychotic-naïve FE patients have also been found to show basal overactivity of the pituitary–adrenal axis and mood disturbances (Ryan *et al.* 2004) and this may explain the observation of larger (by 10 per cent) pituitary volume at the FE (Pariante *et al.* 2004); this has not been consistently observed in chronic schizophrenia patients who also appear to have smaller pituitary volumes relative to healthy individuals, perhaps due to the effects of antipsychotic medication (Pariante *et al.* 2004).

Overall, there is a reasonable amount of data demonstrating that many of the neuronal abnormalities, in particular the NAA reduction in the frontal, temporal and hippocampal regions seen in chronic schizophrenia, are already present at illness onset and may be of developmental origin. These abnormalities, however, appear to respond at least to some degree favourably to antipsychotic treatment and deserve further investigation.

Functional brain abnormalities: nature, course and significance

A number of functional brain abnormalities have been associated with schizophrenia (Callicott 2003). There are only a small number of fMRI or PET studies focusing on which of these abnormalities might already be preset at illness onset. Given that several neural structures/regions show schizophrenia-related volumetric alteration at the illness onset, it is conceivable that activation of neural circuits involving one or more of these structures/regions would also be affected early in the illness. It is also possible that functional abnormalities may be evident even in the absence of structural alterations and that some functions may be taken over by other regions in the event of structural damage in core regions.

The initial study by Braus and colleagues (1999) using fMRI and a left hand sequential finger opposition task had shown a significant reduction in fMRI activity in sensorimotor cortices in FE schizophrenia patients on stable medication with typical, but not atypical, antipsychotics compared to healthy controls. In the same study, both antipsychotics appeared to reduce activation of the SMA compared to the activation seen in neuroleptic-naïve schizophrenia patients and healthy controls. A later study from the same research group using fMRI and the same left hand sequential finger opposition task confirmed normal cortical response during motor stimulation in neuroleptic-naive, FE schizophrenia patients (Braus *et al.* 2000); patients were comparable to controls with respect to laterality, change of signal intensity and spatial extent of activation, primarily in the sensorimotor cortex and supplementary motor area (SMA). The effects did not seem to be related to performance related confounds. These two studies, taken together, convincingly demonstrate that functionally abnormal brain response in the primary motor cortex or the SMA are not stable markers of schizophrenia and, when observed, could be associated with its treatment using antipsychotics.

More recent fMRI studies, focusing on neural circuits implicated in the pathophysiology of schizophrenia described earlier, have found some of the core functional abnormalities to be already present at the illness onset. Support for functional abnormalities in the frontal regions, specifically in the dorsolateral prefrontal cortex, comes from an fMRI study of neuroleptic-naïve FE patients during performance of an A-X version of the Continuous Performance Test (Barch *et al.* 2001). This study demonstrated activation deficits in patients in the dorsolateral prefrontal cortex in task conditions requiring context processing but showed intact activation of posterior and inferior prefrontal cortex.

Confirming the suggestions of Braus and colleagues (1999, 2000), patients also showed intact activation of the primary motor and somatosensory cortex in response to stimulus processing demands. A different study (Braus *et al.* 2002b) has shown reduced activation in the right thalamus, right prefrontal cortex and dorsal visual pathways in the parietal lobe in neuroleptic-naïve FE patients compared to healthy controls, when subjects were presented simultaneously with a moving 6-Hz checkerboard and auditory stimuli and required to look and listen. Finally, a recent fMRI study of FE patients on two occasions 6–8 weeks apart (in partial remission at the second scan) during performance of a working memory task revealed that functional responses of the left dorsolateral prefrontal cortex, left thalamus and right cerebellum were disturbed on both occasions in patients, relative to healthy individuals, whereas the dysfunction of the right dorsolateral prefrontal cortex, right thalamus, left cerebellum and cingulate gyrus normalized, with significant reduction in symptoms on the second occasion (Mendrek *et al.* 2004).

PET and Single Photon Emission Computerized Tomography (SPECT) studies have also detected functional brain changes related to the illness and antipsychotic treatment. Using PET, striatal blood flow is reported to be comparable in neuroleptic-naïve FE patients and healthy controls, with a significant increase in blood flow to the striatum after initiation of antipsychotic treatment (Corson *et al.* 2002). Using SPECT, asymmetrical blood flow patterns in the frontal lobe have been noted in antipsychotic-naïve FE patients compared to controls, and an increase in blood flow in putamen with 6 months of antipsychotic treatment (Scottish Schizophrenia Research Group, 1998). In general, the observations of increased blood flow to striatum with antipsychotic treatment concur with observations of treatment-induced increases in caudate/putamen volumes mentioned earlier.

The data available so far to inform us about the functional brain abnormalities suggest the presence of specific functional brain abnormalities in cortical and subcortical regions at the onset of schizophrenia. Importantly, some of these appear amenable to successful treatment of symptoms.

Conclusion

Investigations of the first psychotic episode have yielded a picture of schizophrenia that is multifaceted. The brain of the person experiencing their first psychotic episode is dynamic rather than static, as shown convincingly by functional but also by structural imaging studies. There is a need to view the brain as a more fluid structure and to consider its vulnerability to extrinsic mediation in early course of the disorder. Similarly, early treatment is likely to reduce much of the suffering of the illness, though the issues about neurotoxicity of psychosis remain controversial currently.

References

Andreasen NC, Paradiso S, O'Leary DS (1998). 'Cognitive dysmetria' as an integrative theory of schizophrenia: a dysfunction in cortical-subcortical-cerebellar circuitry? *Schizophr Bull*, 24: 203–218.

Andreasen NC, Nopoulos P, O'Leary DS, Miller DD, Wassink T, Flaum M (1999). Defining the phenotype of schizophrenia: cognitive dysmetria and its neural mechanisms. *Biol Psychiatry*, 46: 908–920.

Antonova E, Sharma T, Morris R, Kumari V (2004). The relationship between brain structure and neurocognition in schizophrenia: A selective review. *Schizophr Res*, 70 (2–3): 117–145.

Barch DM, Carter CS, Braver TS, Sabb FW, MacDonald A 3rd, Noll DC, Cohen JD (2001). Selective deficits in prefrontal cortex function in medication-naive patients with schizophrenia. *Arch Gen Psychiatry*, 58 (3): 280–288.

Bertolino A, Roffman JL, Lipska BK, van Gelderen P, Olson A, Weinberger DR (2002). Reduced N-acetylaspartate in prefrontal cortex of adult rats with neonatal hippocampal damage. *Cereb Cortex*, 12(9): 983–990.

Bertolino A, Sciota D, Brudaglio F, Altamura M, Blasi G, Bellomo A, Antonucci N, Callicott JH, Goldberg TE, Scarabino T, Weinberger DR, Nardini M (2003). Working memory deficits and levels of N-acetylaspartate in patients with schizophreniform disorder. *Am J Psychiatry*, 160(3): 483–489.

Bertolino A, Weinberger DR (1999). Proton magnetic resonance spectroscopy in schizophrenia. *Eur J Radiol*, 30: 132–141.

Bilder RM, Bogerts B, Ashtari M, Wu H, Alvir JM, Jody D, Reiter G, Bell L, Lieberman JA (1995). Anterior hippocampal volume reductions predict frontal lobe dysfunction in first episode schizophrenia. *Schizophr Res*, 17 (1): 47–58.

Beuler E. *Dementia Praecox or the Group of Schizophrenias*. Reprinted 1950 (trans. and ed. J. Zinkin). 1911. New York: International University Press.

Braus DF, Ende G, Hubrich-Ungureanu P, Henn FA (2000). Cortical response to motor stimulation in neuroleptic-naive first episode schizophrenics. *Psychiatry Res*, 98 (3): 145–154.

Braus DF, Ende G, Weber-Fahr W, Demirakca T, Henn FA (2001). Favorable effect on neuronal viability in the anterior cingulate gyrus due to long-term treatment with atypical antipsychotics: an MRSI study. *Pharmacopsychiatry*, 34 (6): 251–253.

Braus DF, Ende G, Weber-Fahr W, Sartorius A, Krier A, Hubrich-Ungureanu P, Ruf M, Stuck S, Henn FA (1999). Antipsychotic drug effects on motor activation measured by functional magnetic resonance imaging in schizophrenic patients. *Schizophr Res*, 39 (1): 19–29.

Braus DF, Ende G, Weber-Fahr W, Demirakca T, Tost H, Henn FA (2002a). Functioning and neuronal viability of the anterior cingulate neurons following antipsychotic treatment: MR-spectroscopic imaging in chronic schizophrenia. *Eur Neuropsychopharmacol*, 12 (2): 145–152.

Braus DF, Weber-Fahr W, Tost H, Ruf M, Henn FA (2002b). Sensory information processing in neuroleptic-naive first-episode schizophrenic patients: a functional magnetic resonance imaging study. *Arch Gen Psychiatry*, 59 (8): 696–701.

Buchsbaum MS (1990). The frontal lobes, basal ganglia, and temporal lobes as sites for schizophrenia. *Schizophr Bull*, 16, 379–389.

Bustillo JR, Lauriello J, Rowland LM, Thomson LM, Petropoulos H, Hammond R, Hart B, Brooks WM (2002). Longitudinal follow-up of neurochemical changes during the first year of antipsychotic treatment in schizophrenia patients with minimal previous medication exposure. *Schizophr Res*; 58 (2–3): 313–321.

Cahn W, Pol HE, Lems EB, van Haren NE, Schnack HG, van der Linden JA, Schothorst PF, van Engeland H, Kahn RS (2002). Brain volume changes in first-episode schizophrenia: a 1-year follow-up study. *Arch Gen Psychiatry*; 59 (11): 1002–1010.

Callicott JH (2003). An expanded role for functional neuroimaging in schizophrenia. *Curr Opin Neurobiol*; 13 (2): 256–260.

Carlsson A, Hansson LO, Waters N, Carlsson ML (1999). A glutamatergic deficiency model of schizophrenia. *Br J Psychiatry*; 174: 2–6.

Cecil KM, Lenkinski RE, Gur RE, Gur RC (1999). Proton magnetic resonance spectroscopy in the frontal and temporal lobes of neuroleptic naive patients with schizophrenia. *Neuropsychopharmacology*; 20 (2): 131–140.

Chakos MH, Lieberman JA, Bilder RM, Borenstein M, Lerner G, Bogerts B, Wu H, Kinon B, Ashtari M (1994). Increase in caudate nuclei volumes of first-episode schizophrenic patients taking antipsychotic drugs. *American Journal of Psychiatry*; 151 (10): 1430–1436.

Chakos MH, Lieberman JA, Alvir J, Bilder R, Ashtari M (1995). Caudate nuclei volumes in schizophrenic patients treated with typical antipsychotics or clozapine. *Lancet*; 345 (8947): 456–457.

Corson PW, Nopoulos P, Andreasen NC, Heckel D, Arndt S (1999). Caudate size in first-episode neuroleptic-naive schizophrenic patients measured using an artificial neural network. *Biological Psychiatry*; 46 (5): 712–720.

Corson PW, O'Leary DS, Miller del D, Andreasen NC (2002). The effects of neuroleptic medications on basal ganglia blood flow in schizophreniform disorders: a comparison between the neuroleptic-naïve and medicated states. *Biol Psychiatry*; 52 (9): 855–862.

Crespo-Facorro B, Kim JJ, Andreasen NC, O'Leary DS, Magnotta V (2000). Regional frontal abnormalities in schizophrenia: a quantitative gray matter volume and cortical surface size study. *Biological Psychiatry*; 48: 110–119.

Dazzan P, Morgan KD, Orr KG, Hutchinson G, Chitnis X, Suckling J, Fearon P, Salvo J, McGuire PK, Mallett RM, Jones PB, Leff J, Murray RM (2004). The structural brain correlates of neurological soft signs in AESOP first-episode psychoses study. *Brain*; 127 (Pt 1): 143–153.

DeLisi LE, Sakuma M, Ge S, Kushner M (1998). Association of brain structural change with the heterogeneous course of schizophrenia from early childhood through five years subsequent to a first hospitalization. *Psychiatry Res*; 84 (2–3): 75–88.

DeLisi LE, Stritzke PH, Holan V, Anand A, Boccio A, Kuschner M, Riordan H, McClelland J, VanEyle O (1991). Brain morphological changes in first episode cases of schizophrenia: are they progressive? *Schizophr Res*; 5: 206–208.

DeLisi LE, Sakuma M, Tew W, Kushner M, Hoff AL, Grimson R (1997a). Schizophrenia as a chronic active brain process: A study of progressive brain structural change subsequent to the onset of schizophrenia. *Psychiatry Research: Neuroimaging*; 74 (3): 129–140.

DeLisi LE, Sakuma M, Kushner M, Finer DL, Hoff AL, Crow TJ (1997b). Anomalous cerebral asymmetry and language processing in schizophrenia. *Schizophr Bull*; 23: 255–271.

DeLisi LE, Sakuma M, Maurizio AM, Relja M, Hoff AL (2004). Cerebral ventricular change over the first 10 years after the onset of schizophrenia. *Psychiatry Res*; 130 (1): 57–70.

Deicken RF, Johnson C, Pegues M (2000). Proton magnetic resonance spectroscopy of the human brain in schizophrenia. *Rev Neurosci*; 11 (2–3): 147–158.

Deicken RF, Pegues M, Amend D (1999). Reduced hippocampal N-acetylaspartate without volume loss in schizophrenia. *Schizophr Res*, 37: 217–223.

Deicken RF, Zhou L, Schuff N, Weiner MW (1997). Proton magnetic resonance spectroscopy of the anterior cingulate region in schizophrenia. *Schizophr Res*, 27 (1): 65–71.

Ettinger U, Chitnis XA, Kumari V, Fannon DG, Doku V, O'Ceallaigh S, Sharma T (2001). Magnetic resonance imaging of the thalamus in first-episode psychosis. *Am J Psychiatry*, 58: 116–118.

Ettinger U, Chitnis XA, Kumari V, Fannon DG, Sumich AL, O'Ceallaigh S, Doku VC, Sharma T (2002). Magnetic resonance imaging of the thalamus in first-episode psychosis. *American Journal of Psychiatry*, 158 (1): 116–118.

Ettinger U, Kumari V, Chitnis X, Corr PJ, Crawford TJ, Fannon DG, O'Ceallaigh SO, Sumich A, Sharma T (2004). Volumetric neural correlates of antisaccade eye movements: Altered structure-function relationship in first-episode psychosis. *Am J Psychiatry*, 161 (10): 1918–1921.

Fannon D, Chitnis X, Doku V, Tennakoon L, O'Ceallaigh S, Soni W, Sumich A, Lowe J, Santamaria M, Sharma T (2000). Features of structural brain abnormality detected in first-episode psychosis. *Am J Psychiatry*, 157 (11): 1829–1834.

Fannon D, Simmons A, Tennakoon L, O'Ceallaigh S, Sumich A, Doku V, Shew C, Sharma T (2003). Selective deficit of hippocampal N-acetylaspartate in antipsychotic-naive patients with schizophrenia. *Biol Psychiatry*, 54 (6): 587–598.

Geyer MA, Krebs-Thomson K, Braff DL, Swerdlow NR (2001). Pharmacological studies of prepulse inhibition models of sensorimotor gating deficits in schizophrenia: a decade in review. *Psychopharmacology*, 156 (2–3): 117–154.

Gharaibeh WS, Rohlf FJ, Slice DE, DeLisi LE (2000). A geometric morphometric assessment of change in midline brain structural shape following a first episode of schizophrenia. *Biol Psychiatry*, 48(5): 398–405.

Grace AA (1991). Phasic versus tonic dopamine release and the modulation of dopamine system responsivity: a hypothesis for the etiology of schizophrenia. *Neuroscience*, 41 (1); 1–24.

Gray JA (1995). Dopamine release in the nucleus accumbens: the perspective from aberrations of consciousness in schizophrenia. *Neuropsychologia*, 33: 1143–1153.

Gray JA (1998). Integrating schizophrenia. *Schizophr Bull*, 24, 249–266.

Gunduz H, Wu H, Ashtari M, Bogerts B, Crandall D, Robinson DG, Alvir J, Lieberman J, Kane J, Bilder R (2002). Basal ganglia volumes in first-episode schizophrenia and healthy comparison subjects. *Biological Psychiatry*, 51 (10): 801–8.

Gur RE, Maany V, Mozley PD, Swanson C, Bilker W, Gur RC (1998). Subcortical MRI volumes in neuroleptic-naive and treated patients with schizophrenia. *American Journal of Psychiatry*, 155 (12): 1711–1717.

Harte MK, Powell SB, Reynolds LM, Swerdlow NR, Geyer MA, Reynolds GP (2004). Reduced N-acetylaspartate in the temporal cortex of rats reared in isolation. *Biol Psychiatry*, 56 (4): 296–299.

Hirayasu Y, Shenton ME, Salisbury DF, Dickey CC, Fischer IA, Mazzoni P, Kisler T, Arakaki H, Kwon JS, Anderson JE, Yurgelun-Todd D, Tohen M, McCarley RW (1998). Lower left temporal lobe MRI volumes in patients with first-episode schizophrenia compared with psychotic patients with first-episode affective disorder and normal subjects. *American Journal of Psychiatry*, 155 (10): 1384–1391.

Hirayasu Y, Tanaka S, Shenton ME, Salisbury DF, DeSantis MA, Levitt JJ, Wible CG, Yurgelun-Todd D, Kikinis R, Jolesz FA, McCarley RW (2001). Prefrontal gray matter volume reduction in first episode schizophrenia. *Cerebral Cortex*, 11: 374–381.

Ho BC, Alicata D, Ward J, Moser DJ, O'Leary DS, Arndt S, Andreasen NC (2003a). Untreated initial psychosis: relation to cognitive deficits and brain morphology in first-episode schizophrenia. *American Journal of Psychiatry* January; 160 (1): 142–148.

Ho BC, Andreasen NC, Nopoulos P, Arndt S, Magnotta V, Flaum M (2003b). Progressive structural brain abnormalities and their relationship to clinical outcome: a longitudinal magnetic resonance imaging study early in schizophrenia. *Arch Gen Psychiatry*; 60 (6): 585–594.

Hoff AL, Riordan H, O'Donnell D, Stritzke P, Neale C, Boccio A, Anand AK, DeLisi LE (1992). Anomalous lateral sulcus asymmetry and cognitive function in first-episode schizophrenia. *Schizophr Bull*; 18: 257–272.

Hughes C, Kumari V, Soni W, Das M, Binneman B, Drozd S, O'Neil S, Mathew V, Sharma T (2003). Longitudinal study of symptoms and cognitive function in chronic schizophrenia. *Schizophr Res*; 59 (2–3): 137–146.

Javitt DC, Zukin SR (1991). Recent advances in the phencyclidine model of schizophrenia. *Am J Psychiatry*; 148: 1301–1308.

Joyal CC, Laakso MP, Tiihonen J, Syvalahti E, Vilkman H, Laakso A, Alakare B, Rakkolainen V, Salokangas RK, Hietala J (2003). The amygdala and schizophrenia: a volumetric magnetic resonance imaging study in first-episode, neuroleptic-naive patients. *Biol Psychiatry*; 54 (11): 1302–1304.

Kasai K, Shenton ME, Salisbury DF, Hirayasu Y, Onitsuka T, Spencer MH, Yurgelun-Todd DA, Kikinis R, Jolesz FA, McCarley RW (2003). Progressive decrease of left Heschl gyrus and planum temporale gray matter volume in first-episode schizophrenia: a longitudinal magnetic resonance imaging study. *Arch Gen Psychiatry*; 60 (8): 766–775.

Kasai K, McCarley RW, Salisbury DF, Onitsuka T, Demeo S, Yurgelun-Todd D, Kikinis R, Jolesz FA, Shenton ME (2004). Cavum septi pellucidi in first-episode schizophrenia and first-episode affective psychosis: an MRI study. *Schizophr Res*; 71 (1): 65–76.

Kim JJ, Crespo-Facorro B, Andreasen NC, O'Leary DS, Magnotta V, Nopoulos P (2003). Morphology of the lateral superior temporal gyrus in neuroleptic naive patients with schizophrenia: relationship to symptoms. *Schizophr Res*; 60 (2–3): 173–181.

Konicki PE, Kwon KY, Steele V, White J, Fuller M, Jurjus GJ, Jaskiw GE (2001). Prefrontal cortical sulcal widening associated with poor treatment response to clozapine. *Schizophr Res*; 48: 173–176.

Kraepelin E. *Dementia Praecox and Paraphrenia*. 1919. Livingston, Edinburgh.

Lieberman J, Chakos M, Wu H, Alvir J, Hoffman E, Robinson D, Bilder R (2001). Longitudinal study of brain morphology in first episode schizophrenia. *Biol Psychiatry*; 49 (6): 487–499.

McCarley RW, Wible CG, Frumin M, Hirayasu Y, Levitt JJ, Fischer IA, Shenton ME (1999). MRI anatomy of schizophrenia. *Biol Psychiatry*; 45 (9): 1099–1119.

Mendrek A, Laurens KR, Kiehl KA, Ngan ET, Stip E, Liddle PF (2004). Changes in distributed neural circuitry function in patients with first-episode schizophrenia. *Br J Psychiatry*; 185: 205–214.

Middleton FA, Strick PL (1994). Anatomical evidence for cerebellar and basal ganglia involvement in higher cognitive function. *Science*; 266: 458–461.

Molina V, Reig S, Sarramea F, Sanz J, Francisco Artaloytia J, Luque R, Aragues M, Pascau J, Benito C, Palomo T, Desco M (2003). Anatomical and functional brain variables associated with clozapine response in treatment-resistant schizophrenia. *Psychiatry Res*; 124 (3): 153–161.

Molina V, Sanz J, Sarramea F, Benito C, Palamo T (2004). Lower prefrontal gray matter volume in schizophrenia in chronic but not in first episode schizophrenia patients. *Psychiatry Research: Neuroimaging*; 131: 45–56.

Narr KL, Thompson PM, Szeszko P, Robinson D, Jang S, Woods RP, Kim S, Hayashi KM, Asunction D, Toga AW, Bilder RM (2004). Regional specificity of hippocampal volume reductions in first-episode schizophrenia. *Neuroimage*; 21 (4): 1563–1575.

O'Donnell P, Grace AA (1998). Dysfunctions in multiple interrelated systems as the neurobiological bases of schizophrenic symptom clusters. *Schizophr Bull*; 24: 267–283.

Olney JW, Farber NB (1995). Glutamate receptor dysfunction in schizophrenia. *Arch Gen Psychiatry*, 52: 998–1007.

Pae CU, Choe BY, Joo RH, Lim HK, Kim TS, Yoo SS, Choi BG, Kim JJ, Lee SJ, Lee C, Paik IH, Lee CU (2004). Neuronal dysfunction of the frontal lobe in schizophrenia. *Neuropsychobiology*, 50 (3): 211–215.

Pariante CM, Vassilopoulou K, Velakoulis D, Phillips L, Soulsby B, Wood SJ, Brewer W, Smith DJ, Dazzan P, Yung AR, Zervas IM, Christodoulou GN, Murray R, McGorry PD, Pantelis C (2004). Pituitary volume in psychosis. *Br J Psychiatry*, 185: 5–10.

Poland RE, Cloak C, Lutchmansingh PJ, McCracken JT, Chang L, Ernst T (1999). Brain N-acetyl aspartate concentrations measured by H MRS are reduced in adult male rats subjected to perinatal stress: preliminary observations and hypothetical implications for neurodevelopmental disorders. *J Psychiatr Res*, 33 (1): 41–51.

Prasad KM, Rohm BR, Keshavan MS (2004a). Parahippocampal gyrus in first episode psychotic disorders: a structural magnetic resonance imaging study. *Prog Neuropsychopharmacol Biol Psychiatry*, 28 (4): 651–658.

Prasad KM, Patel AR, Muddasani S, Sweeney J, Keshavan MS (2004b). The entorhinal cortex in first-episode psychotic disorders: a structural magnetic resonance imaging study. *Am J Psychiatry*, 161 (9): 1612–1619.

Renshaw PF, Yurgelun-Todd DA, Tohen M, Gruber S, Cohen BM (1995). Temporal lobe proton magnetic resonance spectroscopy of patients with first-episode psychosis. *Am J Psychiatry*, 152 (3): 444–446.

Robinson DG, Woerner MG, McMeniman M, Mendelowitz A, Bilder RM (2004). Symptomatic and functional recovery from a first episode of schizophrenia or schizoaffective disorder. *Am J Psychiatry*, 161(3): 473–479.

Rowland L, Bustillo JR, Lauriello J (2001). Proton magnetic resonance spectroscopy (H-MRS) studies of schizophrenia. *Semin Clin Neuropsychiatry*, 6 (2): 121–130.

Rubin Y, LaPlaca MC, Smith DH, Thibault LE, Lenkinski RE (1995). The effect of N-acetylaspartate on the intracellular free calcium concentration in NTera2-neurons. *Neurosci Lett*, 198: 209–212.

Ryan MC, Sharifi N, Condren R, Thakore JH (2004). Evidence of basal pituitary-adrenal overactivity in first episode, drug naive patients with schizophrenia. *Psychoneuroendocrinology*, 29 (8): 1065–1070.

Salgado-Pineda P, Baeza I, Perez-Gomez M, Vendrell P, Junque C, Bargallo N (2003). Sustained attention impairment correlates to gray matter decreases in first episode neuroleptic-naive schizophrenic patients. *Neuroimage*, 19: 365–375.

Schmahmann JD (1996). From movement to thought: anatomic substrates of the cerebellar contribution to cognitive processing. *Hum Brain Mapp*, 4: 174–198.

Schmahmann JD, Sherman JC (1997). Cerebellar cognitive affective syndrome. *Int Rev Neurobiol*, 41: 433–440.

Scottish Schizophrenia Research Group (1998). Regional cerebral blood flow in first-episode schizophrenia patients before and after antipsychotic drug treatment. *Acta Psychiatr Scand*, 97(6):440–449.

Semkovska M, Bedard MA, Stip E (2001). Hypofrontality and negative symptoms in schizophrenia: synthesis of anatomic and neuropsychological knowledge and ecological perspectives. *Encephale*, 27 (5): 405–415.

Shad MU, Muddasani S, Prasad K, Sweeney JA, Keshavan MS (2004). Insight and prefrontal cortex in first-episode Schizophrenia. *Neuroimage*, 22 (3): 1315–1320.

Shenton ME, Dickey CC, Frumin M, McCarley RW (2001). A review of MRI findings in schizophrenia. *Schizophr Res*, 49: 1–52.

Sigmundsson T, Maier M, Toone BK, Williams SC, Simmons A, Greenwood K, Ron MA (2003). Frontal lobe N-acetylaspartate correlates with psychopathology in schizophrenia: a proton magnetic resonance spectroscopy study. *Schizophr Res;* 64 (1): 63–71.

Sumich A, Chitnis XA, Fannon DG, O'Ceallaigh S, Doku VC, Falrowicz A, Marshall N, Matthew VM, Potter M, Sharma T (2002). Temporal lobe abnormalities in first-episode psychosis. *Am J Psychiatry;* 159 (7): 1232–1235.

Szeszko PR, Bilder RM, Lencz T, Ashtari M, Goldman RS, Reiter G, Wu H, Lieberman JA (2000). Reduced anterior cingulate gyrus volume correlates with executive dysfunction in men with first-episode schizophrenia. *Schizophr Res;* 43: 97–108.

Szeszko PR, Gunning-Dixon F, Ashtari M, Snyder PJ, Lieberman JA, Bilder RM (2003b). Reversed cerebellar asymmetry in men with first-episode schizophrenia. *Biol Psychiatry;* 53 (5): 450–459.

Szeszko PR, Gunning-Dixon F, Goldman RS, Bates J, Ashtari M, Snyder PJ, Lieberman JA, Bilder RM (2003a). Lack of normal association between cerebellar volume and neuropsychological functions in first-episode schizophrenia. *Am J Psychiatry;* 160 (10): 1884–1887.

Szeszko PR, Strous RD, Goldman RS, Ashtari M, Knuth KH, Lieberman JA, Bilder RM (2002). Neuropsychological correlates of hippocampal volumes in patients experiencing a first episode of schizophrenia. *Am J Psychiatry;* 159: 217–226.

Theberge J, Bartha R, Drost DJ, Menon RS, Malla A, Takhar J, Neufeld RW, Rogers J, Pavlosky W, Schaefer B, Densmore M, Al-Semaan Y, Williamson PC (2002). Glutamate and glutamine measured with 4.0 T proton MRS in never-treated patients with schizophrenia and healthy volunteers. *Am J Psychiatry;* 159 (11): 1944–1946.

Theberge J, Al-Semaan Y, Drost DJ, Malla AK, Neufeld RW, Bartha R, Manchanda R, Menon R, Densmore M, Schaefer B, Williamson PC (2004). Duration of untreated psychosis vs. N-acetylaspartate and choline in first episode schizophrenia: a 1H magnetic resonance spectroscopy study at 4.0 Tesla. *Psychiatry Res;* 131 (2): 107–114.

Weinberger DR, Lipska BK (1995). Cortical maldevelopment, anti-psychotic drugs, and schizophrenia: a search for common ground. *Schizophr Res;* 16: 87–110.

Weinberger DR, McClure RK (2002). Neurotoxicity, neuroplasticity, and magnetic resonance imaging morphometry: What is happening in the schizophrenic brain? *Archives of General Psychiatry;* 59: 553–558.

Wood SJ, Berger G, Velakoulis D, Phillips LJ, McGorry PD, Yung AR, Desmond P, Pantelis C (2003). Proton magnetic resonance spectroscopy in first episode psychosis and ultra high-risk individuals. *Schizophr Bull;* 29 (4): 831–843.

Wright IC, Rabe-Hesketh S, Woodruff PW, David AS, Murray RM, Bullmore ET (2000). Meta-analysis of regional brain volumes in schizophrenia. *Am J Psychiatry;* 157 (1): 16–25.

Zipursky RB, Lambe EK, Kapur S, Mikulis DJ (1998). Cerebral gray matter volume deficits in first episode psychosis. *Arch Gen Psychiatry;* 55: 540–546.

Chapter 8

Diagnostic variability in the early course of schizophrenia

Evelyn J. Bromet and Bushra Naz

In the late 1980s, we embarked on an epidemiologic study of the early course of schizophrenia, with a special emphasis on the influence of substance abuse on fluctuations in symptoms and functioning. In designing the study, our methodological goal was to meet the three basic requirements of epidemiologic research:

1 Ascertaining a representative sample so that the findings would be generalizable;

2 Formulating a valid and reliable diagnosis so that the results would be reproducible; and

3 Assembling a cohort that was at an early stage of their illness in order to maximize the utility and interpretation of the follow-up data and minimize the bias associated with treatment-seeking behavior.

Although the topics of sampling and diagnosis represent seemingly separate design issues, in the case of schizophrenia, they are interdependent. This is because under DSM III-R and IV, the classification requires a six month duration of the prodromal, active (presence of delusions, hallucinations, disorganized speech, or grossly disorganized or catatonic behavior), and/or residual phases of the illness. For first-episode or first-admission patients, the follow-up itself often clarifies the diagnosis. Thus, to minimize misclassification, it would be critical to include in the sample patients who either present with, or have for the potential for developing, schizophrenia, e.g., true-positive and false-negative cases. In addition, as this chapter suggests, it is crucial to adopt a longitudinal strategy for diagnosis. These considerations led to an expansion in the focus of the study to psychotic disorders other than schizophrenia and, as described in this chapter, to an examination of the variability and stability of the diagnosis of schizophrenia and its predictors.

Although we currently accept the notion that a longitudinal diagnosis is desirable, and indeed consider it essential for research on first-episode or first-admission samples, when we were designing our study it was uncommon for researchers to adopt a longitudinal perspective on diagnosis. At the time, the best available epidemiologic model was the World Health Organization's *Determinants of Outcome of Severe Mental Disorders*, in which all patients seeking treatment for the first time in their lives from selected catchment areas around the globe were systematically diagnosed and assessed with the same tools over time (Jablensky *et al.* 1992). The diagnosis, however, was made cross-sectionally.

There were three reasons why a cross-sectional diagnosis was the standard method of classification at the time. First, most schizophrenia research was based on consecutive admission samples, rather than first admissions, and thus the longitudinal piece of the diagnosis was built in. Second, the evidence suggested that schizophrenia was a stable diagnosis, with more than 90 per cent of patients receiving the same diagnosis at subsequent admissions (e.g., Babigian *et al.* 1965; Jørgensen and Mortensen 1988; Kendell 1974; Weeke 1984). However, evidence from readmission studies pertains only to the positive predictive value of the diagnosis in patients who are rehospitalized (see below).

Moreover, findings from studies conducted prior to 1990 were based on clinical discharge diagnoses that were formulated after weeks of observation. A reasonable concern in the late 1980s was whether the positive predictive value would be lower in patients who were discharged in a matter of days or weeks. Another concern was whether it would be lower because of the increased prevalence of substance abuse and depression (Burke *et al.* 1991). Most importantly, because there was no prospective evidence on the sensitivity and specificity of the initial diagnosis of schizophrenia in the late 1980s, i.e., follow-ups of patient cohorts regardless of readmission status, the true positive predictive value of the diagnosis of schizophrenia in first-episode or first-admission samples was not known.

The third reason that a longitudinal approach to diagnosis was not in fashion was that epidemiologists, among others, believed that a structured diagnostic interview, particularly in patient populations, provided systematic and sufficient information needed to formulate a valid and reliable differential diagnosis. The psychometric properties of these instruments were established in psychiatric patients and their relatives, and the test–retest reliability coefficients were impressively high. Indeed, as we began developing our study, we too assumed that applying state-of-the-art psychiatric interview methods together with a thorough review of the medical record would ensure that the study diagnosis of schizophrenia would be valid and reliable. We had not originally considered that in addition to 'true-positives' and 'true negatives,' the sample might contain a substantial number of 'false-positives' and 'false-negatives.' Fortunately, as the study protocol was being written, we presented our methodology at a meeting of the Stony Brook outpatient psychiatrists. They raised serious concerns about the validity of a cross-sectional diagnosis, not just because of the six month duration criterion for schizophrenia and the extensive comorbidity of substance abuse and depression, but because in their experience, these patients and their relatives, if available, were often poor informants and poor historians. They suggested that the only way to minimize the degree of misclassification was by creating a systematic, longitudinal method for formulating the study diagnosis. Ultimately, as described below, we developed a consensus procedure that utilized all available clinical and research information obtained from multiple sources at multiple follow-up points.

In this chapter, we describe the design of our epidemiologic study, the Suffolk County Mental Health Project (SCMHP), present data on the sensitivity, specificity, positive predictive value, negative predictive value, and kappa coefficient for the baseline diagnosis of schizophrenia compared to the 'gold standard' longitudinal diagnosis, describe the background and clinical differences between true-positive, false-positive, and false-negative cases of schizophrenia, and then discuss our findings in light of other subsequent prospectively designed studies of diagnostic stability.

Design of the Suffolk County Mental Health Project (SCHMP)

In order to assemble an unbiased, reasonably representative cohort, we established collaborations with all of the inpatient treatment programs in Suffolk County, Long Island, where the State University of New York at Stony Brook is located (Bromet *et al.* 2002). Suffolk County has a population of 1.3 million. In the late 1980s, there were 12 inpatient settings: six community hospitals having psychiatric units ranging from 20–30 beds; two state hospitals—one for adults and one for children; a veterans hospital with multiple psychiatric wards; a 30-bed academic inpatient ward; and two private psychiatric hospitals. (The latter agreed to participate in 1994.) Specifically, from September 1989–December 1995, the head nurse or social worker of each unit (a project staff member in the academic and adult state facility) identified potential study participants using the following criteria:

- age 15–60
- resident of Suffolk County
- clinical evidence of psychosis or a facility diagnosis indicating psychosis or treatment with an antipsychotic agent

+ IQ greater than 70
+ capable of and willing to give informed consent (for adolescents 15–17, the parents needed to provide written consent first)
+ first admission or first lifetime psychiatric hospitalization occurred within six months of index admission
+ no clear organic etiology (except substance abuse)
+ able to converse in English.

By recruiting first-admission patients with definite or possible psychotic symptoms from all of the programs, the sample was designed to be as inclusive and as representative as possible. However, we were not able to include individuals who sought inpatient care outside Suffolk County (unless they were rehospitalized within six months in Suffolk County) or were treated only in the emergency room or jail.

Patients were approached for the study after their psychosis had cleared in order to insure that they had the capacity to understand the consent process. Thus, most interviews took place in the hospital fairly close to the discharge date. The interviewers were experienced, masters level mental health professionals. The consent process covered the interview, along with permissions to audiotape the interview, review the medical record, talk to a significant other, and talk with the treating clinician. Most participants complied fully, but respondents were not excluded if they refused permission for components other than the interview.

After the initial face-to-face interview in the hospital, respondents were interviewed in person at the 6-, 24-, and 48-month follow-up points. Telephone contact was attempted every three months till the 24-month point, and every six months afterwards in order to keep track of the cohort and to ascertain changes in treatment, living arrangements, role functioning, and symptomatology. Many retention strategies were implemented to maintain as high a follow-up rate as possible, including having contact with respondents every three months, updating location information at each major contact with respondents or significant others, offering a financial incentive, scheduling interviews at times and places convenient to the respondent, and dropping by the respondents' homes if necessary to schedule an interview. We routinely mailed out birthday cards and holiday cards as well.

Perhaps the most important and controversial strategy for maintaining the integrity of the cohort was keeping the same interviewer with a respondent over time. Besides wanting as high a follow-up rate as possible, another goal was to obtain accurate information and reconcile discrepancies, rather than confirm in yet another study that people give inconsistent reports about their mental health over time. In fact, the interviewers were explicitly instructed to review previous clinical information so that they could disentangle discrepancies that arose during the follow-up interview. The fact that the follow-up interviews were not done blindly has implications for examining stability of symptoms rated during the interviews and the interviewers' own diagnoses. However, the research diagnosis (see below) was concealed from the interviewers until after the 24-month follow-up interview. Nevertheless, the findings presented here on the sensitivity and specificity of the baseline diagnosis of schizophrenia should be interpreted as reflecting the 'best case scenario.'

Assessment

The heart of the baseline interview was the Structured Clinical Interview for DSM-III-R (SCID) (Spitzer *et al.* 1992). Each face-to-face follow-up also included a SCID update. The SCID was modified by omitting the skip-out rules for the depression and mania modules and adding items on violence, suicidal behavior, and quantity and frequency of substance use. Symptoms were coded as present based on the SCID interview and on notes in the medical record. The interval SCIDs covered the period since previous interview and also inquired about symptoms previously ascertained from other sources (usually the medical record). If symptoms were reported for the first time at a follow-up interview, the interviewer was instructed to ascertain the time of onset and obtain as precise a chronology as possible.

After each face-to-face assessment, the interviewers completed the Brief Psychiatric Rating Scale (BPRS) (Woerner *et al.* 1988), the Scales for the Assessment of Negative (SANS) and Positive (SAPS) Symptoms (Andreasen *et al.* 1995), and the Global Assessment of Functioning (GAF) (Endicott *et al.* 1976) for the best month of the year before index admission and the worst week in the month before each face-to-face follow-up contact.

The interviewers also composed a narrative, summarizing the respondent's symptoms and illness course, occupational and psychosocial functioning, major life events, and treatment experiences. In addition, discharge summaries were requested for all hospitalizations.

Research diagnosis

After the baseline assessment, two research psychiatrists independently completed the SCID-P (psychiatrist diagnostic summary form) using all available information. The Principal Investigator (EB) then compared them.

When a consensus was not reached, the opinion of a third psychiatrist was solicited, but it was unusual for a consensus to be reached. In these cases, the diagnosis was deemed 'unknown.'

After both the 6- and 24-month assessments, two project psychiatrists, at least one of whom had not reviewed the case earlier, reviewed each case independently without knowledge of the baseline research diagnosis. They each assigned a diagnosis and completed a set of DSM criteria checklists developed for the project. Prior to the consensus meeting, the two psychiatrists met to discuss each case to see if they could reach a consensus on the diagnosis and the supporting criteria. Regardless of whether they agreed with one another, all cases were presented at monthly meetings of four or more psychiatrists where primary and comorbid consensus diagnoses were assigned using both DSM-III-R and DSM-IV criteria. A consensus was also reached about whether the diagnosis was definite or probable (meaning the person did not quite reach criteria but everyone agreed that this was the most likely diagnosis). The previous research diagnosis was revealed after the consensus decision was reached. If the new diagnosis was different from the previous one, the psychiatrists then determined what factors accounted for the change (i.e., illness course, new information not previously known, reinterpretation of the same information) (Fennig *et al.* 1994; Schwartz *et al.* 2000).

Analysis

The analysis uses epidemiologic statistics to examine the temporal consistency of the baseline vs. 24-month diagnosis of schizophrenia and schizoaffective disorder (SZ/SA). Specifically, we calculated sensitivity (true-positives divided by true-positive + false-negatives × 100), specificity (true-negatives divided by true-negatives + false-positives × 100), positive predictive value (true-positives divided by true-positives + false-negatives × 100), and negative predictive value (true-negatives divided by true-negatives + false-negatives × 100) (Greenberg *et al.* 2001). The kappa coefficient was also calculated.

Comparisons of the true-positive, false-positive and false-negative groups were conducted using chi square or analysis of variance. In addition to demographic characteristics and the rating scales noted above, the analysis focused on a composite indicator of family history of SZ/SA, based on the Family History RDC (Endicott *et al.* 1985) administered in the 6- and 24-month interview, the significant other interview, or information in the medical record; the Cannon-Spoor measure of premorbid adjustment for pre-teen, early teen, and later adolescence (Cannon-Spoor *et al.* 1982); SCID ratings of Schneiderian symptoms (mind being controlled, thought broadcasting, bizarre delusions);

hospital discharge diagnosis; and length of hospitalization, dichotomized into at/above vs. below the median for the type of hospital (community, public, university) and year hospitalized (1989–1991, 1992–1993, 1994–1995). Repeated measures analysis of variance was used to examine the three age periods of the premorbid adjustment measure and the GAF scores at baseline, 6, 24, and 48-month follow-up.

Results

The initial response rate was 72 per cent, and more than 85 per cent were successfully followed over a two-year period. Of the 675 respondents interviewed at baseline, 47 were excluded because they later proved not to meet the inclusion and exclusion criteria. Among the 628 members of the cohort, 582 (92.7 per cent) received a 24-month longitudinal diagnosis. With one exception (a cohort member who died shortly before the 24-month point), all were successfully contacted either in person, by telephone, or via a significant other at 24-month follow-up.

The 46 lost/refused cases were not significantly different from the analysis sample demographically or clinically except that the lost/refused were older on admission (33.1 + 10.1 vs. 29.4 + 9.6; t = 2.46; p <0.05) and had somewhat lower SANS ratings (1.13 + 0.94 vs. 1.43 + 0.96; t = 1.99; p <.05). Compared to the analysis sample, the baseline diagnostic distribution of the lost/refused was within 10 per cent of the analysis sample with two exceptions: relatively more lost/refused were classified as having psychosis NOS (28.3 per cent vs. 11.9 per cent) and substance induced psychosis (13.0 per cent vs. 3.4 per cent).

Table 8.1 shows the baseline and 24-month classification of SZ/SA, and the resulting sensitivity, specificity, positive predictive value, negative predictive value, and kappa coefficient. Similar to findings from studies of readmitted patients, the positive predictive value (proportion of respondents with a baseline diagnosis who received the same diagnosis at follow-up) was high (88.7 per cent). The specificity of the baseline diagnosis of SZ/SA was also excellent (95.6 per cent), indicating that respondents without this diagnosis at follow-up rarely received the diagnosis at baseline. However, the sensitivity and negative predictive value were considerably lower (56.6 per cent and 78.2 per cent respectively), and the kappa coefficient was also modest (0.56). Thus, the longitudinal perspective was clearly important in establishing an unbiased cohort of individuals with SZ/SA.

Table 8.2 shows the baseline diagnoses of the 96 false-negative cases and the 24-month diagnoses of the 16 false-positives cases. Among the false-negatives, 16 (16.7 per cent) had been given a provisional diagnosis of schizophreniform

Table 8.1 Comparison of baseline research diagnosis of schizophrenia and schizoaffective disorder (SZ/SA) with the 24-month longitudinal diagnosis

Baseline diagnosis	24-month diagnosis		Total
	SZ/SA	**Other**	**Total**
SZ/SA	125 'True-positives'	16 'False-positives'	141
Other	96 'False-negatives'	345 'True-negatives'	441
Total	221	361	582
Sensitivity	125/221 × 100	56.46	
Specificity	345/361 × 100	95.6%	
Positive predictive value	125/141 × 100	88.7%	
Negative predictive value	345/441 × 100	78.2%	
Kappa coefficient		0.56	

disorder at baseline. We note that all together, 32 respondents were given this diagnosis at baseline (Naz *et al.* 2003). The other most frequent diagnosis at baseline was psychosis NOS. Among the false-positives, six individuals' diagnoses became less clear as time went on, while 8 (50 per cent) were later diagnosed with an affective psychosis. In spite of the high level of substance abuse overall (31 per cent of the sample were actively abusing substances around the time of their hospitalization), only one of these respondents was later diagnosed as having a substance induced psychosis.

A six-month research diagnosis was available for 536 of the 582 respondents in the cohort. Fifty-two (56.5 per cent) of the 92 false-negatives were diagnosed

Table 8.2 DSM-IV diagnoses of false-positive (N = 16) and false-negative (N = 96) cases

Diagnosis	24-month diagnosis of false + (N = 16)	Baseline diagnosis of false − (N = 96)
Schizophreniform		16
Psychosis NOS	3	31
Unknown	3	24
Delusional disorder		7
MDD psy	5	10
BP psychosis	3	6
Substance induced	1	2
Non-psychotic dx	1	0

as SZ/SA at after the six-month follow-up. Conversely, 15 of the 16 false-positives received a six-month diagnosis; eight were still diagnosed as SA/SA at that time.

Comparison of true-positive, false-positive, and false-negative cases with SZ/SA

Because of the heterogeneity of the true-negative group, we limited the comparison to the respondents who were diagnosed with schizophrenia at least once (true positives, false-negatives, and false-positives). Demographically, the three groups were similar (Table 8.3) except that the false-positive group included relatively more blacks. In all groups, the majority of patients were male and not in school or working prior to admission. Only a small percentage had a family history of schizophrenia.

The three groups differed markedly, however, in their clinical histories and clinical presentations. The true-positives were most likely to report that on average, their first psychotic symptom occurred two years before admission, to have received antipsychotic treatment before admission, and to exhibit the poorest level of functioning during the year before admission (based on GAF scores for that period). Their premorbid functioning was also poorer (Figure 8.1). More specifically, although for the age period 6–11, the premorbid functioning of the three groups was similar, by the early teen years, the true-positives reported substantially worse functioning than the other two groups, and their functioning continued to decline in late adolescence. The false-negative group showed a parallel change in their functioning, although the overall picture was better. The false-positives had the best functioning in their early and late teens.

Once hospitalized, the true-positives were most likely to have bizarre and Schneiderian delusions (e.g., mind control, thought broadcasting) and to exhibit the most severe negative symptoms. However, the severity ratings on the CGI and SAPS were identical in the true-positive and false-positive groups. Moreover, compared to the false-negatives, the false-positives were more severely ill in the hospital and more likely to have Schneiderian symptoms. Thus, their initial diagnosis was consistent with a diagnosis of SZ/SA. Significantly more of the true-positives were diagnosed by their treating psychiatrist with SZ/SA and remained in the hospital for a longer time than average. Interestingly, the false-negatives had briefer lengths of stay than the false-positives although they were equally likely receive a clinical discharge diagnosis of SZ/SA.

Table 8.3 Comparison of true-positive, false-negative, and false-positive cases of SZ/SA

	True + N = 125	False + N = 16	False − N = 96	Test statistic when p <0.05
Background characteristics				
Age, mean + SD	28.6 + 8.8	29.6 + 8.6	27.4 + 7.9	
Ever in special education %	37.4	12.5	31.2	
Black %	24.8	56.3	11.5	$\chi^2 = 35.4$***
Low SES household %	41.9	50.0	30.5	
Male %	63.2	50.0	65.6	
Out of role before adm %	65.6	56.3	52.1	
Family history of SZ %	17.1	6.3	12.5	
Clinical characteristics				
Received anti-psychotics <adm %	35.5	25.0	17.7	$\chi^2 = 8.6$**
Median days from onset of psychosis to admission	604	297	61	F = 8.15**
GAF best month of year before adm, mean + SD	47.8 + 12.0	52.6 + 14.4	56.8 + 13.6	F = 13.5***
Lifetime substance dx %	47.1	39.6	53.3	$\chi^2 = 7.08$*
Substance dx active <adm %	25.6	31.3	25.0	
SANS, mean + SD	2.0 + 0.9	1.3 + 1.0	1.7 + 0.9	F = 3.53*
SAPS, mean + SD	2.1 + 1.0	2.1 + 0.6	1.7 + 1.0	F = 3.7*
Hamilton, mean + SD	14.5 + 6.6	17.3 + 6.6	13.9 + 6.3	
BPRS CGI, mean + SD	4.8 + 2.0	4.8 + 0.8	4.3 + 1.0	F = 6.8***
SCID: bizarre delusions %	55.0	35.7	18.0	$\chi^2 = 29.5$***
SCID: thought broadcasting %	33.1	21.4	11.0	$\chi^2 = 14.2$***
SCID: mind control % Hospital information	36.2	25.0	11.5	$\chi^2 = 16.0$***
Admitted to public hospital %	41.6	50.0	41.7	
Length of stay >median	72.6	31.3	61.5	$\chi^2 = 11.7$**
Discharge dx of SZ/SA	44.8	25.0	24.0	$\chi^2 = 11.1$**

* p <0.05 ** p <0.01 *** p <0.001

The posthospital functioning is summarized using the GAF scores for the worst week of the month just prior to each contact (Figure 8.2). At baseline, the GAF scores reflect the fact that the sample was in the hospital. By six-months, the true-positives improved somewhat, but were still functioning poorly. They remained at the same level throughout the 48-month period. The false-negatives showed a similar picture, with their GAF scores hovering around

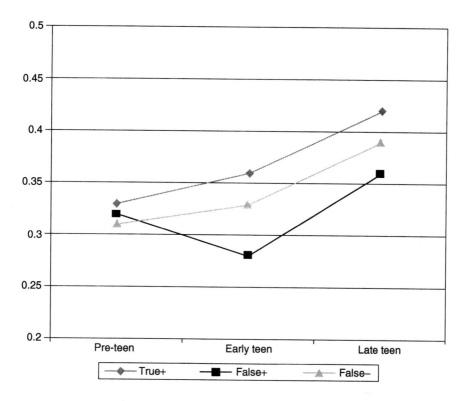

Figure 8.1 Cannon-Spoor Premorbid Adjustment Scales for SZ/SA: comparison of true-positive, false-positive, and false-negative respondents. F (dx) = ns; F (age group) *** (interaction) = ns.

40 at each measurement point. The false-positives, by contrast, continued to improve at each follow-up point. Thus, the longitudinal picture of psychosocial functioning mirrored the diagnostic shifts. Obviously to some extent the quality of overall functioning influenced the diagnostic process, at least through the 24-month point. On the other hand, the 48-month ratings, which were done for the most part by different interviewers because of staff turnover, were similar to those given at the 24-month follow-up.

Discussion

Schizophrenia is a chronic debilitating illness. Using our 24-month longitudinal consensus diagnosis as the gold standard, we diagnosed 221 respondents with schizophrenia or schizoaffective disorder (SZ/SA), or 38.0 per cent of a cohort of 582 first admissions with psychosis. Had we relied only on the baseline diagnosis, we would made the correct diagnosis in 125 cases, and missed the diagnosis in 96 cases. Thus, while the positive predictive value of the baseline diagnosis was excellent, its sensitivity was mediocre.

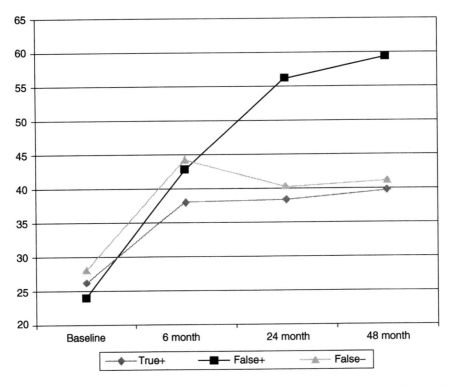

Figure 8.2 GAF functioning in past month: comparison of of true-positive, false-positive, and false-negative SZ/SA respondents. *P* values for all F's are less than 0.001.

In the past decade, several prospective studies have reported the positive-predictive value for other first-admission cohorts. Amin *et al.* (1999) reported on a sample of 168 first-contact admissions with psychosis from Nottingham followed over a three-year period. The positive-predictive values were 83 per cent for DSM-III-R schizophrenia and 33 per cent for schizoaffective disorder. In our sample, the two values were remarkably similar: 88 per cent for schizophrenia and 37 per cent for schizoaffective disorder. Interestingly, over seven year follow-up, the findings from a first-admission sample from Vienna were similar for schizophrenia (86 per cent) but lower for schizoaffective disorder (17 per cent) (Lenz *et al.* 1991). The 25-year follow-up of the Cologne cohort (Maneros *et al.* 1991) provided a similar positive-predictive value for schizophrenia (90 per cent).

The 125 true-positives, or stably diagnosed respondents, had by and large been chronically ill before the hospitalization. Thus the median time from onset of psychosis to hospital admission was almost two years, and most were coded on the WHO onset scale as having an insidious onset.

However, only one third had been treated with antipsychotic medication before being hospitalized. The majority of true-positives were either not working or not in school during the months leading up to the hospitalization, and as a group, they were most likely to receive a hospital discharge diagnosis of SZ/SA.

In contrast, the false-negative respondents were most likely to have an acute onset of relatively short duration and to have been unmedicated before admission. Their symptoms were rated as less severe, and only a small proportion presented with Schneiderian symptoms. Fourteen (14.6 per cent) of the 96 respondents in this group received BPRS clinical global impression ratings of 1–3 (normal, borderline, mild), compared to five or higher (4.0 per cent) of the true-positives and none of the false-positives. Their average GAF score for the best month of the year before admission was the highest of the three groups. In fact, the only variable on which the true-positives and false-positives were in fact similar was in the proportion who had attended special education classes. Jarbin and von Knorring (2003) also reported that those patients who shifted into the diagnosis of schizophrenia had better prepsychotic functioning.

The small false-positive group looked extremely ill at baseline. They more closely resembled the true-positives on the clinical ratings than was true for the false-negatives. However, their length of stay was significantly shorter than was the case for either of the other groups, and they were least likely to report a family history of schizophrenia.

Over the 48-month follow-up, those receiving a 24-month diagnosis of schizophrenia, regardless of whether they received the diagnosis from the very beginning, showed poor functioning that did not improve. The false-positive group continued to do better as time elapsed.

What are the lessons learned from this study? The first question we must ask is whether the labor-intensive rediagnosis efforts were worthwhile. We initially thought that the six-month diagnosis would serve as our principal study diagnosis. Clearly, from the evidence presented above, if we had not proceeded with the 24-month reevaluation, half of the false-positive and false-negative cases would have been misclassified. Misclassification bias is a serious concern for any epidemiologic inquiry, particularly when the disorder is relatively uncommon.

At the 10-year follow-up, DSM-IV diagnoses are updated via structured interview and medical records. In the first third of the sample followed to date, 15 additional participants not previously diagnosed with SZ/SA were given the diagnosis at the ten year point, including seven previously diagnosed with an affective psychosis, three with delusional disorder, two with substance induced psychosis, and one each with psychosis NOS, brief psychosis, and unknown.

In their seminal paper on diagnostic validity, Robins and Guze (1970) listed follow-up research as one of the five key steps to establish the validity of diagnosis. There is now a convergence of evidence that an initial diagnosis of schizophrenia at first admission has high temporal stability, and that a substantial minority of patients with other psychosis diagnoses will be initially misclassified. Given the extensive and expensive research on the biological and genetic underpinnings of schizophrenia, the importance of establishing a valid diagnosis and minimizing misclassification bias is obvious. In the absence of a biological marker, the longitudinal perspective should be brought to bear.

References

Amin S, Singh SP, Brewin J, Jones PB, Medley I, Harrison G (1999). Diagnostic stability of first-episode psychosis: comparison of ICD-10 and DSM-III-R systems. *British Journal of Psychiatry,* 175, 537–543.

Andreasen NC, Arndt S, Alliger R, Miller D, Flaum M (1995). Symptoms of schizophrenia. *Archives of General Psychiatry,* 52, 341–351.

Babigian HM, Gardner EA, Miles HC, Romano J (1965). Diagnostic consistency and change in a follow-up study of 1215 patients. *American Journal of Psychiatry,* 121, 895–901.

Bromet EJ, Mojtabai R, Fennig S (2002). The Suffolk County Mental Health project: an epidemiologic sudy of course and outcome. In R Zipursky and C Schulz (eds) *Early Stages of Schizophrenia,* pp. 33–54. Washington, DC: APA Press.

Burke KC, Burke JD Jr, Rae DS, Regier DA (1991). Comparing age of onset of major depression and other psychiatric disorders by birth cohorts in five US community populations. *Archives of General Psychiatry,* 48, 789–795.

Cannon-Spoor HE, Potkin SG, Wyatt RJ (1982). Measurement of premorbid adjustment in chronic schizophrenia. *Schizophrenia Bulletin,* 8, 470–484.

Endicott J, Andreasen N, Spitzer RL (1985). *Family History – Research Diagnostic Criteria,* New York: Biometrics Research Unit of the New York State Psychiatric Institute.

Endicott J, Spitzer RL, Fleiss JL, Cohen J (1976). The global assessment scale: a procedure for measuring overall severity of psychiatric disturbance. *Archives of General Psychiatry,* 33, 766–771.

Fennig S, Kovasznay B, Rich C, Ram R, Pato C, Miller A, Rubinstein J, Carlson G, Schwartz J, Phelan J, Lavelle J, Craig T, Bromet E (1994). Six-month stability of psychiatric diagnoses in first-admission patients with psychosis. *American Journal of Psychiatry,* 151, 1200–1208.

Greenberg RS, Daniels SR, Flanders WD, Eley JW, Boring JR III (2001). *Medical Epidemiology,* pp. 78–81. New York: Lange Medical Books/McGraw-Hill.

Jablensky A, Sartorius N, Ernberg G, Anker M, Korten A, Cooper JE, Day R, Bertelsen A (1992). Schizophrenia: Manifestations, incidence and course in different cultures: A World Health Organization ten-country study. *Psychological Medicine Monographs,* Supplement 20, 1–97.

Jarbin H, von Knorring AL (2003). Diagnostic stability in adolescent onset psychotic disorders. *European Child and Adolescent Psychiatry,* 12, 15–22.

Jørgensen P, Mortensen PB (1988). Admission pattern and diagnostic stability of patients with functional psychoses in Denmark during a two-year observation period. *Acta Psychiatrica Scandinavica,* 78, 361–365.

Kendell RE (1974). The stability of psychiatric diagnoses. *British Journal of Psychiatry,* 124, 352–356.

Lenz G, Simhandl C, Thau K, Berner P, Gabriel E (1991). Temporal stability of diagnostic criteria for functional psychoses. *Psychopathology*, 24, 328–335.

Maneros A, Deister A, Rohde A (1991). Stability of diagnoses in affective, schizoaffective and schizophrenic disorders: cross-sectional versus longitudinal diagnosis. *European Archives of Psychiatry and Clinical Neuroscience*, 241, 187–192.

Naz B, Bromet, EJ, Mojtabai R (2003). Distinguishing between first-admission schizophreniform disorder and schizophrenia. *Schizophrenia Research*, 62, 51–58.

Robins E, Guze SB (1970). Establishment of diagnostic validity in psychiatric illness: its application to schizophrenia. *American Journal of Psychiatry*, 126, 107–111.

Schwartz JE, Fennig S, Tanenberg-Karant M, Carlson G, Craig T, Galambos N, Lavelle J, Bromet EJ (2000). Congruence of diagnoses two years after a first-admission diagnosis of psychosis. *Archives of General Psychiatry*, 57, 593–600.

Spitzer RL, Williams JBW, Gibbon M, First MB (1992). The Structured Clinical Interview for DSM-III-R (SCID). I. History, rationale, and description. *Archives of General Psychiatry*, 49, 624–629.

Weeke A (1984). Admission pattern and diagnostic stability among unipolar and bipolar manic-depressive patients. *Acta Psychiatrica Scandinavica*, 70, 603–613.

Woerner M, Manuzza S, Kane J (1988). Anchoring the BPRS: an aid to improved reliability. *Psychopharmacology Bulletin*, 24, 112–124.

Chapter 9

Sex differences in schizophrenia: the case for developmental origins and etiological implications

Jill M. Goldstein and Deborah J. Walder

There are numerous studies demonstrating sex differences in the phenomenology and genetic transmission of schizophrenia (for review see Goldstein and Lewine 2000). Although one's sex modifies the phenotypic expression of schizophrenia, there is some debate about whether these differences have etiological implications (Goldstein 1995a, 1995b; Goldstein and Lewine 2000). We have argued that sex differences in incidence, genetic transmission, and brain abnormalities underscore its importance for understanding the etiology of the illness. In this chapter, we will provide further support for this position by providing evidence that sex differences in adulthood in schizophrenia begin during the premorbid period, underscoring the role of one's sex in characterizing the vulnerability for schizophrenia.

Incidence and prevalence

The incidence of schizophrenia ranges from approximately 0.5 to 2.0 per 10 000 population, and the prevalence from 1–12 per cent in different countries. Although early work supported the notion that the incidence did not vary by the individual's sex (Neugebauer *et al.* 1980; Wyatt *et al.* 1988), this was challenged more recently (Sartorius *et al.* 1986; Cooper *et al.* 1987; Castle *et al.* 1991; Iacono and Beiser 1992; Castle *et al.* 1993). The difference in findings between the earlier and later studies can, in part, be explained by the use of different diagnostic criteria. Studies using samples based on DSM-II criteria (American Psychiatric Association 1968) for schizophrenia included more affective psychosis among women and thus attenuated the sex effect for the incidence of schizophrenia, since women were more likely to express affective disorders than men.

An extensive critical review of the literature on incidence and prevalence of schizophrenia from 1980–1994 (Goldstein 1995b) supported the notion that the sex effect on incidence was, in part, highly dependent on the stringency of the diagnostic criteria and the decision of what other related diagnoses were included in the definition of a case, an idea that was empirically tested by Lewine and colleagues (1984), Castle and colleagues (1991, 1993), and Iacono and Beiser (1992). Studies using broader criteria reported no significant sex differences in incidence or prevalence (e.g. Hafner *et al.* 1989; Ring *et al.* 1991) while studies using more stringent diagnostic criteria for schizophrenia showed a significant sex effect on incidence, with men experiencing significantly higher rates than women (Lewine 1984; Castle *et al.* 1991; Iacono and Beiser 1992; Castle *et al.* 1993). Males younger than age 45 years had the highest incidence compared to young females. Women older than age 45 years had a significantly higher incidence of schizophrenia than men older than age 45 (Goldstein *et al.* 1989; Castle *et al.* 1991; Hambrecht *et al.* 1992; Iacono and Beiser 1992; Castle *et al.* 1993). This did not offset the higher incidence among younger males, thus resulting in a significantly higher rate among men when all ages were combined, e.g. male-to-female risk ratio was 1.34 (Castle *et al.* 1991, 1993).

Regarding sex differences in prevalence, studies reported a lower male-to-female rate ratio than did incidence studies (e.g. Halldin 1984; Munk-Jorgensen *et al.* 1986; Freeman and Alport 1987). However, as with incidence studies, male-to-female rate ratios varied from 1.04 (Bamrah *et al.* 1991) to 2.1 (Sikanartey and Eaton 1984), based on diagnostic criteria, sampling frame, and duration of the reported prevalence (i.e. point and period, ranging from two weeks to lifetime) (Goldstein 1995b). Thus, more recent studies of incidence and prevalence demonstrate slightly, and significantly, higher rates among men than women, suggesting an etiological role for one's sex as a risk factor for schizophrenia.

Genetic transmission

Schizophrenia is a familial disorder, with elevated rates among first degree relatives ranging from 3–15 per cent (Tsuang *et al.* 1974; Tsuang and Winokur 1975; Gottesman and Shields 1982; Kendler *et al.* 1985; Kendler and Walsh 1995). Familial studies have demonstrated that the sex of the proband differentially affected the risk of schizophrenia among first degree relatives of probands with schizophrenia (Bellodi *et al.* 1986; Shimizu *et al.* 1987; Goldstein *et al.* 1990; Wolyniec *et al.* 1992; Goldstein 1995a); for a critical review of familial transmission and twin concordance studies (1920–1993), see Goldstein (1995a). These studies have shown that, compared with relatives of men with schizophrenia, relatives of women had higher rates of schizophrenia and related psychotic spectrum disorders, i.e. schizoaffective and schizophreniform disorders. Relatives of men with schizophrenia had significantly higher rates of schizotypal personality disorder and flat affect, respectively, a milder expression and subsyndromal phenomenology of the disorder (Goldstein *et al.* 1990, 1995; Goldstein 1995a).

The few studies that have attempted to explain the effect of sex on familial risk have looked at age at onset, premorbid history, and symptom expression, variables that have been found to differ by sex (Pulver *et al.* 1990; Goldstein *et al.* 1992; Goldstein *et al.* 1995). Some studies have suggested that sex effects may be explained by a pseudoautosomal locus for schizophrenia (Crow 1988), a dominant X-Y model of transmission (Crow *et al.* 1994; DeLisi *et al.* 1994b), genetic heterogeneity (Goldstein *et al.* 1995), and/or an excess of CAG-based, trinucleotide repeat expansions among female cases (Morris *et al.* 1995). Although the exact mechanisms remain unclear, results on the genetic transmission of schizophrenia suggest that one's sex may modify, in some way, the transmission of the disorder, again implicating etiology.

Sex differences in brain abnormalities

Recent research has suggested that there are sex differences in brain abnormalities in schizophrenia (Goldstein *et al.* 2002), which is a reasonable expectation since other neurodevelopmental disorders have shown sex-mediated neurobehavioral and neuroanatomical consequences (Young *et al.* 1982). One question of interest has been whether sex differences in schizophrenia are similar, but exaggerated, normal sex differences in the brain. Evidence from the animal and human literature clearly demonstrates that the development of the brain differs in males and females, due in large part to the genomic and non-genomic regulatory effects of sex steroid hormones. Since schizophrenia is considered, at least in part, a neurodevelopmental disorder (Erlenmeyer-Kimling *et al.* 1984; Marcus *et al.* 1987; Weinberger 1987; Castle and Murray 1991; Murray 1994), it makes sense that the consequences of early insults to, or genetically-determined disruption of, brain development will in some way be influenced by the effects of sex hormones.

Normal sexual dimorphisms

A number of animal and human studies have demonstrated normal sexual dimorphisms of the brain (Allen and Gorski 1986; MacLusky *et al.* 1987; Witelson 1989; Allen and Gorski 1990; Benes *et al.* 1994; Filipek *et al.* 1994; Kulynych *et al.* 1994; Schlaepfer *et al.* 1995; Witelson *et al.* 1995; Caviness *et al.* 1996;

Giedd *et al.* 1996; Paus *et al.* 1996; Harasty *et al.* 1997; Passe *et al.* 1997; Gur *et al.* 1999; Highley *et al.* 1999; Rabinowicz *et al.* 1999). Early work in this area, primarily in rats, focused on the effects of sex steroid hormones on brain morphology during critical periods of early development (reviewed in McEwen 1983; Pilgrim and Hutchison 1994). Postmortem work in humans also identified sexual dimorphisms in brain regions involved in the neural control of sexual and maternal behavior and gonadotropin secretion (Allen and Gorski 1987; Allen *et al.* 1989; Witelson 1989; Allen and Gorski 1990; Highley *et al.* 1999).

In-vivo imaging and postmortem studies of sexual dimorphisms in humans report that the cerebrum is larger in men than women by approximately 8–10 per cent (Filipek *et al.* 1994; Witelson *et al.* 1995; Passe *et al.* 1997; Rabinowicz *et al.* 1999; Nopoulos *et al.* 2000). However, regionally-specific sex differences, relative to size of cerebrum, have been reported, and the direction of the sex effects differs depending on the brain region. These studies have reported, in women, relative to cerebrum size, greater cortical gray matter volume (Gur *et al.* 1999), larger volumes of regions associated with language functions, e.g. Broca's area (Harasty *et al.* 1997) and superior temporal cortex, in particular, planum temporale (Jacobs *et al.* 1993; Schlaepfer *et al.* 1995; Harasty *et al.* 1997), and larger volumes of the hippocampus (Filipek *et al.* 1994; Giedd *et al.* 1996; Murphy *et al.* 1996), caudate (Filipek *et al.* 1994; Murphy *et al.* 1996), thalamic nuclei (Murphy *et al.* 1996), anterior cingulate gyrus (Paus *et al.* 1996), dorsolateral prefrontal cortex (Schlaepfer *et al.* 1995), right inferior parietal lobe (Nopoulos *et al.* 2000), and white matter involved in interhemispheric connectivity (Allen and Gorski 1987; Witelson 1989; Highley *et al.* 1999; Nopoulos *et al.* 2000). Cell packing density, or number of neurons per unit volume, in the planum temporale was also greater in women than men (Witelson *et al.* 1995).

Compared to women, men have been found to have larger volumes, relative to cerebrum size, or differences in neuronal densities in other limbic and paralimbic regions (i.e. amygdala (Giedd *et al.* 1996), hypothalamus (Swaab and Fliers 1985; Allen *et al.* 1989; Zhou *et al.* 1995), and paracingulate gyrus (Paus *et al.* 1996)), larger genu of the corpus callosum (Witelson 1989) and overall white matter volume (Passe *et al.* 1997; Gur *et al.* 1999), and greater cerebrospinal fluid, lateral ventricles (Agartz *et al.* 1992; Kaye *et al.* 1992) or sulcal volume (Gur *et al.* 1999). Some have argued that men have more neurons across the entire cortex (Pakkenberg and Gundersen 1997; Rabinowicz *et al.* 1999) and women, more neuropil (Jacobs *et al.* 1993; Rabinowicz *et al.* 1999). However, these findings are inconsistent with others (Witelson *et al.* 1995; Harasty *et al.* 1997), and suggest that sex differences in neuronal characteristics depend on the brain region and/or cortical layer assessed

(Witelson *et al.* 1995). Thus, the consistency and etiology of sexual dimorphisms in the human brain remain unresolved.

One potential factor involved in human sexual dimorphisms may be the effects of sex steroid hormones on brain development. However, for the most part, this has been demonstrated only in animals (McEwen 1983; Tobet *et al.* 1993; Pilgrim and Hutchison 1994; Park *et al.* 1996; Gorski 2000). Although there are species-specific mechanisms, there may be some that are shared, given recent work demonstrating that the spatial organization of estrogen receptors in human adults in particular brain regions was similar to homologous regions in several other mammalian species (Donahue *et al.* 2000). Although the relative roles of testosterone and estrogen on the sexual differentiation of the human brain are as yet unclear, most likely both will contribute.

One mechanism well studied in animals is the role of aromatization on sexual differentiation (reviewed in Kawata 1995). During critical periods of early development, i.e. mid to late gestation and early postnatal periods, testosterone is, in part, converted to estradiol by the enzyme aromatase. Estradiol has been found to enhance neuronal density and size, maturation and migration, neurite growth and synaptogenesis (McEwen 1983; Miranda and Toran-Allerand 1992), and masculinize the rat brain. During early brain development in rodents, ferrets, and monkeys (MacLusky *et al.* 1987; Clark *et al.* 1988; Miranda and Toran-Allerand 1992; Tobet *et al.* 1993; Park *et al.* 1996), aromatase activity has been found in the hypothalamus and amygdala, where there is the highest concentration of sex steroid receptors, and the hippocampus, thalamic nuclei, specific cortical regions, and the corpus callosum and optic tract (MacLusky *et al.* 1987), the majority of which have been implicated in schizophrenia. Further, animal studies have demonstrated the relationship between differential localization of androgen and estrogen receptors during critical periods of development and brain morphology and behavior (McEwen 1983; Sandhu *et al.* 1986).

In a recent MRI study of normal subjects (Goldstein *et al.* 2001), we demonstrated that there were region-specific sex differences in adult brain volumes, relative to cerebrum size, particularly in the cortex. We raised the hypothesis that these region-specific sex differences in the adult brain may be related to factors affecting *in-utero* and early postnatal sexual differentiation of the brain (McEwen 1983; MacLusky *et al.* 1987; Pilgrim and Hutchison 1994). Independent of our work, this was recently suggested in a study that found sex differences in the distribution of androgen receptors in the adult human hypothalamus (Fernández-Guasti *et al.* 2000). In a preliminary attempt to indirectly examine this hypothesis, we found that cerebral regions implicated in early sexual differentiation in several mammalian species (e.g. amygdala, hypothalamus, hippocampus, orbital, dorsolateral and medial prefrontal cortices, posterior parietal cortex, primary auditory cortex, insula, basal forebrain, cingulate gyrus, medial dorsal thalamus, and basal ganglia), were significantly more likely to retain sexual dimorphisms of adult human cerebral volumes than brain regions that, according to the animal literature, do not have a high density of sex steroid receptors early in development (Goldstein *et al.* 2001). The interpretation that our findings on normal sex differences in the brain implicated fetal and early postnatal factors was underscored by the significant specific cortical sexual dimorphisms, since the density of cortical gonadal receptors recedes dramatically after early postnatal development, demonstrated in rats and monkeys (McEwen 1983; MacLusky *et al.* 1987; Clark *et al.* 1988; Toran-Allerand 1996).

There is precedence, suggested by the animal literature, for the idea that sex steroid hormones during development may relate to sex differences in the brain in adulthood (Shughrue *et al.* 1990; Tobet *et al.* 1993; Pilgrim and Hutchison 1994; Kawata 1995; Park *et al.* 1996). Aromatase activity, occurring during fetal development (see above discussion), is due to epigenetic hormonal factors, e.g., secretion of testicular testosterone, and sex-specific genetic programs affecting early brain development (Beyer *et al.* 1993; Beyer *et al.* 1994; reviewed in Kawata 1995), enhanced or modified by gonadal steroids later in development. In addition, other developmental mechanisms responsible for sexual differentiation may include direct effects of testosterone and differential apoptotic cell death (found to be, in part, regulated by androgens), and 'activational effects' of circulating hormones, occurring later in development (e.g. during puberty), which can potentiate neural circuits laid down during early development (Pilgrim and Hutchison 1994; Kawata 1995). In addition, the co-localization of gonadal receptors with neurotransmitters, such as the monoamines (e.g. Canick *et al.* 1987; Reisert *et al.* 1990; Beyer *et al.* 1991; Stewart *et al.* 1991) and y-aminobutyric acid (GABA) (O'Connor *et al.* 1988; Tobet *et al.* 1999), and growth factors, such as insulin and nerve growth factor (Kawata 1995; Toran-Allerand 1996), may mediate the relationship between receptor density and dimorphism. These findings in animals have potential implications for understanding sex differences in schizophrenia, a neurodevelopmental disorder with fetal and/or early postnatal origins.

Implications of normal sexual dimorphisms for understanding sex differences in schizophrenia

There have been relatively few previous studies designed to test for sex differences in structural brain abnormalities in schizophrenia, and there was a tendency among them to find greater abnormalities among the men (Nopoulos *et al.* 1997). MRI and postmortem studies showed that men had larger lateral and third ventricles (Andreasen *et al.* 1990; Haas *et al.* 1991; Goldstein *et al.* 2002) and anterior temporal horn (Bogerts *et al.* 1990), and smaller medial temporal volume, e.g. hippocampus and amygdala (Bogerts *et al.* 1990; Gur *et al.* 2000b; Goldstein *et al.* 2002), Heschl's gyrus (Reite *et al.* 1997; Rojas *et al.* 1997; Goldstein *et al.* 2002), superior temporal gyrus (Reite *et al.* 1997; Gur *et al.* 2000b), and overall frontal (Andreasen *et al.* 1994) and temporal lobe volumes (Bryant *et al.* 1999) (findings not wholly consistent) (Flaum *et al.* 1995; Lauriello *et al.* 1997). In addition, more left-lateralized abnormalities among men were reported (Bogerts *et al.* 1990; Haas *et al.* 1991; Bryant *et al.* 1999), such as smaller volumes of the left planum temporale (Rossi *et al.* 1991; Falkai *et al.* 1992; Kwon *et al.* 1999; Hirayasu *et al.* 2000), left Heschl's gyrus (Hirayasu *et al.* 2000), left superior temporal gyrus (Falkai *et al.* 1995), and left hippocampus (Bogerts *et al.* 1990; Shenton *et al.* 1992). Other abnormalities more likely found in men with schizophrenia, e.g. greater sulcal volume (Gur *et al.* 1991) and smaller thalamic size (Andreasen *et al.* 1990), suggested somewhat more pervasive brain damage in men than women (Nopoulos *et al.* 1997).

However, recent work has reported smaller volumes among women as well as men, depending on the cortical region assessed (Goldstein *et al.* 2002). Some have reported smaller volumes of heteromodal association areas among women with schizophrenia than men (e.g. dorsolateral prefrontal cortex and superior temporal gyrus (STG) (Schlaepfer *et al.* 1994), and orbital prefrontal cortex (Gur *et al.* 2000a)). However, others found smaller volumes of STG in men (Falkai *et al.* 1995; Barta *et al.* 1997; Reite *et al.* 1997), and similar abnormalities in men and women in dorsolateral prefrontal cortex (Gur *et al.* 2000a). Two recent studies (Gur *et al.* 2000a; Goldstein *et al.* 2002) demonstrated different differences between men and women with schizophrenia compared with their normal counterparts, depending on the particular prefrontal region assessed. The inconsistencies across studies may be, in part, due to methodological and sample size differences and to a relative dearth of conceptual models tested in studies of sex differences.

We recently proposed a heuristic framework for examining sex effects in brain abnormalities in schizophrenia. The premise, based on numerous studies, was that the risk for schizophrenia is initiated during prenatal and perinatal development (McNeil *et al.* 1993; Geddes and Lawrie 1995; Cannon *et al.* 1998; Jones *et al.* 1998; Buka *et al.* 2001a; Dalman *et al.* 1999). Further, animal studies, described above, demonstrated that the critical early period of the sexual differentiation of the brain, so-called organizational effects of gonadal hormones, also occurs in second and third trimester and early postnatal development (for review see Kawata 1995). We thus hypothesized that the organizational effects of gonadal hormones, occurring at the same time as risk factors for schizophrenia, would modify brain abnormalities differentially in males and females who developed schizophrenia. We hypothesized that the cortex would be more vulnerable to sex-specific brain abnormalities, since animal studies have shown that the cortex has a high density of gonadal hormone receptors only during these early critical periods of development, which then primarily recede postnatally (MacLusky *et al.* 1987; Clark *et al.* 1988; Toran-Allerand 1996). The largest adult normal sexual dimorphisms were in the cortex (Goldstein *et al.* 2001). Thus, we hypothesized that factors affecting normal sexual dimorphisms would have implications for understanding brain abnormalities in schizophrenia.

The MRI study (Goldstein *et al.* 2002) tested for sex differences in brain volumes, relative to cerebrum size, in regions found in animal studies to have a high density of sex steroid receptors pre- and perinatally (Pfaff and Keiner 1973; MacLusky *et al.* 1987; Clark *et al.* 1988; Shughrue *et al.* 1990) and found to be abnormal in schizophrenia, which included: middle frontal gyrus, frontomedial and frontoorbital cortices; basal forebrain; anterior, posterior, and paracingulate gyri; insula; parahippocampal gyrus; posterior parietal cortex (angular and supramarginal gyri); primary auditory cortex (Heschl's gyrus); and subcortical regions: amygdala; hippocampus; dorsal medial thalamic nuclei; and the caudate, putamen, and globus pallidum. We hypothesized that significant sex-specific effects in schizophrenia (i.e. disturbed normal sexual dimorphisms) would be more likely in cortical than subcortical regions. We also tested whether sex differences in normal asymmetries, reported in Heschl's gyrus, superior temporal gyrus, planum temporale (PT), and Brocas area (Crow 1990; DeLisi *et al.* 1994a; Shaywitz *et al.* 1995; Reite *et al.* 1997), would be disturbed in schizophrenia.

Our findings showed sex-specific effects in schizophrenia in the hypothesized cortical regions found to be normally sexually dimorphic and abnormal in schizophrenia (frontomedial and frontoorbital cortices, basal forebrain, cingulate gyrus, angular and supramarginal gyrus, Heschl's and planum temporale (PT)). The findings were consistent with, and extended, other work demonstrating sex differences in these brain regions (Hoff *et al.* 1992; Paus *et al.* 1996; Rojas *et al.* 1997; Frederikse *et al.* 2000; Gur *et al.* 2000a; Szeszko *et al.* 2000). Further, abnormal asymmetry of the PT in males was consistent with numerous imaging (Hoff *et al.* 1992; DeLisi *et al.* 1994a; Petty *et al.* 1995;

Barta *et al.* 1997; Kwon *et al.* 1999) and postmortem (Falkai *et al.* 1992; Falkai *et al.* 1995) studies, or in females, with right-sided abnormalities (Hoff *et al.* 1992; DeLisi *et al.* 1994a). We extended previous work by providing a heuristic model for examining sex differences across the entire brain.

Findings suggested that factors that contribute to producing normal sexual dimorphisms may be the same factors that modulate brain abnormalities in schizophrenia. The impact of sex steroid hormones on brain development, particularly during late gestation and early postnatal sexual differentiation of the brain (McEwen 1983; MacLusky *et al.* 1987), may contribute to understanding the mechanisms responsible for the sex-specific cortical effects, since this is the same developmental timing implicated in schizophrenia and the initiation of cortical differentiation. Potential mechanisms were discussed above. Although this study was not a study of developmental mechanisms, the results suggested potential hypotheses about sex effects, timing of insults, and consequences for brain morphology that could be tested in animal models in future studies. Thus, we argued that an understanding of sex-specific brain abnormalities in schizophrenia may lead to etiological clues, in addition to understanding the normal properties of the male and female brain in the face of disease. Further, these sex effects may have their origins during fetal and/or early postnatal development (Goldstein *et al.* 2002), suggesting that one's sex influences the vulnerability for schizophrenia.

Evidence for sex differences in the vulnerability for schizophrenia

Age at onset

One of the most replicated findings in the schizophrenia literature is the age at onset differences between men and women (for reviews, see Lewine 1981; Angermeyer and Kuhn 1988; Lewine 1988). The literature consistently demonstrates that men have an earlier onset age than women, which is specific to schizophrenia, not an artifact of admission practices, and similar across cultures (Lewine 1981; Sartorius *et al.* 1986; Angermeyer and Kuhn 1988; Lewine 1988). The peak period of onset for men is age 18–25 years old and for women, age 25-mid 30 years old (Lewine 1981; Loranger 1984; Lewine 1988; Angermeyer *et al.* 1989; Goldstein *et al.* 1989; Hafner *et al.* 1989). In early adolescence, the onset ratio of men to women is generally 2:1 (Lewine 1981). However, by age 50 and older, two female cases onset for every male case (Loranger 1984; Goldstein *et al.* 1989; Hafner *et al.* 1989; Castle *et al.* 1998). Approximately 3–10 per cent of women onset after age 40 compared to few, if any, men (Lewine 1981; Angermeyer *et al.* 1989; Goldstein *et al.* 1989; Hafner *et al.* 1989; Faraone *et al.* 1994; Castle *et al.* 1998). This sex effect suggests that males are more vulnerable to an earlier age at onset, which, in other studies, has been related to poorer prognosis and course.

Premorbid history

Given that schizophrenia is a disorder characterized by an age at onset, typically not prior to late teens/early adulthood, capturing the premorbid or prodromal period is particularly challenging. Several methodological approaches have been implemented to obtain early developmental data that predate the onset of acute psychosis. As outlined by Walker *et al.* (2002b), these include *prospective studies* that examine individuals who are at behavioral and/or genetic high risk for developing schizophrenia (e.g., first-degree relatives of patients with schizophrenia), *follow-up studies* that examine childhood data of large birth cohorts who went on to develop psychiatric conditions in adulthood, *retrospective studies* that identify adult patients with schizophrenia and examine archival data from their childhoods, and *retrospective studies* that examine information provided by informants (e.g., family members) about patients' premorbid histories.

We conducted a Medline search of studies published between the late 1960s–2002 focused on cognitive, behavioral, neuroendocrine, and neuroanatomic factors in the premorbid history of schizophrenia in general. Key words included schizophrenia, premorbid, high-risk, at-risk, prenatal, sex differences, gender, first-episode, longitudinal, neuropsychological, cognitive, neuroanatomical, and neuromotor. We reviewed all of the relevant literature on this topic in order to examine whether any of the studies mentioned sex effects. Out of the 112 articles reviewed, 35 (31 per cent) examined sex differences and 25/35 (71 per cent) found evidence of sex differences.

It has been consistently demonstrated across time periods that women tend to have a better premorbid history than men with schizophrenia (Gittelman-Klein and Klein 1969; Salokangas 1983; Childers and Harding 1990; Foerster *et al.* 1991b). Women with schizophrenia are more often married (Watt and Szulecka 1979; Ciompi 1980; Wattie and Kedward 1985; Hafner *et al.* 1989) and have better childhood histories, including better school achievement and sociability (Gittelman-Klein and Klein 1969; Preston *et al.* 2002), fewer learning disabilities (Goldstein *et al.* 1994), and higher IQs (Aylward *et al.* 1984). Boys at high risk for schizophrenia have exhibited more neurobehavioral deficits than girls at high risk, regarding attentional deficits and neuromotor abnormalities (Mednick *et al.* 1978; Erlenmeyer-Kimling *et al.* 1984), aggression (John *et al.* 1982; Marcus *et al.* 1987), and physical anomalies (Green *et al.* 1989; Waddington *et al.* 1990) and more likely to have obstetric complications in their history (Lewis and Murray 1987; Foerster *et al.* 1991a). These studies suggest that males are at higher risk for early developmental deficits than females, prior to the onset of illness, thus indicating a poorer premorbid history and greater vulnerability for the illness.

In a recent review Walker *et al.* (2002b) concluded that there are sex differences in the childhood and adolescent behavior of individuals who go on to develop schizophrenia. Males became more disruptive and females became more withdrawn with increasing age. In one retrospective study, Walker *et al.* (1995a, b) had parents rate the behavior of their adult offspring (e.g., those with schizophrenia and same-sex healthy siblings) at four age periods spanning birth to 16 years. After age four, there were higher rates of externalizing and internalizing behavior problems in preschizophrenic (preSZ) males relative to their healthy same-sex siblings. The preSZ females only differed from same-sex siblings in that they showed more internalizing problems after age eight. When directly comparing males to females, the preSZ females had higher rates of internalizing problems than their male counterparts. Moreover, rates of depression were higher in preSZ females than their same-sex siblings and preSZ males. Depression severity increased to a greater extent in the preSZ females during the adolescent period in comparison to all other groups. Walker *et al.* (2002b) note that parallel findings in community samples of adolescent girls (Gjerde and Block 1996) suggest that preSZ individuals experience an exacerbation of what are otherwise typical sex differences in depression. The fact that females with schizophrenia, just as healthy females, may be at higher risk for affective syndromes, was demonstrated even earlier in development than around puberty. In a unique archival study that examined childhood home movies of adult patients with schizophrenia and their siblings, Walker *et al.* (1993) found less expression of positive facial emotion in preSZ females relative to same-sex healthy siblings, preSZ males and non-schizophrenic males, a pattern that emerged in infancy and became more prominent in adolescence. These findings provide further evidence that the vulnerability for schizophrenia begins prior to the onset of psychosis and that it is differentially expressed by males and females.

Differential risks of the male and female brain to early insults

The idea that the brains of males and females may be at different risks for consequences due to insults occurring during early developmental periods is not new. In fact, there are a few animal and human studies examining sex differences in the effects of pre- and perinatal complications on the developing brain. In monkeys, early lesions to the frontoorbital cortex during development resulted in worse performance for males than females on a spatial delayed-response task (Goldman *et al.* 1974). This is consistent with a human study of epileptic patients with early brain lesions, of whom males showed general cognitive deficits in language, memory, and attention, whereas consequences for females were less severe (Strauss 1992). It is also consistent with studies showing that low birthweight boys had increased intra- and periventricular hemorrhage, neurological deficits and educational problems compared with low birthweight girls (Rantakallio and Wendt 1985; Amato *et al.* 1987; Murray *et al.* 1989), suggesting that the same fetal insults may produce more severe consequences for males. In rats, prenatal exposure to insults producing anoxia had more severe consequences for learning and performance in males than in females. Postnatal exposure had similar effects on learning behavior in male and female rats (Grimm and Frieder 1985). It has been suggested that hypoxic and other critical obstetric events in humans have been related to increased lateral and third ventricles, cortical and white matter abnormalities (Liechty *et al.* 1983; Volpe 1987; Lewis 1989; Cannon *et al.* 1998; Silverman *et al.* 1998; Cannon *et al.* 2002b). Increased lateral ventricles and sulcal enlargement have been found in other childhood neurodevelopmental disorders (Bergstrom *et al.* 1984), the majority of which have a higher incidence in males. These findings suggest that insults particularly during the prenatal period relate not only to sex differences in behavior postnatally, but also to structural brain abnormalities in adulthood.

Male and female brain abnormalities in schizophrenia prior to psychosis onset

In schizophrenia, there is some evidence of sex differences in structural brain abnormalities during the premorbid period. Two MRI studies of adolescent offspring of parents with schizophrenia showed reduced left amygdala volume, enlarged third ventricular volume, and smaller overall brain volume than children of normal parents (Keshavan *et al.* 1997). Adolescents and young adults were found to have reduced left hippocampus-amygdala volumes (Lawrie *et al.* 1999). Results also suggested altered NAA/choline ratios in the cingulate gyrus (Keshavan *et al.* 1997). In addition, cortical anomalies found in high risk offspring increased with genetic risk (Cannon *et al.* 1993) and risk associated with a hypoxic-genetic interaction effect (Cannon *et al.* 2002b). Thus, although these high-risk studies did not have the statistical power to investigate differential sex effects, non-psychotic offspring of parents with schizophrenia showed abnormalities in a number of brain regions, found to be normally sexually dimorphic and differentially abnormal in adult men and women with schizophrenia (Goldstein *et al.* 2002). Some evidence for differential sex effects in brain abnormalities during the premorbid period was implied in an MRI and neuropsychological study of first episode patients (Szeszko *et al.* 2002). These authors showed an association between anterior hippocampal volume and executive and motor functioning in male patients, which was not present in females. Moreover, anterior hippocampal volume was more strongly associated with motor functioning among male than female patients (Szeszko *et al.* 2002).

Finally, a number of the brain regions found to be abnormal prior to illness onset have been implicated in the control of the neuroendocrine system, in which deficits have been reported prior to illness onset. Walker and colleagues (reviewed in Walker and Diforio 1997) have been investigating the hypothesis that the etiology for schizophrenia may, at least in part, involve pre- and/ or postnatal insults affecting brain regions associated with the negative feedback system that dampens hypothalamic-pituitary-adrenal (HPA) activity, such as the hippocampus. She suggests that this will result in long-standing dysregulation of the HPA axis (i.e. overproduction of glucocorticoids), which is associated with neuronal dysfunction or death during development and hypersensitivity to stress in childhood and adulthood. In support of this, a number of studies have reported in schizophrenia higher rates of baseline cortisol activity and hyperresponsivity to stress (Roy *et al.* 1986; Breier *et al.* 1988; Risch *et al.* 1992; Walder *et al.* 2000) and associations of heightened cortisol secretion with hippocampal volumetric reductions (Walker *et al.* 2002a) and impaired cognitive performance on tasks associated with hippocampal function (Walder *et al.* 2000). Cortisol release deficits have been associated with a number of other behavioral problems found in high risk offspring of parents with schizophrenia, such as social withdrawal, depression, and social inhibition (reviewed in Walker and Diforio 1997). Elevated levels of cortisol were also found in schizotypal personality disorder patients, underscoring the premise that neuroendocrine dysfunction may be part of the *vulnerability* to schizophrenia, rather than due to the psychosis per se or medication effects (Walker *et al.* 1996; Weinstein *et al.* 1999). Moreover, elevations in cortisol secretion have been linked with more severe symptoms in adolescents with schizotypal personality disorder (Walker *et al.* 2001) and adults with schizophrenia (Walder *et al.* 2000). Finally, some studies have reported that normal males secrete higher levels of cortisol than females

(Schaeffer and Baum 1984; Davis and Emory 1995), suggesting the potential for differential sex effects on this system in males and females with schizophrenia. In fact, there is a high rate of endocrine dysfunction in schizophrenia, associated with the adrenal *and* gonadal systems, with rates of dysfunction reported from 50–75 per cent (Beaumont *et al.* 1974; Ghadirian *et al.* 1982; Sullivan and Lukoff 1990; Reicher-Rossler *et al.* 1994).

Evidence for factors producing differential effects on the male and female brain

A number of studies have demonstrated links between pre- and perinatal obstetric factors and the risk for schizophrenia (Yolken and Torrey 1995; Jones *et al.* 1998), including viral and bacterial infections in mid-pregnancy (Mednick *et al.* 1994; Buka *et al.* 2001a, b; Brown and Susser 2002), famine (Susser *et al.* 1996), maternal illnesses, such as rubella, diabetes, hypertension, and Herpes simplex-2 (Brown *et al.* 2001), and other adverse maternal conditions such as rhesus incompatibility (Hollister *et al.* 1996). In addition, prenatal and labor-and-delivery complications associated with hypoxic and/or ischemic injury have also been associated with increased risk of schizophrenia, measured as apnea or idiopathic respiratory distress syndrome (RDS), low Apgar score, small for gestational age (SGA) at birth (Cannon *et al.* 2002b), pre-eclampsia (Dalman *et al.* 1999), gestational age <33 weeks (Hultman *et al.* 1999), inertia of labor, vacuum extraction (Dalman *et al.* 1999), ponderal index <20 (a measurement of leanness) (Dalman *et al.* 1999; Hulshoff *et al.* 2000) (for review, see Cannon *et al.* 2002a).

A few studies have reported in males and females, differential risks associated with these obstetric factors for schizophrenia. Compared with SGA girls, boys born SGA are at a tenfold increased risk for schizophrenia (Odds Ratio (OR) = 3.2 (CI 1.4 – 7.2) vs. .3 (CI .03 – 2.4) (Hultman *et al.* 1999)), and boys with a small head circumference are at a twofold increased risk for schizophrenia than girls (OR = 2.1 (CI 1.0 –4.5) vs. 0.8 (CI .3 – 2.5) (Dalman *et al.* 1999; Thomas *et al.* 2001)). In addition, boys exposed to pre-eclampsia or asphyxia at birth were also at higher risk for schizophrenia than exposed girls (e.g. Pre-eclampsia: OR = 3.5 (CI 1.8 – 6.6) vs. 1.1 (CI .3 – 4.6); Asphyxia: 1.6 (CI .9 – 2.8) vs. .8 (CI .4 – 1.7) (Dalman *et al.* 1999; Hultman *et al.* 1999; Thomas *et al.* 2001)). Several studies have reported an increased rate of obstetric complications in schizophrenia that is greater for males than females (Foerster *et al.* 1991a; Matsumoto *et al.* 2001), although not in all studies (Verdoux *et al.* 1997; Rosso *et al.* 2000). In a recent study, Caucasian female patients had a lower frequency of hypoxia-associated OCs compared to Caucasian males, although the risk for schizophrenia did not differ by sex (OR = 1.04) (Cannon *et al.* 2000). Not all obstetric factors place males at higher risk for schizophrenia than females. For example, maternal diabetes showed a 13.5 (CI 0.8–239.4) risk ratio for schizophrenia in females (even though the exposure rate was low with large confidence intervals (Hultman *et al.* 1999)). In addition, the relationship between prenatal maternal viral infection and risk for schizophrenia in offspring was shown in one study to be more pronounced in females than males (Murray *et al.* 1992a, b).

Although some studies do not show differential sex effects of OCs on schizophrenia (Verdoux *et al.* 1997; Cannon *et al.* 2000), a number of studies have found males to be more vulnerable to early developmental insults than girls. For example, males with OCs (O'Callaghan *et al.* 1992; Stober *et al.* 1993), have an increased risk for earlier age at onset. Generally, males with a history of OCs had a 3.5 year earlier age at onset of schizophrenia than those without a history of OCs (Kirov *et al.* 1996). As reviewed by Walker *et al.* (2002b), there is evidence of a stronger link between history of OCs and:

1 Neuropsychological deficits in adulthood among adult males with schizophrenia than females (Casar *et al.* 1997);

2 Neurological soft signs in males with schizophrenia, although not restricted to schizophrenia (Lane *et al.* 1996);

3 More soft neurological signs in males (Hadders-Algra *et al.* 1988b); and

4 Greater behavioral deficits in males (Hadders-Algra *et al.* 1988a).

This is consistent with work demonstrating that females have an advantage over males in terms of cognitive recovery from respiratory distress syndrome on tasks of non-verbal intelligence (Lauterbach *et al.* 2001). Similar sex differences for intelligence were found in a study of children with intracranial hemorrhage (Raz *et al.* 1995). These findings suggest that the male brain may be more vulnerable than the female at particular periods of development to adverse obstetric events.

In order to understand the mechanisms explaining these sex effects, the timing of the event may be as important as the nature of the event. For example, the sexual differentiation of the brain does not begin until around mid-gestation. In a study of famine in which the offspring were exposed in the first trimester, there were no significant sex differences in the risk for schizophrenia (Relative risks = 1.9 vs. 2.2) (Susser *et al.* 1996). In contrast, in studies that investigated second and third trimester events, such as pre-eclampsia (see previous discussion), sex effects in morbidity risk were more evident.

We would argue that sex differences in the effects of OCs on the brain would more likely occur during the critical period of the organizational effects of gonadal hormones on the sexual differentiation of the brain.

Conclusions

In summary, we have argued that the impact of one's sex on schizophrenia has important implications for the etiology of schizophrenia. Studies have demonstrated significant sex differences in incidence, genetic transmission, and brain abnormalities with developmental origins, suggesting some impact of one's sex on the risk for the disorder and subsequent consequences to the brain. We have provided indirect evidence in our previous studies that sex differences in brain abnormalities in schizophrenia may be initiated at the time of the early sexual differentiation of the brain, that is, during fetal and early postnatal development. This has support from animal studies demonstrating differential brain abnormalities and behavioral consequences to adult male and female animals, depending on the timing of the insult during fetal and early postnatal brain development. This premise also has support from studies demonstrating significant differential risks for schizophrenia in men and women, given exposure to particular obstetric factors. Finally, the idea that sex differences in schizophrenia define part of the vulnerability for the illness, i.e. have early developmental origins, is underscored by a number of high risk and birth cohort studies demonstrating sex differences in the premorbid histories of individuals who later onset with the illness across multiple domains, including sex differences in behavioural, neurological, psychophysiological, psychiatric, and neuroendocrine histories.

Acknowledgements

This manuscript was written in part, supported by NIMH RO1 MH56956 (to JG), funded by National Institute of Mental Health and, in part, by the Office for Research on Women's Health. DJW was supported by postdoctoral fellowships in Harvard-Partners Consortium in Neuropsychology, Brigham and Women's Hospital, Harvard Medical School, and NiMH Clinical Research Training Program in Biological Psychiatry, Harvard Medical School (NiMHT32MH16259).

References

Agartz I, Sääf J, Wahlund L-O, Wetterberg L (1992). Quantitative estimations of cerebrospinal fluid spaces and brain regions in healthy controls using computer-assisted tissue classification of magnetic resonance images: relation to age and sex. *Magnetic Resonance Imaging,* 10, 217–26.

Allen LS, Gorski RA (1986). Sexual dimorphism of the human anterior commissure [abstract]. *Anatomical Record,* 214, 3A.

Allen LS, Gorski RA (1987). Sex differences in the human massa intermedia [abstract]. *Society for Neuroscience Abstracts,* 13, 46.

Allen LS, Gorski RA (1990). Sex difference in the bed nucleus of the stria terminalis of the human brain. *Journal of Comparative Neurology,* 302, 697–706.

Allen LS, Hines M, Shryne JE, Gorski RA (1989). Two sexually dimorphic cell groups in the human brain. *Journal of Neuroscience,* 9, 497–506.

Amato M, Howald H, Muralt GV (1987). Foetal sex distribution of peri-intraventricular haemorrhage in preterm infants. *European Neurology,* 27, 20.

American Psychiatric Association (1968). *Diagnostic and Statistical Manual of Mental Disorders.* Washington, DC: American Psychiatric Association

Andreasen NC, Ehrhardt JC, Swayze VW *et al.* (1990). Magnetic resonance imaging of the brain in schizophrenia: the pathophysiologic significance of structural abnormalities. *Archives of General Psychiatry,* 47, 35–44.

Andreasen NC, Flashman L, Flaum M *et al.* (1994). Regional brain abnormalities in schizophrenia measured with magnetic resonance imaging. *JAMA,* 272, 1763–69.

Angermeyer MC, Kuhn L (1988). Gender differences in age at onset of schizophrenia. An overview. *European Archives of Psychiatry and Neurological Sciences,* 237, 351–64.

Angermeyer MC, Goldstein JM, Kuhn L (1989). Gender differences in schizophrenia: rehospitalization and community survival. *Psychological Medicine,* 19, 365–82.

Aylward E, Walker E, Bettes B (1984). Intelligence in schizophrenia: meta-analysis of the research. *Schizophrenia Bulletin,* 10, 430–59.

Bamrah JS, Freeman HL, Goldberg DP (1991). Epidemiology of schizophrenia in Salford, 1974–84. Changes in an urban community over ten years. *British Journal of Psychiatry,* 159, 802–10.

Barta P, Pearlson G, Brill LB, II *et al.* (1997). Planum temporale asymmetry reversal in schizophrenia: replication and relationship to gray matter abnormalities. *American Journal of Psychiatry,* 154, 661–7.

Beaumont PJV, Gelder MG, Friesen HG *et al.* (1974). The effects of phenothiazines on endocrine function: I. *British Journal of Psychiatry,* 124, 413–19.

Bellodi L, Bussoleni C, Scorza-Smeraldi R, Grassi G, Zacchetti L, Smeraldi E (1986). Family study of schizophrenia: exploratory analysis for relevant factors. *Schizophrenia Bulletin,* 12, 120–28.

Benes FM, Turtle M, Khan Y, Farol P (1994). Myelination of a key relay zone in the hippocampal formation occurs in the human brain during childhood, adolescence, and adulthood. *Archives of General Psychiatry,* 51, 477–84.

Bergstrom K, Bille B, Rasmussen F (1984). Computed tomography of the brain in children with minor neurodevelopmental disorders. *Neuropediatrics,* 15, 115–19.

Beyer C, Pilgrim C, Reisert I (1991). Dopamine content and metabolism in mesencephalic and diencephalic cell cultures: sex differences and effects of sex steroids. *Journal of Neuroscience,* 11, 1325–33.

Beyer C, Wozniak A, Hutchinson JB (1993). Sex-specific aromatization of testosterone in mouse hypothalamic neurons. *Neuroendocrinology,* 58, 673–81.

Beyer C, Green SJ, Barker PJ, Huskisson NS, Hutchinson JB (1994). Aromatase-immunoreactivity is localised specifically in neurones in the developing mouse hypothalamus and cortex. *Brain Research,* 638, 203–10.

Bogerts B, Ashtari M, Degreef G, Alvir JMJ, Bilder RM, Lieberman JA (1990). Reduced temporal limbic structure volumes on magnetic resonance images in first episode schizophrenia. *Psychiatry Research,* 35, 1–13.

Breier A, Wolkowitz OM, Doran AR, Bellar S, Pickar D (1988). Neurobiological effects of lumbar puncture stress in psychiatric patients and healthy volunteers. *Psychiatry Research,* 25, 187–94.

Brown AS, Susser ES (2002). In utero infection and adult schizophrenia. *Ment Retard Dev Disabil Res Rev,* 8, 51–7.

Brown AS, Cohen P, Harkavy-Friedman J *et al.* (2001). A.E. Bennett Research Award. Prenatal rubella, premorbid abnormalities, and adult schizophrenia. *Biological Psychiatry,* 49, 473–86.

Bryant NL, Buchanan RW, Vladar K, Breier A, Rothman M (1999). Gender differences in temporal lobe structures of patients with schizophrenia: a volumetric MRI study. *American Journal of Psychiatry,* 156, 603–09.

Buka SL, Tsuang MT, Torrey EF, Klebanoff MA, Bernstein D, Yolken RH (2001a). Maternal infections and subsequent psychosis among offspring: a forty year prospective study. *Archives of General Psychiatry,* 58, 1032–37.

Buka SL, Tsuang MT, Torrey EF, Klebanoff MA, Wagner R, Yolken RY (2001b). Maternal cytokine levels during pregnancy and adult psychosis. *Brain, Behavior and Immunity,* 15, 411-20.

Canick JA, Tobet SA, Baum MJ *et al.* (1987). Studies of the role of catecholamines in the regulation of the developmental pattern of hypothalamic aromatase. *Steroids,* 50, 509–21.

Cannon M, Jones P, Murray R (2002a). Obstetric complications and schizophrenia: historical and meta-analytic review. *American Journal of Psychiatry,* 159, 1080–92.

Cannon TD, Mednick SA, Parnas J, Schulsinger F, Praestholm J, Vestergaard A (1993). Developmental brain abnormalities in the offspring of schizophrenic mothers. I. Contributions of genetic and perinatal factors. *Archives of General Psychiatry,* 50, 551–64.

Cannon TD, Rosso IM, Hollister JM, Bearden CE, Sanchez LE, Hadley T (2000). A prospective cohort study of genetic and perinatal influences in the etiology of schizophrenia. *Schizophrenia Bulletin,* 26, 351–66.

Cannon TD, van Erp TGM, Huttunen M *et al.* (1998). Regional gray matter, white matter, and cerebrospinal fluid distributions in schizophrenic patients, their siblings, and controls. *Archives of General Psychiatry,* 55, 1084–91.

Cannon TD, van Erp TG, Rosso IM *et al.* (2002b). Fetal hypoxia and structural brain abnormalities in schizophrenic patients, their siblings, and controls. *Archives of General Psychiatry,* 59, 35–41.

Casar C, Artamendi M, Gutierrez M, Gil P, Garcia MJ, Cvesta MJ (1997). Neuropsychological deficits, obstetric complications and premorbid adjustment in patients with the first psychotic episode. *Actas luso-Espanolas de Neurologia y Psiquiatria Ciencias Afines,* 25, 303–07.

Castle D, Sham P, Murray R (1998). Differences in distribution of ages of onset in males and females with schizophrenia. *Schizophrenia Research,* 33, 179–83.

Castle D, Wessely S, Der G, Murray RM (1991). The incidence of operationally defined schizophrenia in Camberwell, 1965–84. *British Journal of Psychiatry,* 159, 790–94.

Castle DJ, Murray RM (1991). The neurodevelopmental basis of sex differences in schizophrenia. *Psychological Medicine,* 21, 565–75.

Castle DJ, Wessely S, Murray RM (1993). Sex and schizophrenia: effects of diagnostic stringency, and associations with premorbid variables. *British Journal of Psychiatry,* 162, 653–64.

Caviness VS, Kennedy DN, Richelme C, Rademacher J, Filipek PA (1996). The human brain age 7–11 years: a volumetric analysis based upon magnetic resonance images. *Cerebral Cortex,* 6, 726–36.

Childers SE, Harding CM (1990). Gender, premorbid social functioning, and long-term outcome in DSM-III schizophrenia. *Schizophrenia Bulletin,* 16, 309–18.

Ciompi L (1980). Catamnestic long-term study on the course of life and aging in schizophrenics. *Schizophrenia Bulletin,* 6, 606–18.

Clark AS, MacLusky NJ, Goldman-Rakic PS (1988). Androgen binding and metabolism in the cerebral cortex of the developing rhesus monkey. *Endocrinology,* 123, 932–40.

Cooper JE, Goodhead D, Craig T, Harris M, Howat J, Korer J (1987). The incidence of schizophrenia in Nottingham. *British Journal of Psychiatry,* 151, 619–26.

Crow TJ (1988). Sex chromosomes and psychosis: the case for a pseudoautosomal locus. *British Journal of Psychiatry,* 153, 675–83.

Crow TJ (1990). Temporal lobe asymmetries as the key to the etiology of schizophrenia. *Schizophrenia Bulletin,* 16, 433–43.

Crow TJ, DeLisi LE, Lofthouse R *et al.* (1994). An examination of linkage of schizophrenia and schizoaffective disorder to the pseudoautosomal region (Xp22.3). *British Journal of Psychiatry,* 159–64.

Dalman C, Allebeck P, Cullberg J, Grunewald C, Koster M (1999). Obstetric complications and the risk of schizophrenia: a longitudinal study of a national birth cohort. *Archives of General Psychiatry,* 56, 234–40.

Davis M, Emory E (1995). Sex differences in neonatal stress responsivity. *Child Development,* 66, 14–27.

DeLisi LE, Hoff AL, Neale C, Kushner M (1994a). Asymmetries in the superior temporal lobe in male and female first-episode schizophrenic patients: measures of the planum temporale and superior temporal gyrus by MRI. *Schizophrenia Research,* 12, 19–28.

DeLisi LE, Devoto M, Lofthouse R *et al.* (1994b). Search for linkage to schizophrenia on the X and Y chromosomes. *American Journal of Medical Genetics (Neuropsychiatric Genetics),* 54, 113–21.

Donahue JE, Stopa EG, Chorsky RL *et al.* (2000). Cells containing immunoreactive estrogen receptor-α in the human basal forebrain. *Brain Research,* 856, 142–51.

Erlenmeyer-Kimling L, Kestenbaum C, Bird H, Hildoff U (1984). Assessment of the New York high-risk project subjects in Sample A who are now clinical deviants. In Watt N, Anthony EJ, Wynne LC and Rolf JE (eds). *Children at Risk for Schizophrenia: A Longitudinal Perspective,* pp. 227–239. Cambridge: Cambridge University Press.

Falkai P, Bogerts B, Benno G *et al.* (1992). Loss of sylvian fissure asymmetry in schizophrenia: a quantitative post-mortem study. *Schizophrenia Research,* 7, 23–32.

Falkai P, Bogerts B, Schneider T *et al.* (1995). Disturbed planum temporale asymmetry in schizophrenia. A quantitative post-mortem study. *Schizophrenia Research,* 14, 161–76.

Faraone SV, Chen WJ, Goldstein JM, Tsuang MT (1994). Gender differences in the age at onset of schizophrenia: fact or artifact? *British Journal of Psychiatry,* 625–29.

Fernández-Guasti A, Kruijver FPM, Fodor M, Swaab DF (2000). Sex differences in the distribution of androgen receptors in the human hypothalamus. *Journal of Comparative Neurology,* 425, 422–35.

Filipek PA, Richelme C, Kennedy DN, Caviness VS, Jr. (1994). The young adult human brain: an MRI-based morphometric analysis. *Cerebral Cortex,* 4, 344–60.

Flaum M, Swayze VW, II, O'Leary DS *et al.* (1995). Effects of diagnosis, laterality, and gender on brain morphology in schizophrenia. *American Journal of Psychiatry,* 152, 704–14.

Foerster A, Lewis SW, Owen MJ, Murray RM (1991a). Low birth weight and a family history of schizophrenia predict poor premorbid functioning in psychosis. *Schizophrenia Research,* 5, 13–20.

Foerster A, Lewis SW, Owen MJ, Murray RM (1991b). Pre-morbid adjustment and personality in psychosis: Effects of sex and diagnosis. *British Journal of Psychiatry,* 158, 171–6.

Frederikse ME, Lu A, Aylward E, Barta PE, Sharma T, Pearlson GD (2000). Sex differences in inferior parietal lobule volume in schizophrenia. *American Journal of Psychiatry,* 157, 422–27.

Freeman HL, Alport M (1987). Prevalence of schizophrenia in an urban population. *British Journal of Psychiatry,* 149, 603–11.

Geddes JR, Lawrie SM (1995). Obstetric complications and schizophrenia: a meta-analysis. *British Journal of Psychiatry*, 67, 786–93.

Ghadirian AM, Chouinard G, Annable L (1982). Sexual dysfunction and plasma prolactin levels in neuroleptic-treated schizophrenic outpatients. *Journal of Nervous and Mental Disease*, 170, 463–67.

Giedd JN, Snell JW, Lange N *et al.* (1996). Quantitative magnetic resonance imaging of human brain development: ages 4–18. *Cerebral Cortex*, 6, 551–60.

Gittelman-Klein R, Klein DF (1969). Premorbid asocial adjustment and prognosis in schizophrenia. *Journal of Psychiatric Research*, 7, 35–53.

Gjerde PF, Block J (1996). A developmental perspective on depressive symptoms in adolescence: gender differences in autocentric-allocentric modes of impulse regulation. In Cicchetti D and Toth S (eds) *Adolescence: opportunities and challenges*, pp. 167–97. University of Rochester Press, Rochester, NY.

Goldman PS, Crawford HT, Stokes LP, Galkin TW, Rosvold HE (1974). Sex-dependent behavioral effects of cerebral cortical lesions in the developing rhesus monkey. *Science*, 186, 540–42.

Goldstein J, Faraone S, Chen W, Tolomiczenko G, Tsuang M (1990). Sex differences in the familial transmission of schizophrenia. *British Journal of Psychiatry*, 156, 819–26.

Goldstein JM (1995a). Gender and the familial transmission of schizophrenia. In Seeman MV (ed.) *Gender and Psychopathology*, pp. 201–26. Washington, DC: American Psychiatric Press.

Goldstein JM (1995b). The impact of gender on understanding the epidemiology of schizophrenia. In Seeman MV (ed.) *Gender and Psychopathology*, pp. 159–99. Washington, DC: American Psychiatric Association Press.

Goldstein JM, Lewine RRJ (2000). Overview of sex differences in schizophrenia: Where have we been and where do we go from here. In Castle DJ, McGrath JJ and Kulkarni J (eds) *Women and Schizophrenia*, pp. 111–53. Cambridge: Cambridge University Press.

Goldstein JM, Tsuang MT, Faraone SV (1989). Gender and schizophrenia: Implications for understanding the heterogeneity of the illness. *Psychiatry Research*, 28, 243–53.

Goldstein JM, Faraone SV, Chen WJ, Tsuang MT (1992). Gender and the familial risk for schizophrenia. Disentangling confounding factors. *Schizophrenia Research*, 7, 135–40.

Goldstein JM, Faraone SV, Chen WJ, Tsuang MT (1995). Genetic heterogeneity may in part explain sex differences in the familial risk for schizophrenia. *Biological Psychiatry*, 38, 808–13.

Goldstein JM, Seidman LJ, Santangelo S, Knapp P, Tsuang MT (1994). Are schizophrenic men at higher risk for developmental deficits than schizophrenic women? Implications for adult neuropsychological functions. *Journal of Psychiatric Research*, 28, 483–98.

Goldstein JM, Seidman LJ, Horton NJ *et al.* (2001). Normal sexual dimorphism of the adult human brain assessed by in-vivo magnetic resonance imaging. *Cerebral Cortex*, 11, 490–97.

Goldstein JM, Seidman LJ, O'Brien LM *et al.* (2002). Impact of normal sexual dimorphisms on sex differences in structural brain abnormalities in schizophrenia assessed by magnetic resonance imaging. *Archives of General Psychiatry*, 59, 154–64.

Gorski RA (2000). Sexual differentiation of the nervous system. In Kandel ER, Schwartz JH and Jessell TM (eds) *Principles of Neural Science*, pp. 1131–46. New York: McGraw-Hill Health Professions Division.

Gottesman II, Shields J (1982). *Schizophrenia: The Epigenetic Puzzle*. Cambridge: Cambridge University Press.

Green MF, Satz P, Gaier DJ, Gazell S, Kharabi F (1989). Minor physical anomalies in schizophrenia. *Schizophrenia Bulletin*, 15, 91–99.

Grimm VE, Frieder B (1985). Differential vulnerability of male and female rats to the timing of various perinatal insults. *International Journal of Neuroscience,* 27, 155–64.

Gur RC, Turetsky BI, Matsui M *et al.* (1999). Sex differences in brain gray and white matter in healthy young adults: correlations with cognitive performance. *Journal of Neuroscience,* 19, 4065–72.

Gur RE, Cowell PE, Latshaw A *et al.* (2000a). Reduced dorsal and orbital prefrontal gray matter volumes in schizophrenia. *Archives of General Psychiatry,* 57, 761–68.

Gur RE, Turetsky BI, Cowell PE *et al.* (2000b). Temporolimbic volume reductions in schizophrenia. *Archives of General Psychiatry,* 57, 769–75.

Gur RE, Mozley PD, Resnick SM *et al.* (1991). Magnetic resonance imaging in schizophrenia. I. Volumetric analysis of brain and cerebrospinal fluid. *Archives of General Psychiatry,* 48, 407–12.

Haas GL, Sweeney JA, Hien DA, Goldman D, Deck M (1991). Gender differences in schizophrenia [abstract and presentation]. *Schizophrenia Research,* 4, 277.

Hadders-Algra M, Huisjes HJ, Touwen BC (1988a). Perinatal risk factors and minor neurological dysfunction: significance for behaviour and school achievement at nine years. *Developmental Medicine and Child Neurology,* 30, 482–91.

Hadders-Algra M, Huisjes HJ, Touwen BC (1988b). Perinatal correlates of major and minor neurological dysfunction at school age: a multivariate analysis. *Developmental Medicine and Child Neurology,* 30, 472–81.

Hafner H, Riecher A, Maurer K, Loffler W, Munk-Jorgensen P, Stromgren E (1989). How does gender influence age at first hospitalization for schizophrenia? A transnational case register study. *Psychological Medicine,* 19, 903–18.

Halldin J (1984). Prevalence of mental disorder in an urban population in central Sweden. *Acta Psychiatrica Scandinavica,* 69, 503–18.

Hambrecht M, Maurer K, Sartorius N, Hafner H (1992). Transnational stability of gender differences in schizophrenia? An analysis based on the WHO study on determinants of outcome of severe mental disorders. *European Archives of Psychiatry and Clinical Neuroscience,* 242, 6–12.

Harasty J, Double KL, Halliday GM, Kril JJ, McRitchie DA (1997). Language-associated cortical regions are proportionally larger in the female brain. *Archives of Neurology,* 54, 171–76.

Highley JR, Esiri MM, McDonald B, Roberts HC, Walker MA, Crow TJ (1999). The size and fiber composition of the anterior commissure with respect to gender and schizophrenia. *Biological Psychiatry,* 45, 1120–7.

Hirayasu Y, McCarley RW, Salisbury DF *et al.* (2000). Planum temporale and Heschl gyrus volume reduction in schizophrenia. *Archives of General Psychiatry,* 57, 692–99.

Hoff AL, Riordan H, O'Donnell D *et al.* (1992). Anomalous lateral sulcus assymetry and cognitive function in first-episode schizophrenia. *Schizophrenia Bulletin,* 18, 257–72.

Hollister JM, Laing P, Mednick SA (1996). Rhesus incompatibility as a risk factor for schizophrenia in male adults. *Archives of General Psychiatry,* 53, 19–24.

Hulshoff PHE, Hoek HW, Susser E *et al.* (2000). Prenatal exposure to famine and brain morphology in schizophrenia. *American Journal of Psychiatry,* 157, 1170–2.

Hultman CM, Sparén P, Takei N, Murray RM, Cnattingius S (1999). Prenatal and perinatal risk factors for schizophrenia, affective psychosis, and reactive psychosis of early onset: case-control study. *BMJ,* 318, 421–26.

Iacono W, Beiser M (1992). Are males more likely than females to develop schizophrenia? *American Journal of Psychiatry,* 149, 1070–74.

Jacobs B, Schall M, Scheibel AB (1993). A quantitative dendritic analysis of Wernicke's area in humans. II. Gender, hemispheric, and environmental factors. *Journal of Comparative Neurology,* 327, 97–111.

John R, Mednick SA, Schulsinger F (1982). Teacher reports as predictors of schizophrenia and borderline schizophrenia: a Bayesian decision analysis. *Journal of Abnormal Psychology*, 143, 383–8.

Jones PB, Rantakallio P, Hartikainen A-L, Isohanni M, Sipila P (1998). Schizophrenia as a long-term outcome of pregnancy, delivery, and perinatal complications: a 28-year follow-up of the 1996 North Finland general population birth cohort. *American Journal of Psychiatry*, 155, 355–64.

Kawata M (1995). Roles of steroid hormones and their receptors in structural organization in the nervous system. *Neuroscience Research*, 24, 1–46.

Kaye JA, DeCarli C, Luxenberg JS, Rapoport SI (1992). The significance of age-related enlargement of the cerebral ventricles in healthy men and women measured by quantitative computed x-ray tomography. *Journal of the American Geriatrics Society*, 40, 225–31.

Kendler KS, Walsh D (1995). Gender and schizophrenia: Results of an epidemiologically-based family study. *British Journal of Psychiatry*, 167, 184–92.

Kendler KS, Gruenberg AM, Tsuang MT (1985). Psychiatric illness in first-degree relatives of schizophrenic and surgical control patients. A family study using DSM-III criteria. *Archives of General Psychiatry*, 42, 770–79.

Keshavan MS, Montrose DM, Pierri JN *et al.* (1997). Magnetic resonance imaging and spectroscopy in offspring at risk for schizophrenia: preliminary studies. *Progress in Neuro-Psychopharmacology and Biological Psychiatry*, 21, 1285–95.

Kirov G, Jones PB, Harvey I *et al.* (1996). Do obstetric complications cause the earlier age at onset in male than female schizophrenics? *Schizophrenia Research*, 20, 117–24.

Kulynych JJ, Vladar K, Jones DW, Weinberger DR (1994). Gender differences in the normal lateralization of the supratemporal cortex: MRI surface-rendering morphometry of Heschl's gyrus and the planum temporale. *Cerebral Cortex*, 4, 107–18.

Kwon JS, McCarley RW, Hirayasu Y *et al.* (1999). Left planum temporale volume reduction in schizophrenia. *Archives of General Psychiatry*, 56, 142–48.

Lane A, Colgan K, Moynihan F *et al.* (1996). Schizophrenia and neurological soft signs: gender differences in clinical correlates and antecedent factors. *Psychiatry Research*, 64, 105–14.

Lauriello J, Hoff A, Wieneke MH *et al.* (1997). Similar extent of brain dysmorphology in severely ill women and men with schizophrenia. *American Journal of Psychiatry*, 154, 819–25.

Lauterbach MD, Raz S, Sander CJ (2001). Neonatal hypoxic risk in preterm birth infants: the influence of sex and severity of respiratory distress on cognitive recovery. *Neuropsychology*, 15, 411–20.

Lawrie SM, Whalley H, Kestelman JN *et al.* (1999). Magnetic resonance imaging of brain in people at high risk of developing schizophrenia. *Lancet*, 353, 30–33.

Lewine R, Burbach D, Meltzer HY (1984). Effect of diagnostic criteria on the proportion of male to female schizophrenics. *American Journal of Psychiatry*, 141, 84–87.

Lewine RR (1988). Gender and schizophrenia. In Tsuang MT and Simpson JC (eds) *Handbook of Schizophrenia: Nosology, Epidemiology and Genetics of Schizophrenia*, pp. 379–97. Amsterdam: Elsevier Press.

Lewine RRJ (1981). Sex differences in schizophrenia. Timing or subtypes? *Psychological Bulletin*, 90, 432–44.

Lewine RRJ (1984). Stalking the schizophrenia marker: evidence for a general vulnerability model of psychopathology. In Watt NF, Anthony EJ, Wynne LC and Rolf JE (eds) *Children at Risk for Schizophrenia: A Longitudinal Perspective*, pp. 545–50. Cambridge and London: Cambridge University Press.

Lewis S (1989). Congential risk factors for schizophrenia. *Psychological Medicine*, 19, 5–13.

Lewis SW, Murray RM (1987). Obstetric complications, neurodevelopmental deviance, and risk for schizophrenia. *Journal of Psychiatric Research,* 21, 413–21.

Liechty EA, Gilmor RL, Bryson CQ, Bull MJ (1983). Outcome of high risk neonates with ventriculomegaly. *Developmental Medicine and Child Neurology,* 25, 162–68.

Loranger AW (1984). Sex difference in age at onset of schizophrenia. *Archives of General Psychiatry,* 41, 1744–52.

MacLusky NJ, Clark AS, Naftolin F, Goldman-Rakic PS (1987). Estrogen formation in the mammalian brain: possible role of aromatase in sexual differentiation of the hippocampus and neocortex. *Steroids,* 50, 459–74.

Marcus J, Hans SL, Nagler S, Auerbach JG, Mirsky AF, Aubrey A (1987). Review of the NIMH Israeli Kibbutz-City study and the Jerusalem infant development study. *Schizophrenia Bulletin,* 13, 425–38.

Matsumoto H, Takei N, Saito F, Kachi K, Mori N (2001). The association between obstetric complications and childhood-onset schizophrenia: a replication study. *Psychological Medicine,* 31, 907–14.

McEwen BS (1983). Gonadal steroid influences on brain development and sexual differentiation. In Greep R (ed.) *Reproductive Physiology* IV, pp. 99–145. Baltimore, Press University Park.

McNeil TF, Cantor-Graae E, Nordstrum LG, Rosenlund T (1993). Head circumference in 'preschizophrenic' and control neonates. *British Journal of Psychiatry,* 162, 517–23.

Mednick SA, Huttunen MO, Machon RA (1994). Prenatal influenza infections and adult schizophrenia. *Schizophrenia Bulletin,* 20, 263–67.

Mednick SA, Schulsinger F, Teasdale TW, Schulsinger H, Venables PH, Rock DR (1978). Schizophrenia in high-risk children: sex differences in predisposing factors. In Serban G (ed.) *Cognitive Defects in the Development of Mental Illness,* pp. 169–97. New York: Brunner/Mazel Publisher.

Miranda RC, Toran-Allerand D (1992). Developmental expression of estrogen receptor mRNA in the rat cerebral cortex: a nonisotopic *in situ* hybridization histochemistry study. *Cerebral Cortex,* 2, 1–15.

Morris AG, Gaitonde E, McKenna PJ, Mellon JD, Hunt DM (1995). CAG repeat expansions and schizophrenia: associated with disease in females and with early age at onset. *Human Molecular Genetics,* 4, 1957–61.

Munk-Jorgensen P, Weeke A, Jensen EB, Dupont A, Stromgren E (1986). Changes in utilization of Danish psychiatric institutions, II: Census studies 1977 and 1982. *Comprehensive Psychiatry,* 27, 416–29.

Murphy DGM, DeCarli C, McIntosh AR *et al.* (1996). Sex differences in human brain morphometry and metabolism: an in vivo quantitative magnetic resonance imaging and positron emission tomography study on the effect of aging. *Archives of General Psychiatry,* 53, 585–94.

Murray RM (1994). Neurodevelopmental schizophrenia: the rediscovery of dementia praecox. *British Journal of Psychiatry,* suppl 165, 6–12.

Murray RM, Owen MJ, Goodman R, Lewis SW (1990). A neurodevelopmental perspective on some epiphenomena of schizophrenia. In Cazullo CL, Invernizzi G, Sacchetti E and Vita A (eds) *Plasticity and Morphology of the* Central Nervous System, pp. 185–203. Lancaster, MA: MIT Press.

Murray RM, O'Callaghan E, Castle DJ, Lewis SW (1992a). A neurodevelopmental approach to the classification of schizophrenia. *Schizophrenia Bulletin,* 18, 319–32.

Murray RM, Jones P, O'Callaghan E, Takei N, Sham P (1992b). Genes, viruses and neurodevelopmental schizophrenia. *Journal of Psychiatric Research,* 26, 225–35.

Neugebauer R, Dohrenwend PR, Dohrenwend BS (1980). Formulation of hypotheses about the true prevalence of functional psychiatric disorders among adults in the U.S. In Dohrenwend BP, Dohrenwend BS and Gould M (eds) *Mental Illness in the United States: Epidemiological Estimates,* pp. 45–94. New York: Prager.

Nopoulos P, Flaum M, Andreasen NC (1997). Sex differences in brain morphology in schizophrenia. *American Journal of Psychiatry,* 154, 1648–54.

Nopoulos P, Flaum M, O'Leary D, Andreasen NC (2000). Sexual dimorphism in the human brain: evaluation of tissue volume, tissue composition and surface anatomy using magnetic resonance imaging. *Psychiatry Research,* 98, 1–13.

O'Callaghan E, Gibson T, Colohan HA *et al.* (1992). Risk of schizophrenia in adults born after obstetric complications and their association with early onset of illness: a controlled study. *British Journal of Medicine,* 305, 1246–59.

O'Connor LH, Nock B, McEwen BS (1988). Regional specificity of gamma-aminobutryic acid receptor regulation by estradiol. *Neuroendocrinology,* 47, 473–81.

Pakkenberg B, Gundersen HJG (1997). Neocortical neuron number in humans: effect of sex and age. *Journal of Comparative Neurology,* 384, 312–20.

Park J-J, Baum MJ, Paredes RG, Tobet SA (1996). Neurogenesis and cell migration into the sexually dimorphic preoptic area/anterior hypothalamus of the fetal ferret. *Journal of Neurobiology,* 30, 315–28.

Passe TJ, Rajagopalan P, Tupler LA, Byrum CE, MacFall JR, Krishnan KRR (1997). Age and sex effects on brain morphology. *Progress in Neuro-Psychopharmacology and Biological Psychiatry,* 21, 1231–37.

Paus T, Otaky N, Caramanos Z *et al.* (1996). In vivo morphometry of the intrasulcal gray matter in the human cingulate, paracingulate, and superior-rostral sulci: hemispheric asymmetries, gender differences and probability maps. *Journal of Comparative Neurology,* 376, 664–73.

Petty RG, Barta PE, Pearlson GD *et al.* (1995). Reversal of asymmetry of the planum temporale in schizophrenia. *American Journal of Psychiatry,* 152, 715–21.

Pfaff D, Keiner M (1973). Atlas of estradiol-concentrating cells in the central nervous system of the female rat. *Journal of Comparative Neurology,* 151, 121–58.

Pilgrim C, Hutchison JB (1994). Developmental regulation of sex differences in the brain: can the role of gonadal steroids be redefined? *Neuroscience,* 60, 843–55.

Preston NJ, Orr KG, Date R, Nolan L, Castle D (2002). Gender differences in premorbid adjustment of patients with first episode psychosis. *Schizophrenia Research,* 55, 285–90.

Pulver AE, Brown CH, Wolyniec P *et al.* (1990). Schizophrenia: age at onset, gender and familial risk. *Acta Psychiatrica Scandinavica,* 82, 344–51.

Rabinowicz T, Dean DE, Petetot JMC, de Courten-Myers GM (1999). Gender differences in the human cerebral cortex: more neurons in males; more processes in females. *Journal of Child Neurology,* 14, 98–107.

Rantakallio P, Wendt LV (1985). Prognosis for low-birthweight infants up to the age of 14: a population study. *Developmental Medicine and Child Neurology,* 27, 655–63.

Raz S, Lauterbach MD, Hopkins TL *et al.* (1995). A female advantage in cognitive recovery from early cerebral insult. *Developmental Psychology,* 31, 958–66.

Reicher-Rossler A, Hafner H, Stumbaum M, Maurer K (1994). Can estradiol modulate schizophrenic symptomatolgy? *Schizophrenia Bulletin,* 20, 203–14.

Reisert I, Schuster R, Zienecker R, Pilgrim C (1990). Prenatal development of mesencephalic and diencephalic dopaminergic systems in the male and female rat. *Brain Research Developmental Brain Research,* 53, 222–29.

Reite M, Sheeder J, Teale P *et al.* (1997). Magnetic source imaging evidence of sex differences in cerebral lateralization in schizophrenia. *Archives of General Psychiatry,* 54, 433–40.

Ring N, Tantam D, Montague L, Newby D, Black D, Morris J (1991). Gender differences in the incidence of definite schizophrenia and atypical psychosis–focus on negative symptoms of schizophrenia. *Acta Psychiatrica Scandinavica,* 84, 489–96.

Risch SC, Lewine RJ, Kalin NH *et al*. (1992). Limbic-hypothalamic-pituitary-adrenal axis activity and ventricular-to-brain ratio studies in affective illness and schizophrenia. *Neuropsychopharmacology*, 6, 95–100.

Rojas DC, Teale P, Sheeder J, Simon J, Reite M (1997). Sex-specific expression of Heschl's gyrus functional and structural abnormalities in paranoid schizophrenia. *American Journal of Psychiatry*, 154, 1655–62.

Rossi A, Stratta P, Di Michele V, De Cataldo S, Cassacchia M (1991). Lateral ventricular size, educational level and patient subtypes in schizophrenia. *British Journal of Psychiatry*, 159, 443–44.

Rosso IM, Cannon TD, Huttunen T, Huttunen MO, Lonnqvist J, Gasperoni TL (2000). Obstetric risk factors for early-onset schizophrenia in a Finnish birth cohort. *American Journal of Psychiatry*, 157, 801–07.

Roy A, Pickar D, Doran A *et al*. (1986). The corticotropin-releasing hormone stimulation test in chronic schizophrenia. *American Journal of Psychiatry*, 143, 1393–97.

Salokangas RK (1983). Prognostic implications of the sex of schizophrenic patients. *British Journal of Psychiatry*, 142, 145–51.

Sandhu S, Cook P, Diamond MC (1986). Rat cerebral cortical estrogen receptors: male-female, right-left. *Experimental Neurology*, 92, 186–96.

Sartorius N, Jablensky A, Korten A *et al*. (1986). Early manifestations and first-contact incidence of schizophrenia in different cultures. *Psychological Medicine*, 16, 909–28.

Schaeffer M, Baum A (1984). Adrenal cortical response to stress at Three Mile Island. *Psychosomatic Medicine*, 46, 227–37.

Schlaepfer TE, Harris GJ, Tien AY, Peng L, Lee S, Pearlson GD (1995). Structural differences in the cerebral cortex of healthy female and male subjects: a magnetic resonance imaging study. *Psychiatry Research: Neuroimaging*, 61, 129–35.

Schlaepfer TE, Harris GJ, Tien AY *et al*. (1994). Decreased regional cortical gray matter volume in schizophrenia. *American Journal of Psychiatry*, 151, 842–48.

Shaywitz B, Shaywitz SE, Pugh KR *et al*. (1995). Sex differences in the functional organization of the brain for language. *Nature*, 373, 607–09.

Shenton ME, Kikinis R, Jolesz FA *et al*. (1992). Abnormalities of the left temporal lobe and thought disorder in schizophrenia: a quantitative magnetic resonance imaging study. *New England Journal of Medicine*, 327, 604–12.

Shimizu A, Kurachi M, Yamaguchi N, Torii H, Isaki K (1987). Morbidity risk of schizophrenia to parents and siblings of schizophrenic patients. *Japanese Journal of Psychiatry and Neurology*, 41, 65–70.

Shughrue PJ, Stumpf WE, MacLusky NJ, Zielinski JE, Hochberg RB (1990). Developmental changes in estrogen receptors in mouse cerebral cortex between birth and postweaning: studied by autoradiography with 11β-methoxy-16α-[^{125}I]iodoestradiol. *Endocrinology*, 126, 1112–24.

Sikanartey T, Eaton WW (1984). The prevalence of schizophrenia in the Labadi district in Ghana. *Acta Psychiatrica Scandinavica*, 69, 156–61.

Silverman JM, Smith CJ, Guo SL, Mohs RC, Siever LJ, Davis KL (1998). Lateral ventricular enlargement in schizophrenic probands and their siblings with schizophrenia-related disorders. *Biological Psychiatry*, 43, 97–106.

Stewart J, Kühnemann S, Rajabi H (1991). Neonatal exposure to gonadal hormones affects the development of monoamine systems in rat cortex. *Journal of Neuroendocrinology*, 3, 85–93.

Stober G, Franzek E, Beckmann H (1993). Pregnancy and labor complications – their significance in the development of schizophrenic psychoses. *Fortschritte der Neurologie-Psychiatrie*, 61, 329–37.

Strauss E (1992). Sex-related differences in the cognitive consequences of early left-hemispheric lesions. *Journal of Clinical and Experimental Neuropsychology*, 14, 738–48.

Sullivan G, Lukoff D (1990). Sexual side effects of antipsychotic medication: evaluation and interventions. *Hospital and Community Psychiatry*, 41, 1238–41.

Susser E, Neugebauer R, Hoek HW *et al.* (1996). Schizophrenia after prenatal famine. *Archives of General Psychiatry*, 53, 25–31.

Swaab DF, Fliers E (1985). A sexually dimorphic nucleus in the human brain. *Science*, 228, 1112–15.

Szeszko PR, Strous RD, Goldman RS *et al.* (2002). Neuropsychological correlates of hippocampal volumes in patients experiencing a first episode of schizophrenia. *American Journal of Psychiatry*, 159, 217–26.

Szeszko PR, Bilder RM, Lencz T *et al.* (2000). Reduced anterior cingulate gyrus volume correlates with executive dysfunction in men with first-episode schizophrenia. *Schizophrenia Research*, 43, 97–108.

Thomas HV, Dalman C, David AS, Gentz J, Lewis G, Allebeck P (2001). Obstetric complications, age at diagnosis and maternal history of psychosis. *British Journal of Psychiatry*, 179, 409–14.

Tobet SA, Basham ME, Baum MJ (1993). Estrogen receptor immunoreactive neurons in the fetal ferret forebrain. *Brain Research Developmental Brain Research*, 72, 167–80.

Tobet SA, Henderson RG, Whiting PJ, Sieghart W (1999). Special relationship of γ-aminobutyric acid to the ventromedial nucleus of the hypothalamus during embryonic development. *Journal of Comparative Neurology*, 405, 88–98.

Toran-Allerand CD (1996). The estrogen/neurotrophin connection during neural development: is co-localization of estrogen receptors with the neurotrophins and their receptors biologically revelant? *Developmental Neuroscience*, 18, 36–41.

Tsuang MT, Winokur G (1975). The Iowa-500: field work in a 35-year follow-up of depression, mania, and schizophrenia. *Can Psychol Assoc J*, 20, 359–65.

Tsuang MT, Fowler RC, Cadoret RJ, Monnelly E (1974). Schizophrenia among first-degree relatives of paranoid and nonparanoid schizophrenics. *Comprehensive Psychiatry*, 15, 295–302.

Verdoux H, Geddes JR, Takei N *et al.* (1997). Obstetric complications and age at onset in schizophrenia: an international collaborative meta-analysis of individual patient data. *American Journal of Psychiatry*, 154, 1220–27.

Volpe JJ (1987) *Neurology of the Newborn*. Philadelphia, PA: W.B. Saunders.

Waddington J, Youssef H, Kinsella A (1990). Cognitive dysfunction in schizophrenia followed up over 5 years, and its longitudinal relationship to the emergence of tardive dyskinesia. *Psychological Medicine*, 20, 835–42.

Walder DJ, Walker EF, Lewine RJ (2000). Cognitive functioning, cortisol release, and symptom severity in patients with schizophrenia. *Biological Psychiatry*, 48, 1121–32.

Walker E, Weinstein J, Baum K *et al.* (1995a). Antecedents of schizophrenia: moderating influences of age and biological sex. In Hafner H and Gattaz W (eds) *Search for the Cause of Schizophrenia*, pp. 21–42. New York: Springer-Verlag.

Walker E, Davis D, Weinstein J *et al.* (1995b). Modal developmental aspects of schizophrenia across the life-span. In Miller G (ed.) *The Behavioral High-Risk Paradigm in Psychopathology*, pp. 121–57. New York: Springer-Verlag.

Walker EF, Diforio D (1997). Schizophrenia: a neural diathesis-stress model. *Psychological Review*, 104, 667–85.

Walker EF, Walder DJ, Reynolds F (2001). Developmental changes in cortisol secretion in normal and at-risk youth. *Development and Psychopathology*, 13, 721–32.

Walker EF, Bonsall R, Walder DJ (2002a). Plasma hormones and catecholamine metabolites in monozygotic twins discordant for psychosis. *Neuropsychiatry, Neuropsychology, and Behavioral Neurology,* 15, 10–17.

Walker EF, Grimes KE, Davis DM, Smith AJ (1993). Childhood precursors of schizophrenia: Facial expressions of emotion. *American Journal of Psychiatry,* 150, 1654–60.

Walker EF, Walder DJ, Lewine R, Loewy R (2002b). Sex differences in the origins and premorbid development of schizophrenia. In Lewis-Hall F, Williams TS, Panetta JA and Herrerra JM (eds) *Psychiatric Illness in Women,* pp. 193–214. Washington, DC: American Psychiatric Publishing.

Walker EF, Neumann C, Baum KM, Davis D, Diforio D, Bergman A (1996). Developmental pathways to schizophrenia: moderating effects of stress. *Development and Psychopathology,* 8, 647–65.

Watt DC, Szulecka TK (1979). The effect of sex, marriage, and age at first admission on the hospitalization of schizophrenics during two years following discharge. *Psychological Medicine,* 9, 529–39.

Wattie BJS, Kedward HB (1985). Gender differences in living conditions found among male and female schizophrenic patients on a follow-up study. *International Journal of Social Psychiatry,* 31, 205–16.

Weinberger DR (1987). Implications of normal brain development for the pathogenesis of schizophrenia. *Archives of General Psychiatry,* 44, 660–69.

Witelson SF (1989). Hand and sex differences in the isthmus and genu of the human corpus callosum: a postmortem morphological study. *Brain,* 112, 799–835.

Witelson SF, Glezer II, Kigar DL (1995). Women have greater density of neurons in posterior temporal cortex. *Journal of Neuroscience,* 15, 3418–28.

Wolyniec PS, Pulver AE, McGrath JA, Tam D (1992). Schizophrenia: Gender and familial risk. *Journal of Psychiatry Research,* 26, 17–27.

Wyatt RJ, Alexander RC, Egan MF, Kirch DG (1988). Schizophrenia, just the facts. What do we know, how well do we know it? *Schizophrenia Research,* 1, 3–18.

Yolken RH, Torrey EF (1995). Viruses, schizophrenia and bipolar disorder. *Clinical Microbiology Reviews,* 8, 131–45.

Young JG, Cohen DJ, Shaywitz SE *et al.* (1982). Assessment of brain function in clinical pediatric research: behavioral and biological strategies. *Schizophrenia Bulletin,* 8, 205–35.

Zhou JN, Hofman MA, Gooren LJG, Swaab DF (1995). A sex difference in the human brain and its relation to transexuality. *Nature,* 378, 68–70.

Chapter 10

Late-onset schizophrenia: characteristics of patients at the first episode

Philip D. Harvey

There are few aspects of schizophrenia that are more controversial than the existence of late-onset schizophrenia. As recently noted: 'Hardly any psychiatric disorder exists that has been described so inconsistently, defined in such an imprecise manner, and about which we have so little sound empirical knowledge as late onset schizophrenia' (Reicher-Rossler, 1999, p. 3). The debate began around 100 years previously and is still ongoing, fueled by changes in the age of onset criteria for schizophrenia across various editions of the DSM and by epidemiological studies suggesting that some individuals meet the full criteria for schizophrenia and have their first symptoms over the age of 45. More confusion is produced by the fact that there are clearly many psychotic disorders that begin in late life, although they do not present with the full syndrome of schizophrenia, and because many progressive dementing conditions that occur in aging are associated with symptoms that would meet the A criteria for schizophrenia if they did not occur in conjunction with dementia.

Background

As currently defined in the DSM, schizophrenia can have an onset at any age. As a result, any condition that meets the full criteria for schizophrenia should receive that diagnosis. In contrast, the third edition of the DSM (American Psychiatric Association 1980) required that schizophrenia have an onset age of the active phase of illness before age 45. This definition is in direct contrast to the Kraepelinian tradition, where a condition referred to as 'paraphrenia' was diagnosed in cases with late-life onset of the experience of psychotic symptoms. Kraepelin (1919) believed that the critical features of paraphrenia were that affective expression and experience was not impaired and that there was no deteriorating course. As a result, some of the critical features of dementia praecox, from the Karepelinian perspective, were lacking, but the presence of Bluelerian 'accessory' symptoms was the central feature of the illness. This condition was not necessarily believed to be exclusively found in the elderly, in that he believed that any psychotic condition where the onset age was later than dementia praecox (30–50 or later) should be considered for this diagnosis, with the critical differences between paraphrenia and dementia praecox occurring in the dimensions of phenomenological variations and onset age.

This concept has retained its life in Europe, where 'late paraphrenia' is still a commonly applied diagnostic concept, although this diagnostic category has been deleted from the latest editions of the official diagnostic manuals. According to current diagnostic systems in the US, late-onset psychoses that do not meet criteria for schizophrenia should be diagnosed according to their symptomatic characteristics and potential etiological determinants. For instance, according to the DSM-IV delusional disorder patients cannot have prominent hallucinations or evidence of bizarre behavior, thus differentiating them from individuals who meet the full set of criteria for schizophrenia with late onset. If a patient has a suspected denegerative condition, the diagnosis should be psychotic disorder associated with that degenerative condition and hallucinations compared to estimates for younger individuals. Thus, there are a number of psychotic conditions that occur late in life, and the majority of these conditions do not meet full criteria for late-onset schizophrenia. The goal of this chapter is to describe the characteristics of the early course of schizophrenia with late-life onset, in terms of epidemiology, symptom severity, cognitive, and functional characteristics. The issue of the validity of the concept of late-life schizophrenia will also be evaluated, in terms of comparison of the critical associated features of early in the illness schizophrenia across early and late-onset cases.

Epidemiology of late-onset schizophrenia

It is difficult to determine, unless treatment records are used or informants are employed, the age of onset of symptoms in anyone with schizophrenia. One of the reasons that this task is difficult is because of the unawareness of illness that interferes with accurate report on the part of symptoms, as well as because of memory impairments in patients with schizophrenia that render judgments about the timing of events suspect. Aging certainly has the potential to compound this problem. As a result, the best estimates of the prevalence of new cases of schizophrenia will come from catchment-area studies that examine new admissions to treatment for psychotic disorders as a function of age. Although these studies are limited because they, by definition, will miss all cases whose severity of illness is so mild that they never require treatment (e.g., elevating the false-negative rate), they also have the benefit of a comprehensive diagnostic assessment that eliminates the occurrence of false positive cases based on very abbreviated door-to-door assessments or informant reports.

Several community-based studies have examined the prevalence of psychotic symptoms in the elderly. In one study, Christensen and Blazer (1984) reported an incidence of paranoid delusions of around 4 per cent of elderly individuals living in the community, while another study reported a prevalence of hallucinations of about 2–4 per cent in older male community dwellers (Tien 1991). Interestingly, only half of the subjects in the Christensen and Blazer study had ever received mental health attention. Thus, the rate of occurrence of psychotic symptoms in the elderly living in the community is considerably greater than the estimated lifetime prevalence of schizophrenia (about 1 per cent). Consequently, caution is required in generation of prevalence estimates for schizophrenia in later life, because there is a clear elevation in psychosis with advancing age.

Studies that examined the number of new psychiatric contacts in older patients have generated some interesting and challenging data. In a study examining data from the Camberwell case register, a registry of all cases receiving psychiatric services in an inner-city catchment area in London, Castle and Murray (1993) reported that 28 per cent of patients had their first psychotic episode after age 44 and 12 per cent had onset after age 64. Over half of all psychotic episodes that came to clinical attention in individuals over the age of 44 met criteria for schizophrenia while approximately one third of psychotic episodes before age 44 met criteria. They found that the average age of onset for males (31.2) was ten years younger than that of females (41.1) and that the prevalence and associated characteristics of the illness did not differ markedly as a function of the breadth of the schizophrenia criteria that were used. The male/female ratio changed as a function of age of onset, with the ratio at 1.6:1 for onset from age 16 to 25 and 0.2:1 for onset age after 76. Patients with late onset were also much less likely to have a family history of schizophrenia, but some increase in familial prevalence of affective disorders was found in these patients. So, in this study, female gender was an important predictor of later onset age and negative family history predicted later onset age as well.

In a later study, Castle et al. (1997) examined the familial history of schizophrenia in patients who developed schizophrenia-like psychosis after 60. Starting with schizophrenic or healthy index cases (probands), the psychiatric status of relatives was examined. This study has the strength of seeking out relatives for assessment based on the status of probands. For relatives of both schizophrenic patients and of healthy controls, the morbid risk of schizophrenia in relatives was the same. For narrow criteria, the risk was 1.3 per cent for both cases and healthy controls and for broader criteria, the risk was only 0.1 per cent greater for relatives of patients with late-onset psychosis. The conclusion of these investigators was that late-onset psychotic conditions appeared genetically unrelated to earlier-onset schizophrenia.

These findings are in marked contrast to familial risk rates for familial schizophrenia in individuals with an earlier age of onset. In a comparative review, Castle and Howard (1992) found that the rates of schizophrenia in the relatives of early-onset schizophrenic index cases ranged from 4.4 per cent to 19.4 per cent, or 5 to 27 times the population base rate of approximately 0.7 per cent. The data from these studies suggest that there are clear differences in relative risk rates for familial schizophrenia between early and later onset patients with schizophrenia. In addition, the high risk for affective disorders in relatives of late-onset schizophrenia-like psychosis, reported to be as high as 16.3 per cent in one study (Howard *et al.* 1997), raises questions about which group of conditions is more common in the relatives of individuals with late-onset schizophrenia.

In an earlier review paper, Harris and Jeste (1988) examined all studies up to that time that provided adequate information on demographic characteristics and diagnoses. Their review suggested that approximately 15 per cent of patients experiencing a first episode of schizophrenia were over the age of 60 at the time of their first psychiatric admission. In nearly every one of these studies, the proportion of females was greater than that of males in the late-onset schizophrenia cases. They found decreasing prevalence of newly incident cases with age, but 13 per cent, 7 per cent, and 3 per cent of all cases with schizophrenia had onset from ages 40, 50, and 60 or later respectively. Clearly, these data indicate that a substantial number of patients with schizophrenia have an onset of schizophrenia later in their life, raising the issues of their symptomatic presentation, compared to younger patients, and what their premorbid functioning was like.

Symptom characteristics and severity in late onset patients

Patients with late-onset schizophrenia are reported to have a symptom picture similar to that described by Kraepelin in his description of paraphrenia. Hallucinations and delusions are present in most cases, including the presence of bizarre delusions and the 'prototypical' hallucinations that are described in DSM-IV. Some studies have actually suggested that severe prototypical hallucinations were more common in patients with late onset schizophrenia than in early onset cases. In contrast, blunted affect, severe formal thought disorder, and grossly disorganized behavior are typically absent in late onset cases. In studies (Howard *et al.* 1994; Almeida *et al.* 1995a) examining the diagnostic distribution of first episode cases with later-life psychosis, it has been found that two-thirds of the cases where no 'organic' cause could be detected met criteria for schizophrenia and one third for delusional disorder. Interestingly, the older the patient at the time of their first episode, the more likely it was that they would meet criteria for delusional disorder rather than schizophrenia. So, it appears as if patients ranging in age from 45 to 65 or so have a syndrome that appears to be consistent with DSM-IV schizophrenia with predominantly positive symptoms, while even older first episode patients may have exclusively delusional symptoms.

There are several important implications of these findings. Negative symptoms are less severe in late onset patients and negative symptoms have proven less likely to respond to treatment with antipsychotic medications than positive symptoms (see Palmer and Jeste, this volume). At the same time, hallucinations are the symptom of schizophrenia that is most responsive to these same treatments. In addition, functional deficits, as described below, are more strongly related to negative symptoms and cognitive deficits than they are to hallucinations. As a result, the factors that increase vulnerability to severe functional impairment and deterioration in functioning over time are less salient in later onset schizophrenic patients.

Gender differences in symptoms in late-onset schizophrenia

As noted above, females are more likely to develop schizophrenia with later onset than are male patients. In addition, family history is less significant as a predictor of the development of schizophrenia in late-onset patients, implicating environmental or individual-differences factors as vulnerability indicators. When female early and late-onset patients are compared (Lindamer *et al.* 1997), there are several notable clinical differences. First of all, when female late-onset patients are compared to male patients, they have more severe positive symptoms than male patients with similar ages of onset. When compared to female patients with earlier onset, the severity of negative symptoms was much less in female patients with late onset. In contrast, male patients had more severe negative symptoms than the female patients and these male patients did not differ in their negative symptom severity as a function of onset age. Thus, typical gender differences in schizophrenia are preserved in later life (see Goldstein Chapter, this volume). These data also suggest that there may be effects related to hormonal or other menopausal factors that are associated with development of late-onset schizophrenia. While too little research has been conducted to conclusively identify the specific risk factors, the preponderance of female patients with late onset of schizophrenia and age-associated differences in critical schizophrenic symptoms in female patients suggests that this is an important target for later research.

Cognitive and functional status of older patients

There are relatively fewer comparative studies of cognitive functions in adult onset versus later onset older patients with schizophrenia. In one comprehensive study, Jeste *et al.* (1995) found that there were no major differences in either symptom severity or cognitive deficits between patients with late-onset and patients with early-onset schizophrenia. Both late and early-onset patients had notable cognitive deficits compared to healthy controls and there was no difference in either profile or severity of the relative deficits when early-onset and late-onset patients were compared to healthy subjects. The majority of the late-onset patients in this study were among the group described above, whose onset age was earlier than 65 years. Thus, these data suggest that even in patients whose psychotic symptoms develop later, there is similarity to patients with a lifelong history of illness in the specific domains of cognitive impairment.

In a study of patients with more diverse diagnoses, including a large number who did not meet criteria for schizophrenia, Almedia *et al.* (1995b) reported that late-onset psychotic patients had several domains of cognitive functioning where they were no more impaired than healthy comparison subjects. Measures of learning rate and memory span were relatively less impaired than indices of general cognitive ability and executive functioning. These data suggest that the more homogenous the sample of patients with late-life psychosis, particularly if all patients meet criteria for schizophrenia, the more consistent and severe their cognitive impairments were. Thus, consistent with studies of younger patients with schizophrenia at the time of the first episode (Mojtabai *et al.* 2000), more severe cognitive impairments are seen in individuals who meet criteria for schizophrenia than in cases with undifferentiated psychosis or affective psychoses.

Premorbid functioning and other risk factors in late-onset schizophrenia

One of the most consistent findings in late-onset schizophrenia is that premorbid functioning is much less impaired in patients with late-onset schizophrenia than in patients with an earlier age of onset. This level of impairment includes more patients with premorbid employment, more patients with marriage or other evidence of intact social functioning, and higher levels of educational attainment.

Onset age is associated with better premorbid functioning, with patients having onset over age 65 having the most intact premorbid functioning. For instance, in a comprehensive study (Jeste *et al.* 1995) comparing patients with later onset (after age 45) to patients with early-onset schizophrenia and healthy comparison subjects, patients with a later age of onset were found to have higher rates of marriage, employment, and to be more likely to have the paranoid subtype of illness than patients with early-onset schizophrenia. Despite these indicators of better adjustment before the onset of symptoms, symptom severity and cognitive deficits were quite similar. Despite having higher rates of employment and marriage, major indicators of good premorbid adjustment, late-onset patients were still more likely than healthy controls to have had schizoid or paranoid traits during the premorbid period, despite not meeting full criteria for personality disorders. Late-onset patients have been found to be less likely to have children, even if married, than healthy controls (Rabins *et al.* 1984).

In a study focusing on premorbid personality traits, Pearlson *et al.* (1989) found that late-onset patients were more likely than both younger and older early-onset patients to have signs of premorbid schizoid personality traits. These findings are consistent with a number of studies that examined patients who had late-onset psychotic conditions that did not necessarily meet full DSM criteria for schizophrenia. Interestingly, social isolation has repeatedly been reported to be correlate of the development of late-onset paranoid symptoms. While this symptom has often been interpreted as an environmental factor increasing risk for development of paranoid ideation, these findings raise an alternative possibility. It is conceivable that social isolation over the lifetime is a consequence of schizoid personality traits, which lead an individual to prefer isolation and solitary activities, even if they are married and employed.

There are some other potential environmental factors which have been reported to correlate with the development of late-onset psychotic symptoms. Changes in sensory functions, both in terms of hearing and vision, have been reported in late-onset psychotic conditions (e.g., Post 1966; Herbert and Jacobson 1967). Careful follow-up studies have noted that that these sensory impairments may not be specific to late-onset psychosis. Praeger and Jeste (1993) found that psychiatric patients in general, including older patients with late-onset major depression, were more likely to have impairments in both hearing and vision than healthy comparison subjects.

An additional potential risk factor for late-onset schizophrenia, which could not be due to lifelong personality abnormalities, is living alone due to being divorced or widowed in later life. In fact, the results of several studies have suggested that there was an increased prevalence of being widowed or divorced in late-onset psychosis cases relative to a healthy comparison sample (Almeida *et al.* 1995b). These data are inconsistent with the idea of substantial lifelong isolation and indicate that current situational factors could be more important determinants of social isolation than lifelong preferences. Clearly these can be important stressful events for individuals later in their life. At the same time, it is very common to experience becoming widowed in later life, particularly for females, and while the majority of individuals with late-onset psychotic conditions are female, the risk rate for development of psychosis after being widowed is quite small.

It is possible that, compared to early-onset schizophrenia, life events are more likely to precede the development of late-onset psychotic conditions. One of the most commonly applied models of the interactions of stress predisposing factors is the Diathesis-Stress Model (Zubin and Spring 1977). The overall framework of this model suggests that there is a necessary, but not sufficient predisposing factor (i.e., a diathesis) for the illness, combined with a similarly necessary but not sufficient stressor that interacts with the diathesis to lead to the development of the illness (see Cannon chapter this volume). Such a predisposition could be genetically transmitted or acquired environmentally, while the stressor could be psychological or physiological (Harvey *et al.* 1986). Predispositions could have measurable psychological or physiological correlates, with the psychological correlates being in the domains of cognitive deficits, personality traits, or behavioral tendencies. Biological correlates of the predisposition could be found in the domains of abnormal brain structure or function, abnormal patterns of physiological reactivity to environmental stimuli, or the presence of genetic markers associated with susceptibility genes.

One of the problems with the application of this model to later-onset schizophrenia is that it has proven very difficult to identify both the predisposition and stressor. Long-term studies of offspring of schizophrenic parents, the group with the easiest-to-identify predisposition, have failed to identify patterns of environmental experiences that are consistently associated with development of schizophrenia. The most compelling findings in this area (Cannon *et al.* 2000, and see Cannon this volume) suggest that children of schizophrenic parents who experience hypoxia-related obstetrical complications (OCs) have an increased risk for the development of schizophrenia, relative to individuals who have no schizophrenic relatives and experienced OCs, and children of schizophrenic parents born without OCs. In contrast, even rearing by a schizophrenic mother has no impact on risk for schizophrenia in individuals who share genetic predispositions to schizophrenia (Higgins *et al.* 1997).

The data on the risk factors for late-onset schizophrenia does suggest that a lifelong history of schizoid or paranoid traits, combined with environmentally-induced social isolation in later life, may be related to an increased risk for development of late-onset psychosis. The diathesis appears to be marked by lifelong schizoid tendencies, while the stressor appears to be isolation induced by divorce or death of a spouse. While these data have not been collected prospectively, this is a very testable hypothesis that could help to understand some of the inconsistent data collected to date in this area. In fact, if late-onset schizophrenia is the product of schizoid tendencies combined with life stress associated with isolation, intervention possibilities are also quite straightforward.

Summary

Late-onset schizophrenia has several features that contribute to the controversies regarding this diagnostic entity. The presentation of symptoms is somewhat different, with hallucinations most prominent and negative symptoms generally absent. In addition, the gender ratio of the illness is reduced compared to early-onset, with the later the age of onset the greater the female/male ratio. Some data suggest that lifelong schizoid traits and life changes commonly occurring in later life, such as the death of a spouse, are risk factors for late-onset schizophrenia. Later research will need to consider whether lifelong schizoid traits lead to increased vulnerability to schizophrenia following stress exposure, and whether loss of a spouse in late life is a specific stressor linked to the development of psychosis in certain predisposed individuals. Cognitive and functional impairments are seen, but they are reduced considerably in critical areas compared to early-onset cases.

The basis for the argument that late-onset schizophrenia is somehow different from early onset cases lies not just in the phenomenological differences. Genetic differences are the most striking difference between early- and late-onset cases, with schizophrenia largely absent in relatives of late-onset patients, and affective disorder often found to be more common in these relatives than in relatives of healthy comparison subjects. Other differences lie in premorbid functioning, where schizoid symptoms are, if anything, more common in late-onset patients than in early-onset patients prior to the onset of their illness. Other indicators of social and occupational functioning are much more intact than in earlier-onset schizophrenia, again indicating that the early failure to function adequately that is commonly seen in early-onset patients is missing in these patients. As of this point, the major differences between early and late-onset schizophrenia, even when patients who meet full criteria for DSM schizophrenia are compared to earlier-onset patients, will hopefully promote additional research and provoke careful thinking about psychiatric nosology and its late-life implications.

References

Almeida, O., Howard, R.J., Levy, R. and David, A.S. (1995a). Psychotic states arising in late life: Psychopathology and nosology. *British Journal of Psychiatry*, 166, 205–214.

Almeida, O., Howard, R.J., Levy, R., David, A.S., Morris, R.G. and Sahakian, B. (1995b). Clinical and cognitive diversity of psychotic states arising in late life. *Psychological Medicine*, 25, 699–714.

American Psychiatric Association (1980). *Diagnostic and Statistical Manual of Mental Disorders*, 3rd edn. Washington, DC: American Psychiatric Association.

Cannon, T.D., Rosso, I.M., Hollister, J.M., Bearden, C.E., Sanchez, L.E. and Hadley, T. (2000). A prospective cohort study of genetic and perinatal influences in the etiology of schizophrenia. *Schizophrenia Bulletin*, 26, 351–366.

Castle, D.J. and Howard, R. (1992). What do we know about the etiology of late-onset schizophrenia? *European Psychiatry*, 7, 99–108.

Castle, D.J. and Murray, R.M. (1993). The epidemiology of late-onset schizophrenia. *Schizophrenia Bulletin*, 19, 691–700.

Castle, D.J., Wessely, S., Howard, R. and Murray, R.M. (1997). Schizophrenia with onset at the extremes of adult life. *International Journal of Geriatric Psychiatry*, 12, 712–717.

Christenson, R. and Blazer, D. (1984). Epidemiology of persecutory ideation in an elderly population in the community. *American Journal of Psychiatry*, 141, 1088–1091.

Harris, M.J. and Jeste, D.V. (1988). Late-onset schizophrenia: An overview. *Schizophrenia Bulletin*, 14, 39–55.

Harvey, P.D., Walker, E. and Wielgus, M.S. (1986). *Psychological Markers of Vulnerability to Schizophrenia. Progress in Experimental Personality Research*, Vol. 14. New York: Academic Press.

Herbert, M.E. and Jacobson, S. (1967). Late paraphrenia. *British Journal of Psychiatry*, 113, 461–469.

Higgins, J., Gore, R., Gutkind, D., Mednick, S.A., Parnas, J., Schulsinger, F. and Cannon, T.D. (1997). Effects of child-rearing by schizophrenic mothers: a 25-year follow-up. *Acta Psychiatrica Scandanavia*, 96, 402–404.

Howard, R.J., Almeida, O. and Levy, R. (1994). Phenomenology, demography and diagnosis in late paraphrenia. *Psychological Medicine*, 24, 397–410.

Howard, R.J., Castle, D.J., Wessely, S. and Murray, R.M. (1993). A comparative study of 470 cases of late-onset and early-onset schizophrenia. *British Journal of Psychiatry*, 163, 352–357.

Howard, R.J., Graham, C., Sham, P., Dennehey, J., Castle, D.J., Levy, R. and Murray, R. (1997). A controlled family study of late-onset non-affective psychosis (late paraphrenia). *British Journal of Psychiatry*, 170, 511–514.

Jeste, D.V., Harris, M.J., Krull, Kuck, J., McAdams, L.A. and Heaton, R.K. (1995). Clinical and neuropsychological characteristics of patients with late-onset schizophrenia. *American Journal of Psychiatry*, 152, 722–730.

Kraepelin, E. (1919). *Dementia Praecox and Paraphrenia*. Edinburgh: E. and S. Livingstone.

Lindamer, L.A., Lohr, J.B., Harris, M.J. and Jeste, D.V. (1997). Gender, estrogen and schizophrenia. *Psychopharmacology Bulletin*, 33, 221–228.

Mojtabai, R., Bromet, E., Harvey, P.D., Carlson, G., Craig, T. and Fenning, S. (2000). Are there neuropsychological differences between first episode patients with schizophrenia and affective disorder? *American Journal of Psychiatry*, 157, 1453–1460.

Pearlson, G.D., Kreger, L., Rabins, P.V., Chase G.A., Cohen, B., Wirth, J.B., Schlaepfer, T.B. and Tune, L.E. (1989). A chart review study of late-onset and early onset schizophrenia. *American Journal of Psychiatry*, 146, 1568–1574.

Post, F. (1966). *Persistent Persecutory States of the Elderly*. Pergamon Press, Oxford, UK.

Praeger, S. and Jeste, D.V. (1993). Sensory changes in late-life schizophrenia. *Schizophrenia Bulletin*, 19, 755–772.

Rabins, P.V., Pauker, S. and Thomas, J. (1984). Can schizophrenia begin after age 44? *Comprehensive Psychiatry*, 25, 290–293.

Reichler-Rosser, A. (1999). Late onset schizophrenia: the German concept and literature. In Howard, R., Rabins, R. and Castle, D.J. (eds) *Late-onset Schizophrenia*, pp. 3–16. Petersfield, UK: Wrightson Medical.

Tien, A.Y. (1991). Distribution of hallucinations in the population. *Social Psychiatry and Psychiatric Epidemiology*, 26, 287–292.

Zubin, J., Spring, B. (1977). Vulnerability – a new view of schizophrenia. *Journal of Abnormal Psychology*, 86, 103–126.

Section 3

Treatment of early schizophrenia

Chapter 11

Prodromal period: pharmacological and behavioural interventions

Alison R. Yung, Lisa J. Phillips,
and Patrick D. McGorry

Introduction

The prodromal period of schizophrenia is the first manifestation of illness, and refers to a period in which the individual is experiencing symptoms and difficulties, but before the onset of frank psychotic symptoms. Although there is great variability between patients in how their prodromes manifest, certain symptoms and signs have been frequently described. These include depressed mood, anxiety, irritability and aggressive behaviour, suicidal ideation and attempts, and substance use (Yung and McGorry 1996a, 1996b). Consequently many young people experience social withdrawal, and deterioration in role functioning and disruption of peer and family networks. It is not clear at this stage whether these disruptions are primarily biological or psychosocial in origin, or to what extent their trajectory can be altered with intervention. However, it is clear that this early phase is characterized by some level of disability and potentially damaging behaviours.

More proximal to the onset of frank psychotic symptoms, people often experience attenuated or subthreshold forms of psychotic symptoms. These may evolve, at varying rates, into psychotic symptoms. The development of attenuated psychotic symptoms can also have deleterious effects. For example, the belief that others may be thinking badly about or laughing at oneself may result in social withdrawal, non-attendance at school, work or university, and suspiciousness and altered behaviour towards one's family and friends.

Thus the prodromal phase presents two possible targets for intervention:

1 The current symptoms, behaviour or disability, and

2 A preventative focus, that is, treatment which aims to delay, ameliorate or even prevent the progression of disorder, as manifest by the onset of frank psychotic symptoms.

All this seems obvious, and indeed the idea of treatment of the prodromal phase, or 'pre-psychotic intervention', is not new. An earlier generation of psychiatrists were drawn to this notion (Meares 1959; Sullivan 1994). The idea was particularly relevant several decades ago, when safe and effective treatments for schizophrenia were lacking and a great deal of pessimism surrounded the diagnosis. However, these earlier psychiatrists were hampered in their attempts to put pre-psychotic intervention into practice. One of the main challenges was the problem of false positives and their implication for preventive intervention. This issue is still pertinent, but as we discuss below, strategies have recently been developed which assist in reducing this problem. Together with the development of new treatment options, which are safer and more effective than ever before, trialing of pre-psychotic treatments can now begin.

While there are some challenges to overcome, the pre-psychotic phase now offers a tantalizing focus for treatment. This chapter will explore the conceptual issues that underlie pre-psychotic intervention, and discuss the current state of knowledge of both pharmacological and psychological treatments.

Conceptual issues

The term 'the prodromal period of schizophrenia' needs discussion. Prodrome is a retrospective concept, which cannot be deemed to have occurred until after the onset of full-blown psychotic symptoms indicative of definitive psychotic disorder (Yung et al. 1996). A psychotic prodrome (i.e. impending psychotic disorder) cannot be 'diagnosed' with any certainty based on the presence of, for example, depression, anxiety and social isolation. These symptoms may indicate the presence of a threshold or subthreshold mood disorder, substance use, a physical illness or just a reaction to circumstances. A first episode of psychosis cannot even be predicted from the presence of attenuated psychotic symptoms. This is because these symptoms too can resolve before a full-blown psychotic disorder develops, as evidenced by the finding that attenuated psychotic symptoms and 'psychotic-like experiences' are commonly found in the general population, at far higher rates than psychotic disorders (Eaton et al. 1991; van Os et al. 2001). This indicates that at least some attenuated psychotic symptoms must either resolve without full-blown psychosis ensuing, or that they can persist without developing into a full-blown psychotic disorder. Thus the problem of false positives arises.

Use of the term prodrome should therefore be discouraged. We have coined the alternative term 'at-risk mental state' (ARMS) (McGorry and Singh 1995; Yung et al. 1996) to indicate that the person has some mental state features suggestive of a high degree of risk for onset of psychotic disorder, but that full-blown psychosis is not inevitable. The difficulty with referring to individuals as 'prodromal' is that this implies incipient psychosis, when this may not be the case. This becomes highly relevant when preventative intervention is considered. The ARMS concept acknowledges current limitations in our knowledge and understanding about psychosis. It also has ethical advantages in underlining the reality of false positive 'cases' (McGorry *et al.* 2003).

A second issue of terminology is the use of the term 'schizophrenia'. Not all patients with an ARMS will develop a full blown first episode of psychosis, and not all patients with a first episode of psychosis will develop schizophrenia. In the field of pre-psychotic intervention the aim is to prevent a first episode of *psychosis*. This target is more proximal and therapeutically salient than schizophrenia, which can be considered a subtype to which additional patients can graduate distal to the first episode of psychosis.

The advantages and disadvantages of pre-psychotic intervention

Pre-psychotic intervention has two therapeutic goals. The first goal is the treatment of the patient's current problems. As noted, a substantial amount of the disability that develops in schizophrenia occurs in the prodromal phase (Hafner *et al.* 1994; Yung and McGorry 1996b). Some of this disability may persist even after resolution of positive psychotic symptoms and this may create a ceiling for eventual recovery in some patients (Häfner *et al.* 1995; Agerbo *et al.* 2003). Even the young people not 'destined' to develop a psychotic disorder (the false positives) are referred to clinical services due to troubling symptoms or behaviours, which may be legitimate targets for intervention. The second goal is the aim of preventing, ameliorating or delaying the onset of the first psychotic episode.

Other benefits of pre-psychotic intervention include the capacity to research the onset phase of illness and examine the processes (biological and psychosocial) which occur around the time of transition from the subthreshold state to fully-fledged disorder. Risk factors such as substance use, stress, and the underlying neurobiology can be studied. The delineation of this discrete phase, the boundaries of which are often difficult to precisely map, is of great heuristic and practical value (McGorry *et al.* 2003).

A number of disadvantages of pre-psychotic intervention should also be noted. As in all preventive research, the main difficulty is accurately identifying those individuals who will develop full-blown disorder in the absence of intervention, and distinguishing them from phenotypically similar individuals who are not truly at risk of the disorder; that is, the problem of false positives. There is also a group we have called the false false positives (Yung *et al.* 2003). These are people with an ARMS who would have developed a psychotic disorder, except that some alteration in their circumstances prevented this from occurring. At baseline assessment it is impossible to determine to which group a young person belongs. Inevitably, some individuals will be 'diagnosed', followed up and treated as if they were at high risk of developing a psychotic disorder, when this may not be true. These falsely identified individuals may be harmed by being labelled as having an at risk mental state, and/or receiving treatment at this stage. For example they may become anxious or depressed about the possibility of developing schizophrenia, stigmatized by others or themselves or both (Yung *et al.* 2004), and they may avoid developmentally appropriate challenges (Heinssen *et al.* 2001), for fear of increasing their 'stress' level and risking precipitation of psychosis. Similarly, these falsely identified individuals may be exposed to drug or other therapies with potential adverse reactions without gaining any benefit. These issues have been reviewed in detail previously (Cornblatt *et al.* 2001; McGlashan 2001; McGorry *et al.* 2001; Yung and McGorry 1997; Yung *et al.* 2004). Concerns about the risk/benefit balance of early intervention strategies lie at the heart of this controversy, and need to be addressed by an evidence-based approach (Bentall and Morrison 2002; Yung and McGorry 2003a).

The false positive problem and the 'close-in' strategy as a key methodological advance

Overcoming the non-specific nature of prodromal symptoms and the difficulty of predicting who will progress from an ARMS to full-blown psychosis are the major challenges for attempts at pre-psychotic intervention. We have applied a 'multiple-gate screening' and 'close in' strategy, as first described by Bell (1992) to address this issue. Multiple-gate screening is a form of sequential screening that involves putting in place a number of different screening measures to concentrate the level of risk in the selected sample. In other words, an individual must meet a number of conditions to be included in the high-risk sample rather than just one, as in the traditional the genetic high-risk studies approach (Erlenmeyer-Kimling *et al.* 1995; Hodges *et al.* 1999). Close-in follow-up involves shortening the period of follow-up necessary to observe the transition to psychosis, by commencing the follow-up period close to the age of maximum incidence of psychotic disorders. In order to improve the accuracy of identifying the high-risk cohort further, Bell (1992) also recommended using signs of behavioural difficulties in adolescence as selection criteria, such as the inclusion of clinical features. This also allows the approach to become more *clinical*, to move away from traditional screening paradigms and to focus on troubled young people seeking help, who are therefore highly 'incipient' and frankly symptomatic. To maximize the predictive power as well as enabling the engagement of the patient to be well justified on immediate clinical grounds, the timing is critical. Patients should really be as 'incipient' as possible, yet this is difficult to measure and consistently sustain. Transition rates to full psychosis in samples may therefore vary on this basis, and also because of variation in the underlying proportions of true and false positives who enter the sample (McGorry *et al.* 2003). It should be emphasized that young people involved in this strategy have clinical problems, and help is being sought either directly by them or on their behalf by concerned relatives.

This strategy was first translated into practice in Melbourne, Australia in 1994 at the PACE (Personal Assessment and Crisis Evaluation) clinic (Yung *et al.* 1995) in parallel with the development of the EPPIC program (Edwards *et al.* 1994; McGorry 1993; McGorry *et al.* 1996). This approach has now been adopted in a number of other clinical research programmes across the world (e.g. Cornblatt *et al.* 2002b; Morrison *et al.* 2002). These studies have been referred to as 'ultra' high-risk (UHR) studies to differentiate them from the traditional high-risk studies that rely on family history as the primary inclusion criteria. Intake criteria for such studies were initially developed from information gleaned from literature reviews and clinical experience with first episode psychosis patients, and have been evaluated and reviewed in the PACE clinic over the past eight years.

Thus this model for detecting individuals who are putatively experiencing a prodrome that underpins this new wave of studies is a significant departure from earlier endeavours at identifying high-risk cohorts. In contrast to the genetic high risk approach (Erlenmeyer-Kimling *et al.* 1995; Hodges *et al.* 1999) the new approach focuses on patients who have manifest symptoms and impaired functioning, and demonstrate a substantially increased short term risk of psychosis onset. The development of this alternative high-risk strategy has the advantages of a higher rate of transition to psychosis, a lower false positive rate and a shorter follow-up period.

Although the UHR studies ostensibly seek to identify individuals experiencing an initial psychotic prodrome, infallible criteria have not yet been developed towards this end. It should be noted that participants in the UHR model are voluntary and help-seeking: they are concerned about changes in their mental state and functioning and are requesting some assistance to address these changes. Hence, while some turn out to be false positives for subsequent psychotic disorder, they are all 'cases' in the sense of a need for care (McGorry *et al.* 2003). In many cases, the young people are overtly concerned about the possibility that they may be developing a psychotic disorder.

The UHR criteria

UHR criteria currently in operation at the PACE clinic require that a young person aged between 14 and 30 is referred for health care to the service and meets criteria for one or more of the following groups:

+ *Attenuated Psychotic Symptoms Group*: have experienced subthreshold, attenuated positive psychotic symptoms during the past year;
+ *Brief Limited Intermittent Psychotic Symptoms Group (BLIPS)*: have experienced episodes of frank psychotic symptoms that have not lasted longer than a week and have been spontaneously abated; or
+ *Trait and State Risk Factor Group*: have a first-degree relative with a psychotic disorder or the identified patient has a schizotypal personality disorder and they have experienced a significant decrease in functioning during the previous year.

These criteria are described in more detail elsewhere (Yung *et al.* 2003, 2004). As well as meeting the criteria for at least one of these groups, subjects must not have experienced a previous psychotic episode and must live in the Melbourne metropolitan area. Thus, the UHR criteria identify young people who are in the age range of peak incidence of onset of a psychotic disorder (late adolescence/early adulthood) who additionally describe mental state changes that are suggestive of an emerging psychotic process, or who may have a strong family history of psychosis. They must be seeking help, or have been identified by some one else as being in need of a clinical service. It is recognized that some subthreshold cases, in particular those meeting BLIPS criteria, might meet criteria for DSM-IV Brief Psychotic Disorder. However, the meaning of the diagnosis of Brief Psychotic Disorder is unclear in terms of prognosis and need for treatment. We believe a better approach is to conceptualize a brief transient psychotic episode as a possible risk factor for more severe, disabling and chronic course of psychotic disorder. Follow-up of patients who present in this manner enables the critical examination of this syndrome and investigation into whether it is a valid diagnostic entity.

Criteria have also been developed to define the onset of frank psychotic disorder in the UHR group. These are not identical to DSM-IV criteria, but are designed to define the minimal point at which antipsychotic treatment is indicated. This definition is arbitrary, but does at least have clear treatment implications, and applies equally well to substance-related symptoms, symptoms that have a mood component–either depression or mania–and schizophrenia spectrum disorders. The predictive target is first episode psychosis that is judged to require antipsychotic medication, arbitrarily defined by the persistence of frank psychotic symptoms for over one week.

Using these criteria, we found that it was possible to detect and engage a subset of young people who were subthreshold for fully fledged psychotic disorder, yet who have demonstrable clinical needs and other syndromal diagnoses, and who appear to be at incipient risk of frank psychosis (Yung *et al.* 1996, 1998, 2003, 2004). The rate of transition to psychosis within 12 months in this cohort was about 35 per cent (Yung *et al.* 2003, 2004), a rate several thousand-fold over the expected incidence rate for first episode psychosis in the general population. This occurred despite the provision of minimal supportive counselling, case management and SSRI medication if required. The primary diagnostic outcome of the group who developed psychosis was schizophrenia (65 per cent) (Yung *et al.* 2003). These results cannot be easily generalized to the wider population as a whole, or even to individuals who have a family history of psychosis but who are asymptomatic. Participants recruited to research at the PACE clinic are a selected sample, characterized perhaps by high help-seeking characteristics or other non-specific factors. It undoubtedly includes only a minority of those who proceed to a first episode of psychosis, and a possibly unstable proportion of false positives, depending on sampling and detection factors, which in turn are difficult to define and measure, but which can affect the base rate of true positives in the sample. Hence the transition rate may vary and needs to be validated and monitored, because the UHR criteria are not the only variable involved. However, these criteria are now being utilized in a number of other settings around the world, with preliminary results indicating that they predict equally well in the US, UK, and Norway as in Melbourne, Australia (Larsen 2002; Miller *et al.* 2002; Morrison *et al.* 2002). Undoubtedly, there are other clinical features and non-clinical variables which need to be identified and incorporated into future definitions of the UHR state.

Hence it can be seen that by applying the multiple-gate screening and close-in strategy the issue of false positives has been reduced, but not eliminated. Nonetheless, it was felt that with such a high rate of onset of psychotic disorder within this population, examination of preventative interventions in the UHR group was justified. This position gained subsequent support from a landmark publication addressing contemporary conceptualizations of preventive approaches to mental illness. Mrazek and Haggerty (1994) wrote that the current lack of definitive knowledge about the aetiology and risk factors for psychotic disorders, particularly schizophrenia, meant that developing universal (targeting the entire population) and selective (targeting groups whose risk of developing psychosis is significantly higher than average) preventive interventions is not currently possible. Rather they suggested that indicated prevention–targeting individuals who exhibit subthreshold signs and symptoms of psychosis–was the most appropriate at this point in time. They further suggested that combining known risk factors provides the best chance for identifying high-risk individuals – i.e. the multiple-gate screening approach. The theoretical basis for this drew on the work of Eaton (Eaton *et al.* 1995) who was looking at subthreshold clinical features as a form of proximal risk factor for full clinical disorder, in this case depression, and it opened up the whole notion of 'onset' of disorders and what actually constitutes an initial 'case'. Acquisition, intensification and coherence of symptoms and syndromes are necessary but perhaps insufficient dimensions for 'caseness' (Eaton *et al.* 1995). Other variables such as distress, additional comorbidity, functional impairment, and other variables including perceived and objective 'need for care', also need to be considered as necessary features or alternatively as 'risk factors for caseness'. Clearly greater precision is necessary for defining the onset of mental disorders, not only schizophrenia and psychotic illnesses (McGorry *et al.* 2003).

Other clinical high-risk approaches

The German approach to detection of individuals experiencing the prepsychotic phase draws upon a long-standing observation that cognitive, affective and social disturbances often occur years before the first psychotic episode and are often recognized by the person affected at this early stage. These self-experienced deficits were described as 'basic symptoms' (BS) in detail in the 1960s by Huber and colleagues, and have significantly influenced concepts of schizophrenia in German-speaking countries (Gross 1989, 1997; Huber and Gross 1989; Koehler and Sauer 1984). In the prospective Cologne Early Recognition (CER) study (Klosterkotter *et al.* 2001) 160 individuals who were suspected of being in the onset phase of schizophrenia were assessed with the Bonn Scale for Assessment of Basic Symptoms (BSABS) (Klosterkotter *et al.* 1997). Seventy-nine patients developed schizophrenia over the follow-up period, which averaged 9.6 years, on average 1.9 (± 2.5) years after the first examination: 77 of these 79 participants and 33 who did not develop schizophrenia, had reported at least one BS at first examination indicating reasonably good prognostic accuracy of BS.

Interventions in the pre-psychotic phase

Both pharmacological and psychological interventions have been evaluated with individuals who have been identified as being at UHR. These will be considered in turn.

Pharmacological interventions

Some controversy surrounds the proposal of providing pharmacological treatment for individuals in the pre-psychotic phase of illness (Bentall and Morrison 2002). This centres around the belief that psychosis is not necessarily harmful, and, due to possible side effects of antipsychotic medication, that the treatment of subthreshold psychotic symptoms may actually increase an individual's morbidity without providing benefit. As we have argued previously (Yung and McGorry 2003a) when young people are seeking help for distressing symptoms then treatment may be justified, both for symptomatic management and prevention of future ill health. As discussed below, side effects have been found to be minimal. However, debate should continue around this issue and other treatment options explored to maximize choice and benefits for individuals at risk of psychotic disorder. The following treatments have been proposed thus far as possible therapeutic options in the pre-psychotic phase.

Anti-psychotic medication

One treatment that has been suggested is anti-psychotic medication. The rationale behind this proposal is straightforward: anti-psychotic medication has demonstrated efficacy with psychotic populations, and this efficacy might translate to the pre-psychotic phase. Opponents of this approach state that the transition rates to psychosis in the UHR and BS groups are not sufficiently high to warrant provision of treatments with known side-effects, as the false positive rate is too great (Bentall and Morrison 2002). One strategy for reconciling this impasse is to provide anti-psychotic medication within a well-monitored clinical trial environment. Results of two such trials have been released.

The first randomized controlled trial with a high risk cohort was conducted at PACE between 1996–9 (McGorry *et al.* 2002). In this trial, the impact of a combined intensive cognitively-oriented psychological treatment plus very low dose atypical antipsychotic (risperidone) medication (Specific Preventive Intervention or SPI: N = 31) was compared with the effect of supportive therapy (Needs-Based Intervention or NBI: N = 28) on the development of acute illness in the high-risk group. At the end of the six month treatment phase, significantly more subjects in the NBI group had developed an acute psychosis than in the SPI group ($p = 0.026$). This difference was no longer significant at the end of a post-treatment six month follow-up period ($p = 0.16$), though it did remain significant for those members of the SPI group who were compliant with their risperidone treatment. This result suggests that it is possible to delay the onset of acute psychosis in the SPI group compared to the NBI group. Both groups experienced a reduction in global psychopathology and improved functioning over the treatment and follow-up phases, compared to entry levels. Longer-term follow-up of the participants in this study is now taking place. The relative benefits of the medication and psychological treatments also need to be disentangled. With this in mind, a second randomized trial commenced at PACE in 2000. This is a more sophisticated study with three treatment groups and blind randomization to these groups. The three groups are: (a) risperidone (up to 2 mg) and cognitive behavioral therapy, (b) placebo and cognitive behavioural therapy and (c) placebo and befriending. All treatments are offered for 12 months and participants are then monitored for a further 12 months to determine the long-term impact of the treatment.

Results of the first trial using anti-psychotic medication alone with blind randomization to the treatment group at PRIME have recently been revealed (McGlashan *et al.* 2004). This study randomly allocated participants who met prodroma criteria to receive either olanzapine (N = 31) or placebo (N = 29) for 12 months followed by a 12-month monitoring period. Of the total sample of 60 participants, 16 (26.6 per cent) developed an acute psychosis during the treatment period. Five of those who developed a psychosis were in the olanzapine group and 11 from the placebo group. All of the olanzapine 'converters' became psychotic during the first month of treatment. Over the second 12-month period, an additional three from the olanzapine group and two from the placebo group developed psychosis. These results are similar to the PACE trial indicating that provision of a specific anti-psychotic medication could delay the onset of psychosis.

However, although antipsychotic medication is an obvious therapy, other interventions may be more appropriate for early stages of illness (Kane *et al.* 2003; Yung and McGorry 2003). Indeed, frank psychotic symptoms may just be 'noise' around an underlying disease process that could respond to something quite different from anti-psychotic medication (Yung and McGorry 2003). The use of antipsychotics in the high risk group, even in those truly experiencing emerging psychosis, may be analagous to treating a person's angina pectoris with glycerol trinitrite (GTN); the patient feels better, but the underlying disease process (ischaemic heart disease) is not treated and continues unabated, leaving the person at risk of relapse. Indeed, the next episode may be more severe and less amenable to treatment, since the underlying disease has progressed (Yung 2003). Neuroprotective agents, antidepressants and non-pharmacologic therapies may be of more benefit in the UHR group.

Other agents

Other agents may also be effective in preventing, ameliorating or delaying the onset of psychotic disorder. One suggestion has been that neuroprotective agents might be of benefit to young people in the pre-psychotic phase. It is suggested that dysfunctional regulation of the growth and degeneration in some brain areas might explain neurodevelopmental abnormalities seen in early psychosis (Berger *et al.* 2003). Neuroprotective strategies counteracting the loss or supporting the generation of progenitor cells may therefore be a potent therapeutic avenue to explore. Candidate therapies including lithium (Manji *et al.* 1999), eicosapentanoic acid (EPA) (Fenton *et al.* 2000), and glycine (Javitt *et al.* 2001) might therefore have a role in preventing the onset of illness in the UHR population. Open labelled studies using lithium, glycine and EPA are now underway in Melbourne and Yale (Woods, personal communication, Colorado Springs, 2003, Hawkins, personal communication, Sydney, 2003).

Other treatment options have yet to be tested in the UHR population. One candidate treatment is corticotrophin releasing hormone (CRH) receptor agonists (Corcoran *et al.* 2001). A recent study has suggested that estrogen may be effective as an adjunctive treatment to atypical anti-psychotic medications in reducing the psychotic symptoms experienced by women with established psychosis (Kulkarni *et al.* 2001, 2002). Estrogen might therefore have a role in the treatment of UHR women.

Investigators at the Hillside Recognition and Prevention (Hillside-RAP) clinic in New York believe that the development of specific preventive interventions is premature at present. Instead they have chosen a 'naturalistic' approach to study the appropriateness and efficacy of various potential treatments for UHR young people. Thus, they have surveyed the treatment provided to young people meeting RAP criteria by psychiatrists, but have not sought to direct the type of treatment provided. The mental state of over 80 per cent of the patients recruited to RAP has either improved or stabilized over time (Cornblatt *et al.* 2002b). Over 80 per cent of patients received a pharmacological treatment, either anti-psychotic medication or an anti-depressant, with both demonstrating clinical improvements (Cornblatt *et al.* 2002b). The authors of this study suggest that this indicates that anti-depressants may be effective in treating the underlying vulnerability of schizophrenia, and should be considered when developing preventive interventions. It should be noted that many of these young people– particularly the group labelled as experiencing a 'schizophrenia-like psychosis' or SLP–would be seen as already psychotic within the PACE framework.

Other pharmacological interventions may also be indicated in the UHR group, depending on the young person's presentation and current problems. For example, specific treatment for syndromes such as depression and anxiety may include medication.

Psychological interventions

The benefits of psychological intervention, particularly cognitive-behavioural strategies, in the treatment of established psychotic disorders have been well documented. In 1952, Aaron T. Beck published results of a study describing cognitive interventions for delusional beliefs (Beck 1952). Over the following decades a number of randomized controlled trials have demonstrated the efficacy of this form of treatment with individuals with both long-standing and first-episode populations (e.g. Drury *et al.* 1996; Kuipers *et al.* 1997; Sensky *et al.* 2000; Tarrier *et al.* 1998). It has also been demonstrated that cognitive-behavioural monitoring of 'warning signs' can facilitate early intervention and relapse prevention or amelioration (Birchwood 1989), and provision of cognitive therapy to people at risk of relapse significantly reduces relapses and hospital admissions (Gumley *et al.* 1999). Importantly, it has been demonstrated that the value of cognitive-behavioural therapy (CBT) translates from clinical trials to community settings (Turkington *et al.* 2002). CBT also appears to be very acceptable to patients, with reported drop out rates across studies of only 12–15 per cent, and is relatively safe with no evidence of increasing suicidal ideation, agitation or violence in any study to date. Although further studies are required, with larger sample sizes, longer follow-up and more rigorously controlled comparison treatments, one review has concluded that to withhold CBT for psychosis would be unethical (Rector 2001).

Other psychological treatment approaches have also been evaluated in psychotic populations. These include family psychoeducation, psychoanalytically-oriented therapy and group-based therapy (Gleeson *et al.* 2003). Psychologically-oriented treatments do not only target positive psychotic symptoms, but can also assist in promoting medication compliance and can be effective in comorbid syndromes such as depression, anxiety and substance use (Gleeson 2003).

The well-documented efficacy and acceptability of psychological treatment for people with established psychosis suggests that these strategies might also be useful in treating people who are experiencing the pre-psychotic or prodromal phase of illness (French and Morrison 2004). Psychological strategies might aid individuals in this phase of illness to develop strategies to cope with symptoms experienced during this early phase, as well as possibly preventing further symptom development, functional decline and the onset of acute psychosis. Cognitive-behaviour therapy is an obvious approach to evaluate with this patient group. However, it is also thought that the provision of simple supportive therapy along with basic stress-management and problem-solving might also have merit with this population. Some researchers have suggested that, as criteria do not yet exist for the infallible identification of young people during the prodromal phase of illness, and due to the known high risk of side-effects associated with anti-psychotic medication, psychological interventions should be the only treatment provided for this group of patients at the current time (Bentall and Morrison 2002; French and Morrison 2004).

To date, three centres have described psychologically oriented treatment approaches targeted at people who are thought to be experiencing the onset phase of a first psychotic illness.

PACE clinic

Psychological treatment has been a cornerstone of the treatment provided at PACE since its inception. In the intervention trials that have been conducted at PACE, the impact of supportive psychotherapy has been compared with cognitively oriented psychotherapy. Both approaches have their virtues: both focus on engagement and on the formation of a strong, collaborative and respectful relationship between the therapist and the patient, and both aim towards the development of effective coping skills.

The cognitively oriented therapy developed at PACE for the high-risk group utilizes strategies developed for acutely unwell and recovering populations. Cognitive therapy with individuals experiencing psychotic illnesses involves exploring cognitive/reasoning biases and appraisals of the self and the illness. In keeping with this, the core symptoms of psychosis are thought to derive from basic disturbances in information processing resulting in perceptual abnormalities and disturbed experience of the self. Cognitive biases, inaccurate appraisals and core self-schema maintain these maladaptive interpretations (Frith 1992; Garety *et al.* 1994, 2000). The aim of cognitively oriented therapy is to assist people in developing an understanding of the cognitive processes that influence their thoughts and emotions, and to develop more realistic and positive views of themselves and events around them. The underlying goal of the cognitive therapy offered at the PACE Clinic is to strengthen the individual's coping resources, thereby reducing their vulnerability to developing further, or more severe, symptoms. This may ultimately avert the onset of a psychotic episode but also aims to ameliorate presenting symptomatology and reduce distress. Therefore it fits well within a stress-vulnerability framework. The therapy was designed to be provided on an individual basis but could potentially be adapted to suit a group-treatment situation. Young people can currently attend PACE for a maximum of 12 months, with session frequency varying from weekly to fortnightly and even monthly in the final stages depending on client need.

A wide range of psychological symptoms has been attributed to the onset phase of illness. A formulation about the issues faced by the patient is derived through a comprehensive assessment. In order to respond flexibly to the variation in presenting symptoms and problems experienced by PACE patients, a range of modules were developed targeting specific groups of symptoms. The modules are: stress management, depression/negative symptoms, positive symptoms and other comorbidity. Assessment of the client's presenting problems, as well as their own goals, assists in determining which modules should be utilized. Although the therapy is comprised of individual modules targeting specific symptom groups, it may not be appropriate to target one group of symptoms in isolation of other presenting difficulties, i.e., any individual therapy session may incorporate aspects of more than one module. Elements of the stress management module are provided to all patients, in keeping with the stress-vulnerability model of psychosis. This module has the added advantage of providing an easily understood introduction to cognitive behavioural principles, which sets the direction of future sessions. Detailed descriptions of the individual modules are provided in (Phillips and Francey in press). Strategies that are utilized include normalization of experiences, reality testing, challenging maladaptive thoughts, stress management techniques such as relaxation, psychoeducation, goal setting and motivational interviewing around substance use.

More recently the cognitive therapy provided at PACE has been broadened to include a focus on personality and social issues. It is thought that the therapy will develop further as a better understanding of risk factors of psychosis, and the psychological pathways leading to the development of psychosis, are better understood.

FETZ

The FETZ (FrühErkennungs- und Therapie Zentrum for Psychische Krisen) Centre was established in Cologne, Germany in 1997 with its own criteria for identifying the putatively prodromal population, focusing on the presence of

Basic Symptoms. The psychological treatment provided to clients attending the FETZ programme in Cologne includes both individual and group based components. Like the therapy provided at PACE, a manual has been written describing the treatment, which is based primarily on fundamentals of CBT therapy and incorporates intervention strategies that have demonstrated efficacy with first episode or recurrent schizophrenia, as well as for patients with anxiety disorders or depressive symptoms. The therapy is individually tailored to clients following an assessment phase during which symptoms and difficulties experienced by the young person are identified.

The assessment phase is followed by individual sessions. A combination of psychoeducation, symptom, stress and crisis management modules are adapted to the specific needs of each patient. In addition to targeting specific psychological symptoms, the treatment focuses on each individual's attributional styles that underpin those symptoms. Psychoeducation and cognitive techniques are utilized to challenge self-stigmatization and self-stereotypes, helping the person to protect and enhance self-esteem, and to enhance understanding of the context within which symptoms have arisen. In keeping with studies of first-episode schizophrenia patients, it is thought that a focus on attributional style can have a positive effect on self esteem, depressive and anxiety symptoms and social integration (Drury 1996; Jackson *et al.* 1998).

In the next phase, small groups work together with a therapist to address typical problems and deficits of prodromal patients. This includes elements of CBT (for depression, anxiety etc.), the training of social competence and problem solving abilities. There is a focus on social anxiety and social skills development.

The interventions conclude further individual sessions, which use the tools mentioned above to work more individually on symptoms and deficits. In addition, psychoeducation is provided to families in brief multifamily groups.

EDDIE

The Early Detection and Intervention Evaluation (EDDIE) group in Manchester UK have described a cognitive model of the pre-psychotic phase of illness. This model has led to the development of a cognitively-oriented treatment approach. Both the model and the treatment are influenced by existing literature on anxiety disorders, as many of the cognitive processes that have been well-documented in anxiety disorders, such as misinterpretations, selective attention and metacognition, are also thought to occur in the early stages of psychosis (French and Morrison 2004).

The psychological treatment provided at EDDIE draws upon the model of the onset of psychosis that was developed by Morrison (Morrison 2001). Briefly, this model proposes that individuals who develop psychosis experience intrusive thoughts, which they interpret in a culturally maladaptive way. There also seems to be an inability to generate alternative (culturally acceptable) explanations for internal or external events, which might be associated with a lack of supportive social relationships, which would otherwise enhance the development of more appropriate interpretations. Unhelpful cognitions and behavioural responses, such as selective attention, dysfunctional thought control strategies and avoidance are thought to maintain these misinterpretations and the distress associated with them. Individuals experiencing the pre-psychotic phase of illness described a wide range of symptoms–both psychotic and non-psychotic. As Morrison's model incorporates many of the elements underlying non-psychotic symptoms such as panic, obsessions, social phobia and depression, it is particularly suited to the pre-psychotic population.

The therapy provided at EDDIE is formulation driven and collaborative. It is goal-directed, with specific goals derived from discussion with the client. The specific strategies and techniques introduced by the therapist incorporate the client's life experiences, current environment, self and social knowledge, intrusions and their interpretations of intrusions, and their emotional, behavioural, cognitive and physiological responses. Therefore a thorough assessment precedes the active 'change' phase of the treatment. The 'change strategies' that are employed include normalization, generating and evaluating alternative explanations for events, focusing on metacognitions, identifying and challenging maladaptive core events and identifying and changing inappropriate behavioural responses to events (French and Morrison 2004).

EDDIE have compared the impact of cognitively-oriented psychotherapy with monitoring alone (that is, no psychological treatment) on the rate of transition to psychosis in 23 young people meeting UHR criteria (French *et al.* 2002; Morrison *et al.* 2002). After 26 sessions of Cognitive Therapy only one of the 13 participants (8 per cent) in this group had developed psychosis. This compared to four of the 11 in the monitoring group (36 per cent) (French *et al.* 2002). These results are encouraging as they suggest that pharmacological treatment might not be necessary to assist all young people in the pre-psychotic phase of illness.

Social treatments

Young people with UHR mental states may also benefit from case management and a range of general social treatments, including vocational and family counselling, social skills programmes and assistance in developing strategies to cope with subthreshold psychotic symptoms. Families are often involved in the mangement of UHR young people and usually require psychoeducation and support.

Current recommendations

Further research is required to determine which treatment strategies are effective in reducing the burden of symptoms and disability experienced by individuals with an at-risk mental state, and in reducing the risk of progression to a psychotic disorder. This research must meet the highest ethical standards applicable to all medical research. Patients must be given genuine informed consent and be free to withdraw from research at any time. Non-participation in research must not affect access to appropriate clinical care (Yung *et al.* 2004).

Research should be lead by local clinicians and researchers so that culturally normal experiences and behaviours are not misconstrued as signs and symptoms of illness. Further research is needed into both pharmacological and psychosocial treatments for this patient population, using larger sample sizes with a higher proportion of true positive cases (McGlashan *et al.* 2004).

Anti-psychotic medication should not generally be considered as the first treatment option for the UHR group at present, in recognition of the need for further evaluation of the appropriateness and efficacy of this treatment. Exceptions may include the situation when there is rapid deterioration of mental state, when severe suicidal risk is present and treatment of depression has proved ineffective, or when aggression or hostility are increasing and proving a threat to others. If antipsychotic medication is considered, low-dose atypical medication should be used. However, optimal dose and duration have not yet been determined. We have currently recommended that if there is benefit and resolution of symptoms after six weeks, the medication can be continued for between six months and two years with the patients' consent. After this period, if there has been a good recovery and the patient is agreeable, the medication should be gradually withdrawn. If there has been no or limited response to one atypical antipsychotic medication, another can be trialled if the above indications still exist (Yung *et al.* 2004).

Conclusion

The current state of knowledge regarding pharmacological and psychological treatment for individuals suspected of being in the prodromal phase of a psychotic disorder has been reviewed. This area is still in its infancy and needs constant evaluation. The uncertainty of the outcome of an ARMS needs to be balanced against patients' distress and need for treatment of their current problems. We believe that interventions in this group should be applied and investigated in an evidence-based manner, in the context of methodologically sound and ethical clinical trials.

References

Beck, A.T. (1952) Successful outpatient psychotherapy of a chronic schizophrenic with a delusion based on borrowed guilt. *Psychiatry*, 15, 305–312.

Bell, R.Q. (1992) Multiple-risk cohorts and segmenting risk as solutions to the problem of false positives in risk for the major psychoses. *Psychiatry*, 55, 370–381.

Bentall, R.P. and Morrison, A.P. (2002) More harm than good: The case against using anti-psychotic drugs to prevent severe mental illness. *Journal of Mental Health*, 11, 351–356.

Berger, G. E., Wood, S. and McGorry, P.D. (2003) Incipient neurovulnerability and neuroprotection in early psychosis. *Psychopharmacology Bulletin*, 37, 79–101.

Birchwood, M., Smith, J., Macmillan, F., Hogg, B., Prasad, R., Harvey, C., and Bering, S. (1989) Predicting relapse in schizophrenia: The development and implementation of an early signs monitoring system using patients and families as observers: A preliminary investigation. *Psychological Medicine*, 19, 649–656.

Corcoran, C., Gallitano, A., Leitman, D. and Malaspina, D. (2001) The neurobiology of the stress cascade and its potential relevance for schizophrenia. *Journal of Psychiatric Practice*, 7, 3–14.

Cornblatt, B., Lencz, T. and Obuchowski, M. (2002a) The schizophrenia prodrome: Treatment and high-risk perspectives. *Schizophrenia Research*, 54, 177–186.

Cornblatt, B., Lencz, T., Correll, C., Authour, A. and Smith, C. (2002b) Treating the prodrome: Naturalistic findings from the RAP Program. *Acta Psychiatrica Scandinavica Supplementum*, 106, 44.

Cornblatt, B.A., Lencz, T. and Kane, J.M. (2001) Treatment of the schizoporenia prodome: It is presently ethical? *Schizophrenia Research*, 51, 31–38.

Drury, V., Birchwood, M., Cochrane, R. and MacMillan, F. (1996) Cognitive therapy and recovery form acute psychosis: A controlled trial I. Impact on psychotic symptoms. *British Journal of Psychiatry*, 169, 593–601.

Eaton, W.W., Badawi, M. and Melton, B. (1995) Prodromes and precursors: epidemiologic data for primary prevention of disorders with slow onset. *American Journal of Psychiatry*, 152, 967–972.

Eaton, W.W., Romanoski, A., Anthony, J.C. and Nestadt, G. (1991) Screening for psychosis in the general population with a self-report interview. *J Nerv Ment Dis*, 179, 689–693.

Edwards, J., Francey, S.M., McGorry, P.D. and Jackson, H.J. (1994) Early psychosis prevention and intervention: Evolution of a comprehensive community-based specialised service. *Behaviour Change*, 11, 223–233.

Erlenmeyer-Kimling, L., Squires-Wheeler, E., Adamo, U.H., Bassett, A.S. *et al.* (1995) The New York High-Risk Project. *Archives of General Psychiatry*, 52, 857–865.

Fenton, W.S., Hibbeln, J. and Knable, M. (2000) Essential fatty acids, lipid membrane abnormalities, and the diagnosis and treatment of schizophrenia. *Biological Psychiatry*, 47, 8–21.

French, P. and Morrison, A.P. (2004) *Early Detection and Cognitive Therapy for People at High Risk of Developing Psychosis*. Wiley and Sons, New York.

French, P., Morrison, A.P., Walford, L., Knight, A. and Bentall, R. (2002) Cognitive therapy for preventing transition to psychosis in high-risk individuals: A single case study. In A.P. Morrison (ed.) *A Casebook of Cognitive Therapy for Psychosis*, pp. 219–235. Brunner-Routledge, New York.

Frith, C.D. (1992) *The Cognitive Neuropsychology of Schizophrenia.* Lawrence Erlbaum, Hove.

Garety, P.A. and Hemsley, D.R. (1994) *Delusions: Investigations into the psychology of delusional reasoning.* Oxford University Press, Oxford.

Garety, P.A., Fowler, D. and Kuipers, E. (2000) Cognitive-behavioral therapy for medication-resistant symptoms. *Schizophrenia Bulletin*, 26, 73–86.

Gleeson, J., Larsen, T.K. and McGorry, P. (2003) Psychological treatment in pre- and early psychosis. *Journal of the American Academy of Psychoanalysis and Dynamic Psychiatry*, 31, 229–245.

Gross, G. (1989) The 'basic' symptoms of schizophrenia. *British Journal of Psychiatry*, 155 (suppl. 7), 21–25.

Gross, G. (1997) The onset of schizophrenia. *Schizophrenia Research*, 28, 187–198.

Gumley, A., White, C. A. and Power, K. (1999) An interacting cognitive subsystems model of relapse and the course of psychosis. *Clinical Psychology and Psychotherapy*, 6.

Hafner, H., Maurer, K., Loffler, W., Fatkenheuer, B., Van Der Heiden, W., Riecher, R.A., Behrens, S. and Gattaz, W.F. (1994) The epidemiology of early schizophrenia. Influence of age and gender on onset and early course. *British Journal of Psychiatry* (supplement 23), 164, 29–38.

Hodges, A., Byrne, M., Grant, E. and Johnstone, E. (1999) People at risk of schizophrenia. *British Journal of Psychiatry*, 174, 547–553.

Huber, G. and Gross, G. (1989) The concept of basic symptoms in schizophrenic and schizoaffective psychoses. *Recenti Prog Med*, 80, 646–652.

Jackson, H., McGorry, P., Edwards, J., Hulbert, C., Henry, L., Francey, S., Maude, D., Cocks, J., Power, P., Harrigan, S. and Dudgeon, P. (1998) Cognitively-oriented psychotherapy for early psychosis (COPE): Preliminary results. *British Journal of Psychiatry*, 172, 93–100.

Javitt, D.C., Silipo, G., Cienfuegos, A., Shelley, A.M., Bark, N., Park, M., Lindenmayer, J.P., Suckow, R. and Zukin, S.R. (2001) Adjunctive high-dose glycine in the treatment of schizophrenia. *International Journal of Neuropsychpharmacology*, 4, 385–391.

Klosterkotter, J., Gross, G., Huber, G., Wieneke, A., Steinmeyer, E.M. and Schultze-lutter, F. (1997) Evaluation of the 'Bonn Scale for the Assessment of Basic Symptoms – BSABS' as an instrument for the assessment of schizophrenia proneness: A review of recent findings. *Neurology, Psychiatry and Brain Research*, 5, 137–150.

Klosterkotter, J., Hellmich, M., Steinmeyer, E.M. and Schultze-Lutter, F. (2001) Diagnosing schizophrenia in the initial prodromal phase. *Archives of General Psychiatry*, 58, 158–164.

Koehler, K. and Sauer, H. (1984) Huber's basic symptoms: Another approach to negative psychopathology in schizophrenia. *Comprehensive Psychiatry*, 25, 174–182.

Kuipers, E., Garety, P., Fowler, D.F., Dunn, G., Bebbington, P., Freeman, D. and Hadley, C. (1997) London-East Anglia randomised controlled trial of cognitive-behavioural therapy for psychosis. *British Journal of Psychiatry*, 171, 319–327.

Kulkarni, J., Riedel, A., de Castella, A.R., Fitzgerald, P.B., Rolfe, T.J., Taffe, J. and Burger, H. (2001) Estrogen: A potential treatment for schizophrenia. *Schizophrenia Research*, 48, 137–144.

Kulkarni, J., Riedel, A., de Castella, A.R., Fitzgerald, P.B., Rolfe, T.J., Taffe, J. and Burger, H. (2002) A clinical trial of adjunctive oestrogen treatment in women with schizophrenia. *Archives of Women's Mental Health*, 5, 99–104.

Manji, H.K., Moore, G.J. and Chen, G. (1999) Lithium at 50: Have the neuroprotective effects of this unique cation been overlooked? *Biological Psychiatry*, 46, 929–940.

McGlashan, T.H. (2001) Psychosis treatment prior to psychosis onset: Ethical issues. *Schizophrenia Research*, 51, 47–54.

McGlashan, T.H., Zipursky, R.B., Perkins, D.O., Addington, J., Woods, S.W., Miller, T.J. and Lindborg, S. (2004) Olanzapine versus placebo for prodromal schizophrenia. *Schizophr Res*, 67/1S, 6.

McGorry, P.D. (1993) Early psychosis prevention and intervention centre. *Australasian Psychiatry*, 1, 32–34.

McGorry, P.D., Edwards, J., Mihalopoulos, C., Harrigan, S.M. and Jackson, H.J. (1996) EPPIC: An evolving system of early detection and optimal management. *Schizophrenia Bulletin*, 22, 305–326.

McGorry, P.D. and Singh, B.S. (1995) Schizophrenia: risk and possibility. In G.D. Burrows (ed.) *Handbook of Preventive Psychiatry*, pp. 492–514. Elsevier, Amsterdam.

McGorry, P.D., Yung, A. and Phillips, L. (2001) Ethics and early intervention in psychosis: Keeping up the pace and staying in step. *Schizophrenia Research*, 51(1) Aug 2001, Netherlands.

McGorry, P.D., Yung, A.R., and Phillips, L.J. (2003) The "close-in" or Ultra High Risk Model: a safe and effective strategy for research and clinical intervention in prepsychotic mental disorder. *Schizophrenia Bulletin*, 29, 771–790.

McGorry, P.D., Yung, A.R., Phillips, L.J., Yuen, H.P., Francey, S., Cosgrave, E.M., Bravin, J., Adlard, S., MacDonald, T., Blair, A. and Jackson, H. (2002) Randomized controlled trial of interventions designed to reduce the risk of progression to first episode psychosis in a clinical sample with subthreshold symptoms. *Archives of General Psychiatry*, 59, 921–928.

Meares, A. (1959) The diagnosis of prepsychotic schizophrenia. *Lancet*, i, 55–59.

Morrison, A.P. (2001) The interpretation of intrusions in psychosis: An integrative cognitive approach to hallucinations and delusions. *Behavioural and Cognitive Psychotherapy*, 29, 257–276.

Morrison, A.P., Bentall, R.P., French, P., Walford, L., Kilcommons, A., Knight, A., Kreutz, M. and Lewis, S.W. (2002) Randomised controlled trial of early detection and cognitive therapy for preventing transition to psychosis in high-risk individuals. Study design and interim analysis of transition rate and psychological risk factors. *British Journal of Psychiatry – Supplementum*, 43, S78–S84.

Mrazek, P.J. and Haggerty, R.J. (eds) (1994) *Reducing Risks for Mental Disorders: frontiers for preventive intervention research*. National Academy Press, Washington D.C.

Rector, N.A. and Beck, A.T. (2001) Cognitive behavioral therapy for schizophrenia: an empirical review. *Journal of Nervous and Mental Disease*, 189, 278–287.

Sensky, T., Turkington, D., Kingdon, D., Scott, J.L., Scott, J., Siddle, R., O'Carroll, M. and Barnes, T.R. (2000) A randomised controlled trial of cognitive-behavioural therapy for persistent symptoms in schizophrenia resistant to medication. *Archives of General Psychiatry*, 57, 165–172.

Sullivan, H.S. (1994) The onset of schizophrenia. *American Journal of Psychiatry*, 151, 135–139.

Tarrier, N., Yusopoff, L., Kinney, C., McCarthy, E., Gledhill, A., Haddock, G. and Morris, J. (1998) Randomised controlled trial of intensive cognitive behaviour therapy for patients with chronic schizoprhenia. *British Medical Journal*, 317, 303–307.

Turkington, D., Kingdon, D. and Turner, T. (2002) Effectiveness of a brief cognitive-behavioural therapy intervention in the treatment of schizophrenia. *British Journal of Psychiatry*, 180, 523–527.

van Os, J., Hanssen, M., Bijl, R.V. and Vollebergh, W. (2001) Prevalence of psychotic disorder and community level of psychotic symptoms: An urban-rural comparison. *Archives of General Psychiatry*, 58, 663–668.

Yung, A. and McGorry, P. (2003) Keeping an open mind: Investigating options for treatment of the pre-psychotic phase. *Journal of Mental Health*, 12, 341–343.

Yung, A.R. and McGorry, P.D. (1996a) The initial prodrome in psychosis: Descriptive and qualitative aspects. *Australian and New Zealand Journal of Psychiatry,* 30, 587–599.

Yung, A.R. and McGorry, P.D. (1996b) The prodromal phase of first episode psychosis: past and current conceptualisations. *Schizophrenia Bulletin,* 22, 353–370.

Yung, A.R. and McGorry, P.D. (1997) Is pre-psychotic intervention realistic in schizophrenia and related disorders? *Australian and New Zealand Journal of Psychiatry,* 31, 799–805.

Yung, A.R., McGorry, P.D., McFarlane, C.A., Jackson, H.J. and *et al.* (1996) Monitoring and care of young people at incipient risk of psychosis. *Schizophrenia Bulletin,* 22, 283–303.

Yung, A.R., McGorry, P.D., McFarlane, C.A. and Patton, G. (1995) The PACE Clinic: Development of a clinical service for young people at high risk of psychosis. *Australasian Psychiatry,* 3, 345–349.

Yung, A.R., Phillips, L.J. and McGorry, P.D. (2004) *Treating Schizophrenia in the Pre-psychotic Phase.* Dunitz, London.

Chapter 12

Treatment of schizophrenia at the first episode

Delbert G. Robinson

Overview

Why focus upon treatment of the initial phase of schizophrenia? Treatment studies with first-episode patients are of interest for clinical reasons and also for our understanding of the actions of antipsychotic medications. The most basic clinical need for first episode treatment studies arises from the fact that first-episode patients by definition do not have an established response to treatment. Thus, treatment recommendations to first-episode patients and their families must be based upon research findings and not, as is the case with multi-episode patients, the patient's past individual response to treatment. In addition, data (McGlashan 1988) suggest that much of the deterioration associated with schizophrenia occurs during the first years of the illness. The development through research of better treatments for this period of the illness offers the promise of improving long-term course. Finally, if some forms of schizophrenia involve a neurodegenerative process (Lieberman *et al.* 1997), treatment response may change over the course of the illness. If this is the case, studies of treatment response during the initial, middle and later stages of the illness are needed to guide development of optimal treatment recommendations for each stage of the illness.

Besides its direct applicability to the treatment of first episode patients, treatment research with first episode patients is important for understanding the general effects of antipsychotic medications. Most treatment study samples contain largely chronic patients who have had multiple episodes of illness; these study samples may be systematically enriched in patients who are not fully responsive to treatment or not compliant with treatment (or both). Results from these studies may underestimate the effects of the medications tested.

The potential extent of the selection biases in usual studies with multi-episode subjects is demonstrated by the registration trials for risperidone (Chouinard *et al.* 1993; Marder and Meibach 1994), olanzapine (Beasley *et al.* 1996a, 1996b) and quetiapine (Arvanitis *et al.* 1997; Small *et al.* 1997). Table 12.1 shows the demographic characteristics of the 1657 subjects in these trials. Their average age is between 36 and 38 years old. They had been ill, on average, for more than 15 years. Many trial participants had experienced very frequent hospitalizations or episodes of illness. This degree of chronicity and associated refractoriness to treatment is not surprising. Patients who are doing well on their current medications are unlikely to volunteer for treatment with experimental medications. Do these trials provided us with an assessment of the potential full range of effects of these medications? The hypothesis that 38-year old patients with schizophrenia who have been ill for 15 years and experienced multiple hospitalizations are at least partially unresponsive to treatment is an untested and not directly testable hypothesis. However, the nature of the subjects strongly suggests an underrepresentation of responsive subjects in these trials.

First-episode patients have no or minimal previous exposure to treatment. First episode samples are therefore not subject to potential recruitment biases related to subjects' prior responses to treatment. First-episode samples may therefore be more representative of the full spectrum of treatment response in schizophrenia.

Table 12.1 Subject characteristics in registration trials

Study	N	Mean age	Age of onset	Prior hospitalizations/ episodes of illness
Risperidone				
Chouinard 1993	135	37	21	Mean (SD) of 7 (6) hospitalizations
Marder 1994	388	37	22	Mean (SD) of 9.1 (8.6) hospitalizations
Olanzapine				
Beasley 1996a	152	38	22	30.6% with 50 or more episodes
Beasley 1996b	335	36	22	30.4% with more than 20 episodes
Quetiapine				
Arvanitis 1997	361	37	22	30% with 6–10 hospitalizations; 26% with 11 or more hospitalizations
Small 1997	286	37	–	44% with more than 8 hospitalizations[1]

[1]Trial conducted in Europe and the US; data on hospitalizations collected on subjects (N = 169) from centers in US only.

Limitations of first episode studies

Conceptual limitations

Schizophrenia is an extremely complex disorder manifest by abnormalities in cognition, brain structure and function, social/vocational functioning as well as the clinical signs and symptoms of the disorder. The concept of a 'first episode' is usually defined by the first appearance of substantial clinical signs and symptoms of the disorder, by the first hospitalization for the disorder or by the initiation of first antipsychotic treatment. This is an arbitrary distinction from the point of view of the disorder as a whole. Abnormalities in cognition, brain function and social/vocational functioning may precede, sometimes by a long period, the onset of overt symptoms. Even considering only symptoms, many patients have depression, anxiety or other nonpsychotic symptoms before the onset of the classical symptoms of psychosis. Once severe psychotic symptoms appear, follow-up studies have found a substantial percentage of patients have a pattern of persistent, as opposed to episodic, symptoms. This combined with the persistence of abnormalities in cognition, brain function and social/vocational functioning even at times of symptom remission raises questions about the validity of the concept of illness episodes in schizophrenia. Nonetheless, the initiation of antipsychotic treatment is an important event in the clinical course of patients. 'First episode' is a useful concept from this perspective although one must be mindful that it may not accurately characterize the course of the multidimensional deficits found in schizophrenia.

Study design limitations

Although of interest for clinical and scientific reasons, first episode studies are difficult to perform due to the small number of potential subjects available. Compared with the large number of patients with multi-episode schizophrenia, there are relatively few new cases of schizophrenia each year. Because schizophrenia is usually a chronic disorder, these few new cases are enough to maintain the high prevalence of the disorder. Because of its low incidence, studies of first episode schizophrenia typically either have small sample sizes that limit interpretation of the results or take a long time to finish due to the time needed to collect adequate samples. In this case, we often lack data on the most recently introduced treatments. This is especially true for studies examining long-term outcomes with newer treatments. Unfortunately, long-term studies are precisely the studies that are the most informative for making treatment decisions about chronic disorders such as schizophrenia.

The gap between the data that are available and the data that are needed is particularly glaring at this time for first episode studies. Given data from studies with multi-episode subjects that the second generation agents have lower risks than the older agents of causing tardive dyskinesia, the second generation agents quickly replaced the older medications as first-line treatments in many parts of the world. Several first episode studies using the second generation antipsychotics that follow subjects for several years are about to be completed or have been completed but have not yet published. Over the next few years, these studies will provide the data for understanding the effects of the second generation agents in first episode populations. In the meantime, data from long-term studies with the older agents provide a basis for answering many basic questions about the treatment of first episode schizophrenia and also a benchmark for treatment outcomes to compare with the results for the second generation agents.

This chapter will present data on treatment response during the initial phase of schizophrenia. First, response of the first episode will be discussed followed by consideration of strategies for relapse prevention and improvement of long-term outcome.

Treatment of the first episode

On the whole, response rates for the first episode are high. Antipsychotic treatment trials lasting several weeks have reported response rates averaging around 60 per cent (e.g. Scottish Schizophrenia Research Group 1987; Kopala *et al.* 1996; McCreadie 1996) with both first and second generation antipsychotics. Although this degree of response is better than that usually reported for treatment with multi-episode patients, the response rate of first episode patients to more extended treatment is even better.

In a long-term study at our center (Robinson *et al.* 1999a), 118 patients with first episode schizophrenia or schizoaffective disorder were assessed at baseline, treated according to a standardized medication algorithm and assessed prospectively. Subjects progressed from one medication in the algorithm to the next until they responded. The sequence of medications were: fluphenazine; haloperidol; haloperidol plus lithium; either molindone or loxapine; clozapine. Adjuvant medications for mood stabilization and side effects were used as clinically warranted. The sample was 52 per cent male, had a mean (SD) age of 25.2 (6.6) years, was 41 per cent white, 37 per cent African-American, 12 per cent hispanic, 7 per cent asian and 3 per cent mixed racial or ethnic background. There was a range of socioeconomic classes and educational levels, but a predominance of middle class and below (mean SES on the Hollingshead Redlich Scale (Hollingshead and Redlich 1958) was 3.4 (1.3)).

Patients had been ill for an extended period, a mean of 143 (205) weeks since the onset of first behavioral changes related to the illness and 71 (150) weeks since the onset of first psychotic symptoms. At study entry they were severely ill with a mean (SD) Clinical Global Impression Scale (CGI) (Guy 1976) score of 5.5 (1.0) and a Global Assessment Scale (GAS) (Endicott *et al.* 1976) score of 27.1 (9.0). Diagnoses, based upon Research Diagnostic Criteria (Spitzer *et al.* 1977), were schizophrenia, N = 83 (53 per cent paranoid, 11 per cent undifferentiated, 4 per cent disorganized, 2 per cent catatonic subtypes) and schizoaffective disorder, N = 35. Seventy-three percent had no antipsychotics prior to admission; 16 per cent had less than two weeks of medication; and 11 per cent had between 2 and 12 weeks of exposure.

The cumulative percentage of patients responding by one year was 87 per cent. This response rate is very remarkable given that the response criterion was more stringent than those used in most treatment trials in schizophrenia. To be classified as a responder, subjects could not have active delusions, hallucinations or thought disorder. Emphasizing the need for prolonged treatment in some subjects before response, the median time to response was nine weeks.

Despite the overall good response to treatment, some first episode patients are refractory to treatment from the onset of their illness. Of our original sample of 118 subjects, ten subjects failed to meet response criteria despite being treated for one year or longer. They were followed in the study for 12 to 76 months and had persistent severe positive symptoms throughout. Seven of the ten had a trial of clozapine. Clozapine was discontinued in three due to non-response and continued in four patients long-term; these four patients were better able to remain in the community despite continued positive symptoms. Two patients also received ECT and two were eventually placed in state hospital facilities. Development of novel treatment strategies for patients who fail initial treatment is clearly needed.

Besides fulfilling the clinical need to help a severely ill patient population, studies of patients with treatment resistance from illness onset may also be interesting as a means to study the mechanisms of treatment resistance. Given the small number of treatment-resistant subjects in our study, we had a limited ability to find correlates of nonresponse. However, it was striking that all but two of the subjects were men and all were diagnosed as having schizophrenia whereas 30 per cent of the entire sample were diagnosed with schizoaffective disorder. Also of note was that some first episode subjects did not respond to clozapine, either after having had trials of other antipsychotics or in another study at our center using clozapine as a first treatment.

Predictors of response to treatment of the initial episode have been identified. In our study, the following variables were significantly associated (p <0.01) with less likelihood of response to treatment: male gender, subjects' birth complicated by obstetric complications, more severe hallucinations and delusions and poorer attention at baseline, and the development of Parkinsonism during antipsychotic treatment. In addition, longer duration of psychotic symptoms prior to treatment may be associated with poorer response to antipsychotics. Duration of untreated psychosis was significantly associated with treatment response in an interim analysis of our study (Loebel *et al.* 1992); the association was at the trend level using data from the full sample (Robinson *et al.* 1999a). Unlike most of the identified correlates of non-response that are not changeable, duration of untreated psychosis is a potential risk factor for non-response which can be modified. Most centers have found that patients have psychotic symptoms for a year or longer before obtaining treatment. For example, our subjects had active psychotic symptoms for a mean of 71 weeks before entering the study (Robinson *et al.* 1999a). If longer duration of psychosis before treatment is actively toxic, shortening the duration of symptoms before initiating treatment may increase the chance of response. This interpretation of the data is attractive as it suggests a practical method to modify illness course, given that long duration of symptoms in the community could be decreased by community education and outreach. However, this hypothesis needs to be studied and confirmed. An alternate explanation of the data is that delay in seeking treatment is part of an overall process that is associated with a poor treatment response. For example, being part of a family that tolerates a child having psychotic symptoms for a long period before seeking treatment may itself have a poor effect on outcome. In this case, efforts to shorten the duration of symptoms before obtaining treatment would be commendable for reducing patient suffering but would not necessarily modify long term course.

Maintenance treatment and relapse prevention

In contrast to the favorable clinical response for treatment of the initial episode, relapse is frequent during the first years of the illness and may be associated with clinical deterioration (McGlashan 1988). Previous studies have used different definitions of relapse, employed a variety of treatments, and reported a range of relapse rates. Despite this variability, some general trends are evident. In the first year, relapse rates in published studies (Rabiner *et al.* 1986; Kane *et al.* 1982; Linszen *et al.* 1994) are relatively low. The highest rate (Kane *et al.* 1982) was 41 per cent in patients (N = 17) taking placebo.

In contrast, only 17 per cent of patients relapsed over 15 months in the study by Linszen and colleagues with a larger sample (N = 69) receiving treatment. After the first year, relapse rates (Crow *et al.* 1986; Rajkumar and Thara 1989; Leff *et al.* 1990; Scottish Schizophrenia Research Group 1992; Geddes *et al.* 1994; Linszen *et al.* 1994; Zhang *et al.* 1994) rise substantially with published rates of between 35 per cent after 18 months (Zhang *et al.* 1994) and 74 per cent after 5 years of follow-up (Scottish Schizophrenia Research Group 1992).

Long term follow-up (Robinson *et al.* 1999b) of the Hillside sample described above confirmed and expanded the results of these studies. The cumulative rate for first relapse was 82 per cent during the five year follow-up period. Many subjects had multiple relapses. The cumulative rate for a second relapse among subjects who responded from a first relapse was 78.0 per cent after five years. Similarly, the cumulative rate for a third relapse was 86.2 per cent (95 per cent C.I. 61.5 per cent, 100 per cent) by the end of four years among the patients who recovered from their second relapse.

Stopping antipsychotic medication substantially increased the risk of relapse. The risks of relapse for both the first and second relapse were almost five times greater off than on medication (hazard ratio for the first relapse = 4.89; for the second relapse, hazard ratio = 4.57).

How long should maintenance treatment last? So far, maintenance studies have not found a point at which maintenance treatment is not beneficial. Placebo-controlled first episode studies (Kane *et al.* 1982; Crow *et al.* 1986) have shown significant benefits for antipsychotic maintenance during one and two years of follow-up. Our study using a treatment algorithm design also showed significant benefits for maintenance treatment during the first two years of follow-up. Data for maintenance treatment after two years is limited. In our study, we had only 15 patients who relapsed for the first time after 2 years of stability; eight of these patients had discontinued medication when they relapsed, suggesting the continued importance of maintenance medication.

Patients (and often their families) are very eager to know if they are among the very few who can stop maintenance antipsychotics for prolonged periods without relapsing. Unfortunately, first episode research has identified very few predictors of relapse besides stopping antipsychotics, despite examining many candidate variables. For example, diagnosis, obstetric complications, duration of psychotic illness prior to treatment, severity of index episode symptoms and motor findings, homovanillic acid and growth hormone measures, psychotic symptom activation to methylphenidate, neuropsychological and MR measures, and the presence of residual symptoms after the initial episode were not related to time to relapse in our sample. Time to response of the initial episode was also not predictive of relapse. This later finding is important because of the widely held, but incorrect, perception that patients who respond quickly during their first episode have a good prognosis and may not 'need' antipsychotics. This clinical perception is false.

In our sample, we did find that subjects with poor premorbid adaptation to school and premorbid social withdrawal relapsed earlier. An earlier Hillside first episode study (Kane *et al.* 1982) also found a significant association between social isolation in childhood and adolescence and relapse for first episode patients on placebo maintenance. Although subjects with good premorbid functioning were less likely to relapse in both studies, the difference in relapse risk between subjects with poor and good premorbid social adjustment is not large enough to be useful clinically to identify patients who might safely stop antipsychotic maintenance treatment.

Treatment adherence

Because there are no clinically useful methods to determine who might be able to stop antipsychotic maintenance treatment, enhancing adherence with antipsychotic treatment is the only practical method available to prevent patients from having multiple relapses. Thus methods to enhance patient adherence to treatment are of great interest. Studies with primarily multi-episode patients (recently reviewed in Fenton *et al.* 1997; Kampman and Lehtinen 1999) have identified several consistent correlates of medication refusal. These include: more severe psychopathology, lack of insight, comorbid substance abuse, presence of medication side effects, an absence of social supports from family or friends, and practical barriers such as inability to afford medications.

Despite the numerous studies of medication adherence in schizophrenia, information specifically about first episode patients is very limited. Separate studies with first episode patients are of interest because first episode patients and their families lack experience with antipsychotics and with the chronic and relapsing course of schizophrenia. Their assessment of the benefits versus liabilities of antipsychotics may differ from those of multi-episode patients who have experienced the adverse consequences associated with repeated relapses.

To explore medication adherence by subjects in the Hillside study, we examined (Robinson *et al.* 2002) two periods, the first year after initiating antipsychotic treatment for the initial episode and the period following a first relapse of illness. We defined medication discontinuation as failure to take prescribed medication for one week or longer. This definition was chosen because stopping medication for a week clearly indicates a problem with acceptance of antipsychotic treatment (as opposed to 'just forgetting' a dose) and would in most cases prompt a major effort by a clinical team to encourage a patient to resume antipsychotics.

Treatment refusal during the first year

Of the 118 patients entering the study, six patients were not eligible for the analyses because we could not determine if medication discontinuation against medical advice (e.g. subjects who transferred their care to another facility) occurred during the first year. Of the remaining 112 subjects, 29 patients stopped antipsychotic medication for one week or longer against our advice during the first year of the study. The great majority of these subjects refused antipsychotics for a substantial period. Patients who stopped antipsychotics within the first year had poorer estimated premorbid cognitive ability than patients who consistently took medication. The two groups did not differ on demographic characteristics, premorbid social functioning, delay in starting treatment after the onset of psychosis, diagnosis, severity of clinical symptoms, presence of motor side effects to treatment or family member attitudes.

Treatment refusal after the first relapse

Sixty-three patients recovered from their first relapse and continued in the study for at least 100 days following recovery. Forty-four (22 men, 22 women) continued on antipsychotics during their remaining time in the study; nineteen (7 men, 12 women) stopped antipsychotics.

The following variables significantly predicted medication discontinuation after response to the first relapse: lower parental social class, less education, stopping antipsychotics during the first year of the study, depressive symptoms during the first relapse, Parkinsonism during treatment of the first relapse and executive dysfunction. Patients with worse overall course as measured by the highest Global Assessment Scale score obtained after the first relapse were also more likely to discontinue medication but the hazard ratio failed to reach significance ($p = 0.08$). In subsequent multivariate analyses, Parkinsonism (hazard ratio = 41.22; 95 per cent CI = 2.30, 737.89; $p = 0.01$) continued to predict medication discontinuation and better executive function (hazard ratio = 0.40; 95 per cent CI = 0.18, 0.88; $p = 0.02$) continued to predict medication adherence.

Clinical implications of the findings

Medication discontinuation is a major problem in the treatment of first episode patients; twenty-six percent of our patients stopped antipsychotics during the first year of treatment and thirty per cent stopped antipsychotics during maintenance treatment following the first relapse. Our predictor analyses suggest that factors associated with treatment adherence may change over the early illness course. Regarding potential interventions to enhance adherence, our results would encourage clinicians to have a low threshold for treating depression and extrapyramidal side effects. Our cognitive findings also imply that the relationship between cognitive deficits and stopping medication may be more complex than just 'forgetting to take medication' as frequently reported by patients. In particular, our analyses highlighted the association of executive function deficits and medication discontinuation. Executive function deficits may compromise patients' ability to organize complex medication regimens. Simplifying complex medication regimes may be important to enhance adherence for subjects with executive deficits.

Other outcomes

Although acute treatment response and relapse are core measures of treatment outcome, other domains are also crucial in evaluating outcome and should not be overlooked. A striking example of this is the persistence of cognitive deficits in patients whose symptoms respond to treatment. After stabilization of the initial psychotic episode, 94 of the Hillside subjects (Bilder *et al.* 2000) were tested with a comprehensive cognitive battery which included 41 tests. Tests were grouped to characterize six domains: language, memory, attention, executive, motor and visuospatial function. Compared with a healthy control group, every cognitive scale was more impaired in the patient group, with mean effect sizes (in z-score units, reflecting the number of standard deviations below the comparison group means) ranging from −1.11 to −1.75. The overall profile mean was −1.53, indicating a generalized deficit of approximately 1.5 standard deviations. Comparing the different scales, executive functioning and memory were the most impaired and language functioning the least impaired.

An important outcome for patients and their families is social and vocational functioning. As with cognition, social and vocational deficits may be present despite improvement in clinical symptoms. By five years in follow-up, only 25.5 per cent of the Hillside sample (95 per cent CI = 16.1 per cent, 34.7 per cent) had sustained good social functioning for two years or more as defined by fulfillment of age-appropriate role expectations, performance of daily living tasks without supervision, and engagement in social interactions.

Future directions

In summary, most patients have a robust response to treatment of the first episode with antipsychotic medications. However, relapse is the rule and is often the consequence of medication refusal. The cumulative effect is that most patients are not able to achieve a sustained good clinical outcome during the initial years of treatment. Given possible advantages treating cognition and negative symptoms and different side effect profiles, the second generation agents have the potential to improve these outcomes. Will the second generation agents fulfill this promise? So far, several short-term studies comparing second generation and first generation agents in first episode populations have been published. The study with the largest number of subjects was reported by Emsley and colleagues (Emsley and the Risperidone Working Group 1999). The study compared six-week outcomes in 183 first episode subjects assigned to haloperidol (mean end point daily dose 5.6 mg) or risperidone (mean end point daily dose 6.1 mg). Response rates, defined by a 50 per cent reduction in total Positive and Negative Syndrome Scale (PANSS) (Kay *et al.* 1987) scores, did not differ between the groups. Response rates for the haloperidol and risperidone treated groups were 56 per cent and 63 per cent, respectively. For olanzapine, the largest published study is a post hoc analysis by Sanger and colleagues (1999) of 83 first episode subjects who participated in a previously reported 6 week long study with 1996 subjects comparing haloperidol and olanzapine treatment. Inclusion in the first-episode analysis was based upon the subject being in their first episode of psychosis. Prior antipsychotic treatment varied widely within the first-episode subsample. Fifty-nine first episode subjects were assigned to olanzapine (mean modal dose 11.6 mg) and 24 to haloperidol (mean modal dose 10.8 mg). Response rates, based upon a 40 per cent improvement in Brief Psychiatric Rating Scale (BPRS) (Overall and Gorham 1962) total scores derived from a PANSS interview, were 67.2 per cent for olanzapine-treated subjects and 29.2 per cent for haloperidol-treated subjects. Although the study found a large advantage for olanzapine treatment, interpretation of the Sanger *et al.* study is limited by its post hoc nature and the use of high doses of haloperidol. Of note also is the extremely low response rate of the haloperidol-treated subjects in the Sanger *et al.* study in comparison with the response rates obtained in other studies using first generation antipsychotics.

Because acute treatment response rates can be high with first generation agents but relapse is common and long-term adherence a problem, studies longer than six weeks are clearly needed to address the primary clinical challenges confronting the field. The field anxiously awaits the results of longer studies with the second generation antipsychotics to find if they can surpass the long-term outcomes from first generation agents. The importance of a long-term perspective was shown by a study (Robinson *et al.* 1997) performed at our center, subsequent to the large study using first generation agents previously discussed. Our reasoning was that clozapine may be the 'most powerful' antipsychotic currently available given its efficacy in treatment-resistant schizophrenia. Would long-term outcome be better if patients took clozapine from the beginning of their illness instead of the usual practice of reserving clozapine for patients with the most severe forms of schizophrenia? To answer this question, 34 subjects with first episode schizophrenia or schizoaffective disorder were treated with clozapine as their first antipsychotic treatment. The study design was the same as our previous study except for the substitution of clozapine as the initial medication. Mean time in follow-up was 114 weeks. The response rate to acute treatment was no higher than in our earlier study. Further, only 6 of the 19 subjects who responded acutely to clozapine were still taking clozapine when they ended study participation. This low rate of adherence to clozapine prevented assessment of whether long-term clozapine treatment would result in better outcomes. Clozapine has unique barriers (e.g. frequent blood collections) to long-term adherence. Thus outcomes with clozapine treatment may not generalize to treatment with other second generation agents. However, our clozapine outcomes do highlight that even the best antipsychotics cannot help patients who do not take the medications. Thus, we may need not only better medications but also better ways to enhance adherence if we are to succeed in the goal of improving the lives of patients in the early course of schizophrenia.

References

Arvanitis LA, Miller BG and the Seroquel Trial 13 Study Group (1997). Multiple fixed doses of 'Seroquel' (quetiapine) in patients with acute exacerbation of schizophrenia: A comparison with haloperidol and placebo. *Biological Psychiatry*, 42, 233–46.

Beasley CM, Jr., Sanger T, Satterlee W, Tollefson G, Tran P, Hamilton S and The Olanzapine HGAP Study Group (1996a). Olanzapine versus placebo: results of a double-blind, fixed-dose olanzapine trial, *Psychopharmacology*, 124, 159–67.

Beasley CM, Jr., Tollefson G, Tran P, Satterlee W, Sanger T, Hamilton S and The Olanzapine HGAD Study Group (1996b). Olanzapine versus placebo and haloperidol. Acute phase results of the North American double-blind olanzapine trial. *Neuropsychopharmacology*, 14, 111–23.

Bilder RM, Goldman RS, Robinson D, Reiter G, Bell L, Bates JA, Pappadopulos E, Willson DF, Alvir JM, Woerner MG, Geisler S, Kane JM, Lieberman JA (2000). Neuropsychology of first-episode schizophrenia: Initial characterization and clinical correlates. *American Journal of Psychiatry*, 157, 549–559.

Chouinard G, Jones B, Remington G, Bloom D, Addington D, MacEwan GW, Labelle A, Beauclair L, Arnott W (1993). A Canadian multicenter placebo-controlled study of fixed doses of risperidone and haloperidol in the treatment of chronic schizophrenic patients. *Journal of Clinical Psychopharmacology*, 13, 25–40.

Crow TJ, Macmillan JF, Johnson AL, Johnstone EC (1986). A randomised controlled trial of prophylactic neuroleptic treatment. *British Journal of Psychiatry*, 148, 120–7.

Emsley RA and the Risperidone Working Group (1999). Risperidone in the treatment of first-episode psychotic patients: a double-blind multicenter study, *Schizophrenia Bulletin*, 25, 721–9.

Endicott J, Spitzer RL, Fleiss JL, Cohen J (1976). The Global Assessment Scale: a procedure for measuring overall severity of psychiatric disturbance. *Archives of General Psychiatry*, 33, 766–71.

Fenton WS, Blyler CR, Heinssen RK (1997). Determinants of medication compliance in schizophrenia: empirical and clinical findings. *Schizophrenia Bulletin*, 23, 637–51.

Geddes J, Mercer G, Frith CD, MacMillan F, Owens DGC, Johnstone EC (1994). Prediction of outcome following a first episode of schizophrenia. A follow-up study of Northwick Park first episode study subjects. *British Journal of Psychiatry*, 165, 664–8.

Guy W (1976). *ECDEU Assessment Manual for Psychopharmacology*, revised. DHEW Publication No. (ABM) 76–338, pp. 217–22. US Government Printing office, Washington DC.

Hollingshead AB, Redlich FC (1958). *Social Class and Mental Illness; a Community Study*. Wiley, New York.

Kampman O, Lehtinen K (1999). Compliance in psychoses. *Acta psychiatrica Scandinavica*, 100, 167–75.

Kane JM, Rifkin A, Quitkin F, Nayak D, Ramos Lorenzi J (1982). Fluphenazine vs placebo in patients with remitted, acute first-episode schizophrenia. *Archives of General Psychiatry*, 39, 70–73.

Kay SR, Fiszbein A, Opler LA (1987). The positive and negative syndrome scale (PANSS) for schizophrenia. *Schizophrenia Bulletin*, 13, 261–76.

Kopala LC, Fredrikson D, Good KP, Honer WG (1996). Symptoms in neuroleptic-naive, first-episode schizophrenia: Response to risperidone. *Biological Psychiatry*, 39, 296–98.

Leff J, Wig NN, Bedi H, Menon DK, Kuipers L, Korten A, Ernberg G, Day R, Sartorius N, Jablensky A (1990). Relatives' expressed emotion and the course of schziophrenia in Candigarh. A two-year follow-up of a first-contact sample. *British Journal of Psychiatry*, 156, 351–6.

Lieberman JA, Sheitman BB, Kinon BJ (1997). Neurochemical sensitization in the pathophysiology of schizophrenia: deficits and dysfunction in neuronal regulation and plasticity. *Neuropsychopharmacology*, 17, 205–29.

Linszen DH, Dingemans PM, Lenior ME (1994). Cannabis abuse and the course of recent-onset schizophrenic disorders. *Archives of General Psychiatry*, 51, 273–9.

Loebel AD, Lieberman JA, Alvir JM, Mayerhoff DI, Geisler SH, Szymanski SR (1992). Duration of psychosis and outcome in first-episode schizophrenia. *American Journal of Psychiatry*, 149, 1183–8.

Marder SR, Meibach RC (1994). Risperidone in the treatment of schizophrenia. *American Journal of Psychiatry*, 151, 825–35.

McCreadie RG (1996). Managing the first episode of schizophrenia: the role of new therapies. *European Neuropsychopharmacology*, 6 (2), S3–S5.

McGlashan TH (1988). A selective review of recent North American long-term follow up studies of schizophrenia. *Schizophrenia Bulletin*, 14, 515–42.

Overall JE, Gorham DR (1962). The Brief Psychiatric Rating Scale. *Psychological Reports*, 10, 799–812.

Rabiner CJ, Wegner JT, Kane JM (1986). Outcome study of first episode psychosis: I. Relapse rates after 1 year. *American Journal of Psychiatry*, 143, 1155–8.

Rajkumar S and Thara R (1989). Factors affecting relapse in schizophrenia. *Schizophrenia Research*, 2, 403–9.

Robinson DG, Lieberman JA, Sheitman B, Alvir JM, Kane JM (1997). Pilot study of atypical antipsychotic agents in first episode schizophrenia. *Schizophrenia Research*, 24, 196.

Robinson D, Woerner M, Alvir J Ma J, Geisler S, Koreen A, Sheitman B, Chakos M, Mayerhoff D, Bilder R, Goldman R, Lieberman JA (1999a). Predictors of treatment response from a first episode of schizophrenia or schizoaffective disorder. *American Journal of Psychiatry*, 156, 544–9.

Robinson D, Woerner M, Alvir J, Ma J, Bilder R, Goldman R, Geisler S, Koreen A, Sheitman B, Chakos M, Mayerhoff D, Lieberman JA (1999b). Predictors of relapse following response from a first episode of schizophrenia or schizoaffective disorder. *Archives of General Psychiatry*, 56, 241–7.

Robinson DG, Woerner MG, Alvir J, Ma J, Bilder RM, Hinrichsen GA, Lieberman JA (2002). Predictors of medication discontinuation by patients with first-episode schizophrenia and schizoaffective disorder. *Schizophrenia Research*, 57, 209–19.

Sanger TM, Lieberman JA, Tohen M, Grundy S, Beasley C Jr, Tollefson GD (1999). Olanzapine versus haloperidol treatment in first-episode psychosis. *American Journal of Psychiatry*, 156, 79–87.

Scottish Schizophrenia Research Group (1987). The Scottish first episode schizophrenia study. II. Treatment: pimozide versus flupenthixol. *British Journal of Psychiatry*, 150, 334–8.

Scottish Schizophrenia Research Group (1992). The Scottish First Episode Schizophrenia Study VIII: Five-year follow-up: Clinical and psychosocial findings. *British Journal of Psychiatry*, 161, 496–500.

Small JG, Hirsch SR, Arvanitis LA, Miller BG, Link CG and the Seroquel Study Group (1997). Quetiapine in patients with schizophrenia. *Archives of General Psychiatry*, 54, 549–57.

Spitzer RL, Endicott J, Robins E (1977). *Research Diagnostic Criteria (RDC) for a Selected Group of Functional Disorders*, New York Biometrics Research Division, New York.

Zhang M, Wang M, Li J, Phillips MR (1994). Randomised-control trial of family intervention for 78 first-episode male schizophrenia patients. An 18-month study in Suzhou, Jiangsu. *British Journal of Psychiatry*, 165 (suppl. 24), 96–102.

Chapter 13

Treatment of late-life schizophrenia

Gauri V. Nayak, David P. Folsom,
Elizabeth W. Twamley, and Dilip V. Jeste

There have been major advances in the treatment of schizophrenia during the past decade. A large part of the research, however, has been focused on younger patients with early (i.e., typical) onset of the illness. More recently, there has been an increasing awareness of the needs of older patients with schizophrenia. This population includes older patients with early-onset schizophrenia, as well as patients with late-onset schizophrenia (LOS), who first experienced psychotic symptoms in the later part of their lives, i.e., after age 40. It has been estimated that 23.5 per cent of individuals with schizophrenia have an onset of illness after age 40 (Harris and Jeste 1988), with only a small proportion experiencing symptoms for the first time after 60 years of age (Howard et al. 1993).

Late-onset schizophrenia (LOS) is not a novel phenomenon. Manfred Bleuler (1943) recognized and documented cases wherein symptoms of the illness first emerged after 40 years of age. Despite the early recognition of LOS, DSM-III diagnostic criteria for schizophrenia included symptom onset prior to age 45 (American Psychiatric Association 1980). Although existing classification systems (i.e., DSM-IV and ICD-10) no longer have this age criterion, they do not include separate diagnostic criteria for LOS. Recently, an international consensus formally acknowledged the existence of LOS (illness onset after 40 years) and very-late-onset schizophrenia-like psychosis (illness onset after 60 years) (Howard et al. 2000). The report characterized these distinct diagnostic categories and proposed guidelines for treatment. The recognition of these categories is vital for directing research toward treatment strategies for LOS. This is especially important to avoid a misdiagnosis of dementia, which has quite different treatment guidelines from those for LOS.

Clinicians face a common challenge of adapting treatment protocols that are effective in younger patients for the treatment of older patients. In addition, the symptom profile and treatment for patients with LOS are different from those for older patients who have been ill for many years. Older patients with earlier onset tend to have both positive and negative symptoms for decades and have been on neuroleptic medication for extended periods of time, while age-comparable patients with LOS have primarily positive symptoms and have functioned without any signs of the illness for most of their adult lives. Most clinical studies of older patients with schizophrenia include both early and late onset of illness. In this chapter, we will discuss the pharmacological as well as psychosocial treatments that have been adapted for use with patients with LOS as well as older patients with early-onset illness.

Presentation of late-onset schizophrenia (LOS)

The purpose of discussing epidemiology and symptom picture of LOS is twofold: to suggest that LOS is 'true' schizophrenia, and at the same time, to indicate that it has distinctive features that call for somewhat different treatment considerations from those for early-onset schizophrenia. Studies comparing patients with early and late onset schizophrenia have found some similarities between the two groups, such as a predominance of auditory hallucinations and persecutory delusions (Kay and Roth 1961; Rabins *et al.* 1984; Jeste *et al.* 1995b) and significant neuropsychological impairment compared to normal subjects on measures of executive functioning, learning, and psychomotor skills (Jeste *et al.* 1995b). However, the early onset patients tend to have more severe negative symptoms (e.g., emotional blunting, Harris and Jeste 1988), more disorganized thought and speech (e.g., incoherence and circumstantiality, Kay and Roth 1961), and more abnormal personality traits (e.g., reclusiveness and suspiciousness, Castle and Howard 1992; Kay and Roth 1961). Patients with LOS are frequently characterized by the paranoid subtype, and have less severe negative symptoms (Jeste *et al.* 1995b). Although patients with LOS may have some difficulties with premorbid interpersonal functioning, they are more likely to be married and have children and better occupational adjustment prior to illness (Owen and Castle 1999).

LOS is also consistently found to be more prevalent in women (Harris and Jeste 1988; Castle and Murray 1993), and several studies have implicated the possible role of estrogen, which may modulate the dopamine system prior to menopause (Seeman *et al.* 1996). In addition, some major problems associated with the presence of comorbid physical conditions include exacerbation of existing chronic illness, e.g., cardiovascular disease and diabetes mellitus; and drug–drug interactions (Sciolla and Jeste 1998; Owen and Castle 1999). Clinicians must also be aware that regardless of the age of onset, there is a high risk of suicide in schizophrenia patients in the first ten years after illness-onset (Heilä *et al.* 1997; Radomsky *et al.* 1999). There are a few reports of remission of late-onset schizophrenia. Jeste *et al.* (2000) published a case report of an individual who developed schizophrenia-like psychosis at age 52, which remitted after six years of antipsychotic medication therapy. Four years after remission, he continued to function independently, without psychotropic medication, and no relapse of psychiatric symptoms.

Course of early-onset schizophrenia in late life

In contrast to the Kraepelinian concept of dementia praecox, the course of schizophrenia in late life is variable and is generally much more benign than that of a dementing disorder. Jeste *et al.* (2003b) studied the relationship of age to clinical features, psychopathology, movement abnormalities, quality of well-being, and everyday functioning in normal comparison subjects and patients with schizophrenia. The findings suggested aging-associated improvement in overall psychopathology and positive symptoms. The investigators also found that older patients benefited from lower daily doses of neuroleptics medication than younger patients; the reason for this may be that aging is associated with reductions in dopamine, norepinephrine, and serotonin levels and receptor sensitivity. Older patients are also at a greater risk for neuroleptics-induced extra-pyramidal symptoms (EPS) and tardive dyskinesia (TD) (Jeste *et al.* 2003b).

Treatment

Early studies of LOS included treatment with electroconvulsive therapy (ECT), sometimes adjunctive with chlorpromazine or another phenothiazine, which was found to produce temporary remission (Post 1966). Research on conventional neuroleptics found that phenothiazines such as trifluoperazine and thioridazine were more effective than non-neuroleptic medications. More recent studies have found that conventional neuroleptics including haloperidol, which block dopamine receptors, increase the risk for EPS, TD, and other severe side effects in older patients (Sciolla and Jeste 1998; Jeste *et al.* 1999b). Anticholinergic medications are used to treat EPS; however, in older patients, these medications may cause or worsen cognitive impairment, delirium, confusion, sedation, constipation, blurred vision, and increased heart rate. It is important to note that very few treatment studies that focused on patients with LOS have been published. As a result, most of the discussion below is extrapolated from studies of older schizophrenia patients, regardless of age of onset. It is known, however, that patients with LOS require lower daily doses of antipsychotics than similarly aged persons with early onset schizophrenia.

Atypical antipsychotic agents, which act on both dopamine and serotonin receptors, are useful in the management of psychosis and severe behavioral disturbances in the elderly. These drugs include clozapine, risperidone, olanzapine, quetiapine, ziprasidone, and aripiprazole. Atypical antipsychotics are the first-line treatments for older patients with schizophrenia because they are associated with a significantly lower incidence of EPS and TD compared to conventional neuroleptics (Jeste *et al.* 1995a). There is mixed evidence that the atypical antipsychotic medications may produce mild improvements in some of the neurocognitive impairments found in patients with schizophrenia.

Clozapine

Clozapine was considered to be a 'wonder drug' when it was first introduced in 1988. It was found to be superior in managing treatment-resistant psychotic symptoms and severe TD (Sajatovic *et al.* 1998). In a review of literature on the effects of atypical antipsychotics on cognition in schizophrenia, Meltzer and McGurk (1999) found evidence that clozapine improved attention and verbal fluency. Most studies, however, were conducted with younger patients, and clozapine's clinical utility is somewhat limited in older patients with schizophrenia. The risk of agranulocytosis is the most serious side effect of clozapine, and the risk of fatal agranulocytosis is higher in older patients than in younger adults. Other side effects of clozapine that may be more clinically relevant for older patients include postural hypotension, sedation, anticholinergic effects, and lowering of the seizure threshold (Sciolla and Jeste 1998). A number of case studies have reported an increased risk of metabolic side effects such as weight gain, type 2 diabetes mellitus, and hyperlipidemia with clozapine (as well as with olanzapine and some other atypical antipsychotics) (Jin *et al.* 2002). Clozapine is, therefore, not the drug of choice for most elderly patients with LOS.

Risperidone

Risperidone has been the most commonly used atypical antipsychotic in older patients with schizophrenia. Double-blind studies comparing risperidone with haloperidol indicated that risperidone had better efficacy and tolerability in younger adult patients. Studies in older adults showed significantly lower risk of EPS and TD with risperidone than with typical neuroleptics (Jeste *et al.* 1999a, b). At the same time, it should be pointed out that higher doses of risperidone are associated with increased risks of EPS, postural hypotension, and hyperprolactinemia. A recent large multisite international double-blind study by Jeste *et al.* (2003a) involved a comparison of risperidone and olanzapine effects in 176 elderly patients with schizophrenia. The researchers found that, over an eight-week period, both drugs significantly reduced the severity of psychotic and extrapyramidal symptoms and had a relatively low risk of side effects.

The optimal median doses of risperidone and olanzapine were 2 and 10 mg/day, respectively. Patients taking olanzapine gained significantly more weight than those treated with risperidone. Psychotic symptoms in older patients tend to respond to lower doses of risperidone than those in younger patients, and doses must be raised with caution, as the risk of EPS and other side effects is dose-related.

Olanzapine

Olanzapine is another atypical antipsychotic that is frequently used in older patients with schizophrenia. Kennedy *et al.* (2003) compared six-week clinical response and safety profiles of haloperidol versus olanzapine in elderly schizophrenia patients in a double-blind, randomized controlled study. The investigators found that patients taking olanzapine had significantly greater improvement in positive and negative symptoms as well as anxiety and depression-related symptoms than patients treated with haloperidol. They also found that olanzapine was better tolerated in terms of EPS, and it was equivalent to haloperidol for anticholinergic side effects (Kennedy *et al.* 2003). As mentioned above, Jeste *et al.* (2003a) compared olanzapine and risperidone in elderly patients with chronic schizophrenia, and found that the two drugs were comparable in therapeutic efficacy and most side effects (except for weight gain). In patients with LOS, olanzapine may be useful because of its favorable safety profile in terms of EPS and TD, but its metabolic effects such as weight gain and type 2 diabetes mellitus should be monitored. A typical starting dose of olanzapine in older patients is 5 mg, with 7.5–12.5 mg/day as the usual maintenance dose.

Quetiapine

McManus *et al.* (1999) examined the effects of quetiapine in elderly patients with different psychotic disorders including schizophrenia, and found that it was well-tolerated, and resulted in symptom improvement. The most common adverse effects were somnolence, postural hypotension, and dizziness. Quetiapine has a very low risk of EPS and TD, and is also not anticholinergic. However, sedation is a common side effect with higher doses. The recommended dose of quetiapine in elderly patients with schizophrenia may range from 50 to 200 mg/day.

Ziprasidone and aripiprazole

Ziprasidone and aripiprazole are the newest of the atypical antipsychotics, only recently introduced for clinical use in schizophrenia patients. Their pharmacological profiles seem to be beneficial for older patients, as they both have a low incidence of EPS, weight gain, and anticholinergic side effects (Sable and Jeste 2002). Ziprasidone is known to cause QT prolongation. Aripiprazole is believed to be different from other atypical antipsychotics in that it is a partial dopamine agonist. There are no published clinical trials of either of these newest antipsychotic medications in older patients with schizophrenia; therefore, treatment recommendations for use in patients with LOS must await further data on the optimal dosing.

Regardless of the choice of antipsychotic medication, treating physicians should begin with relatively low doses in order to reduce the risks of side effects associated with age-related pharmacodynamic and pharmacokinetic changes (Owen and Castle 1999). Dose titration should be gradual, and response to treatment should be carefully monitored. Various short-term and long-term adverse effects need to be monitored closely.

One barrier to the successful treatment of schizophrenia is lack of adherence to antipsychotic medications (Dolder *et al.* 2003). Lacro *et al.* (personal communication, December 2003) are currently testing an intervention called Medication Adherence Therapy, which uses cognitive, affective, and behavioral techniques to improve treatment adherence.

Adjunctive treatment

Many older patients with schizophrenia have depressive symptoms (Jin *et al.* 2001). Such symptoms are associated with increased functional impairment. Adjunctive treatment with citalopram and other antidepressants may help reduce the severity of depression in these patients (Kasckow *et al.* 2001).

Neuropsychological impairment predicts functional outcome in patients with schizophrenia (Bellack *et al.* 1994, 1999; Green 1996; Green and Neuchterlein 1999; Twamley *et al.* 2002; McGurk *et al.* 2000), explaining 20–60 per cent of the variance in measured outcomes (Green *et al.* 2000). Although there is evidence that atypical antipsychotic drugs may produce mild improvement in some areas of cognition (Bilder *et al.* 2002; Keefe *et al.* 1999; Harvey and Keefe, 2001; McGurk 1999; Purdon 1999), patients continue to experience considerable residual cognitive deficits (Rund and Borg 1999). Furthermore, the antipsychotics have only limited effect on negative symptoms of schizophrenia. Thus, a number of investigators have pursued non-pharmacological means of improving residual cognitive and functional deficits in patients with schizophrenia. Some of these interventions include Cognitive Behavioral Social Skills Training (CBSST) (Granholm *et al.* 2002; McQuaid *et al.* 2000), Functional Adaptation Skills Training (FAST) (Patterson *et al.* 2003), cognitive training (Twamley *et al.* 2003b), and vocational rehabilitation (Twamley *et al.* 2003b).

Cognitive behavioral social skills training

Although there has been growing evidence of the efficacy of cognitive behavior therapy (CBT) and social skills training (SST) in younger adults with schizophrenia, there had been no published investigations of interventions specifically designed for older schizophrenia patients. Cognitive Behavioral Social Skills Training (CBSST) was developed to meet this need. Randomized controlled trials were conducted to evaluate the efficacy of CBSST to augment regular pharmacotherapy. The intervention involves training in challenging false beliefs, reconstructing maladaptive thoughts, problem-solving, and communication skills. To tailor the intervention specifically for older adults, training includes age-related problem-solving skills and role-plays. Presentation of information through multiple modalities and training in the use of mnemonic strategies help compensate for age-related cognitive decline found in older patients (Granholm *et al.* 2002). CBSST may improve patients' functioning by increasing their ability to cope with stressors and increasing their adherence to treatment (McQuaid *et al.* 2000). CBSST may be especially well received by patients with LOS because of their better premorbid functioning and more intact cognitive abilities. Also, patients with LOS are more likely to have unique stressors that they experience for the first time at an older age, such as impairment in occupational and interpersonal functioning.

Functional Adaptation Skills Training (FAST)

The FAST intervention was developed to increase the independence and quality of life of older patients of chronic psychotic disorders (Patterson *et al.* 2003). The areas of everyday functioning targeted for intervention include medication management, social skills, communication skills, organization and planning, transportation, and financial management. Preliminary findings indicate global improvements in measures of everyday functioning, both immediately after the completion of the intervention and at a three-month follow-up evaluation (Patterson *et al.* 2003). The investigators have acknowledged that despite its strengths, the ecological validity of FAST is still limited due to its reliance on performance-based measures. It is difficult to predict how the patients' behavior will be affected by FAST when faced with real-world complexities and challenges. Patients with LOS tend to have less severe negative symptoms than older patients with early-onset schizophrenia. Yet, the LOS patients must cope with many of the same problems of everyday functioning that persons with early-onset schizophrenia face, and moreover, their lives often change radically with the late emergence of psychosis after decades of near-normal premorbid functioning. Some of the skills provided by FAST can help them adapt to their changing environment, specifically in terms of managing their medication and generating social support networks to aid in their recovery.

Cognitive training

Cognitive training (CT), also known as cognitive rehabilitation and cognitive remediation, is a psychosocial intervention that aims to help patients improve their thinking and memory abilities. In a literature review of 17 randomized controlled trials of CT in younger adults, Twamley *et al.* (2003a) concluded that CT has potential for improving cognitive performance, symptoms, and everyday functioning in patients with schizophrenia. CT can be implemented on an individual basis or in groups. The interventions usually involve task practice via repeated drills and/or strategy coaching, and sometimes include computerized training. It remains unclear whether CT is helpful in reversing cognitive impairment (as argued by the restorative model) or in helping individuals learn new strategies or modify their environments to 'work around' their cognitive deficits (as posited by the compensatory model). Twamley and colleagues are currently conducting an investigation of a manualized CT intervention targeting prospective memory, attention, learning, and problem-solving in middle-aged and older patients with primary psychotic disorders.

Work rehabilitation

One of the tragic consequences of schizophrenia, both for affected individuals and for the society as a whole, is the functional decline in ability to maintain employment. Remaining active in work is frequently cited as a primary component of successful aging, and many 'normal' people now continue to work into their 60s, 70s, and even 80s. Yet, the vast majority of middle-aged and older people with schizophrenia are unemployed, even though many of them want to work or to volunteer. Preliminary research suggests that this population can benefit from work rehabilitation programs, but existing programs do not target older people with psychiatric disabilities, who are typically assumed to have little potential for returning to meaningful work.

In an ongoing randomized controlled trial, Twamley and colleagues are comparing an evidence-based work rehabilitation intervention called Individual Placement and Support (IPS) (Becker and Drake, 1993) to conventional vocational rehabilitation (CVR). IPS is a 'place then train' approach that emphasizes rapid, individualized job placement, training on the job, integrated mental health and vocational treatment, and time-unlimited follow-along support from a vocational specialist. CVR, in contrast, emphasizes the 'train then place' approach, which focuses on prevocational job readiness training and does not feature the other elements of IPS. In a recent review and meta-analysis (Twamley *et al.* 2003b), of the 11 randomized controlled trials of work rehabilitation in younger adult patients (nine of which were trials examining IPS interventions), outcomes strongly favored the experimental groups in terms of the percentage of participants who worked at any point during the studies (weighted mean effect size = 0.66). In the five investigations comparing IPS to CVR services, 51 per cent of the participants receiving IPS worked competitively, versus 18 per cent of those in the comparison groups (weighted mean effect size = 0.79).

Summary

The studies of late-life schizophrenia suggest some important distinctions and implications for treatment of older patients with this disorder. Many of the published studies of older patients with schizophrenia include patients with both early and late onset; most treatment recommendations are, therefore, tailored to older patients rather than to patients with late onset of illness. Available data show that older patients with schizophrenia do better with atypical antipsychotics compared to conventional neuroleptics, and respond to lower doses of medication compared to younger patients. Late-onset patients need even lower doses than age-comparable patients with early-onset schizophrenia. Treating clinicians must be aware of the fact that older patients have a higher incidence of medication side effects with antipsychotic medication, usually have other comorbid medical illnesses, which the antipsychotic medication may worsen, and often take multiple medications increasing the risk of adverse drug–drug interactions. Adjunctive psychosocial treatment has the potential to benefit older patients with schizophrenia, and lead to better functioning in daily life.

References

American Psychiatric Association (1980). *Diagnostic and Statistical Manual of Mental Disorders*, 3rd edn, American Psychiatric Press, Washington, DC.

Becker DR and Drake RE. (1993). *A Working Life: The Individual Placement Support (IPS) Program*, New Hampshire-Dartmouth Psychiatric Research Center, Concord, NH.

Bellack AS, Gold JM and Buchanan RW. (1999). Cognitive rehabilitation for schizophrenia: Problems, prospects, and strategies. *Schizophrenia Bulletin*, 25, 257–274.

Bellack AS, Sayers M, Meuser KT and Bennett M. (1994). An evaluation of social problem solving in schizophrenia. *Journal of Abnormal Psychology*, 103, 371–378.

Bilder RM, Goldman RS, Volavka J *et al.* (2002). Neurocognitive effects of clozapine, olanzapine, risperidone, and haloperidol in patients with chronic schizophrenia or schizoaffective disorder. *American Journal of Psychiatry*, 159, 1018–1028.

Bleuler M. (1943). Late schizophrenic clinical pictures. *Fortschritte der Neurologie-Psychiatrie*, 15, 259–290.

Castle DJ and Howard R. (1992). What do we know about the aetiology of late-onset schizophrenia? *European Psychiatry*, 7, 99–108.

Castle DJ and Murray RM. (1993). The epidemiology of late-onset schizophrenia. *Schizophrenia Bulletin*, 19, 691–700.

Dolder CR, Lacro JP, Leckband S *et al.* (2003). Interventions to improve antipsychotic medication adherence. *Journal of Clinical Psychopharmacology*, 23, 389–399.

Granholm E, McQuaid JR, McClure FS, Pedrelli P and Jeste DV. (2002). A randomized controlled pilot study of cognitive behavioral social skills training for older patients with schizophrenia. *Schizophrenia Research*, 53, 167–169.

Green MF. (1996). What are the functional consequences of neurocognitive deficits in schizophrenia? *American Journal of Psychiatry*, 153, 321–330.

Green MF, Kern RS, Braff DL and Mintz J. (2000). Neurocognitive deficits and functional outcome in schizophrenia: Are we measuring the 'right stuff'? *Schizophrenia Bulletin*, 26, 119–136.

Green MF and Neuchterlein KH. (1999). Should schizophrenia be treated as a neurocognitive disorder? *Schizophrenia Bulletin*, 25, 309–318.

Harris MJ and Jeste DV. (1988). Late-onset schizophrenia: An overview. *Schizophrenia Bulletin*, 14, 39–55.

Harvey PD and Keefe RSE. (2001). Studies of cognitive change in patients with schizophrenia following novel antipsychotic treatment. *American Journal of Psychiatry*, 158, 176–184.

Heilä H, Isometsä ET, Henriksson MM *et al.* (1997). Suicide and schizophrenia: A nationwide psychological autopsy study on age- and sex-specific clinical characteristics of 92 suicide victims with schizophrenia. *American Journal of Psychiatry*, 154, 1235–1242.

Howard R, Castle D, Wessely S and Murray RM. (1993). A comparative study of 470 cases of early and late-onset schizophrenia. *Brit J Psychiat*, 163, 352–357.

Howard R, Rabins PV, Seeman MV, Jeste DV and the International Late-Onset Schizophrenia Group. (2000). Late-onset schizophrenia and very-late-onset schizophrenia-like psychois: An international consensus. *American Journal of Psychiatry*, 157, 172–178.

Jeste DV, Barak Y, Madhusoodanan S, Grossman F and Gharabawi G. (2003a). An international multisite double-blind trial of the atypical antipsychotic risperidone and olanzapine in 175 elderly patients with chronic schizophrenia. *American Journal of Geriatric Psychiatry*, 12, 638–647.

Jeste DV, Caligiuri MP, Paulsen JS, *et al.* (1995a). Risk of tardive dyskinesia in older patients: A prospective longitudinal study of 266 patients. *Archives of General Psychiatry*, 52, 756–765.

Jeste DV, Harless KA and Palmer BW. (2000). Chronic late-onset schizophrenia-like psychosis that remitted: Revisiting Newton's psychosis? *American Journal of Psychiatry*, 157, 444–449.

Jeste DV, Harris MJ, Krull A *et al.* (1995b). Clinical and neuropsychological characteristics of patients with late-onset schizophrenia. *American Journal of Psychiatry*, 152, 722–730.

Jeste DV, Lacro JP, Bailey A *et al.* (1999a). Lower incidence of tardive dyskinesia with risperidone compared with haloperidol in older patients. *Journal of the American Geriatric Society*, 47, 716–719.

Jeste DV, Twamley EW, Eyler Zorrilla LT *et al.* (2003b). Aging and outcome in schizophrenia. *Acta Psychiatrica Scandinavica*, 107, 336–343.

Jeste DV, Rockwell E, Harris MJ, Lohr JB and Lacro J. (1999b). Conventional vs. newer antipsychotics in elderly patients. *American Journal of Geriatric Psychiatry*, 7, 70–76.

Jin H, Meyer JM and Jeste DV. (2002). Phenomenology of and risk factors for new-onset diabetes mellitus and diabetic ketoacidosis associated with atypical antipsychotics: An analysis of 45 published cases. *Annals of Clinical Psychiatry*, 14, 59–64.

Jin H, Zisook S, Palmer BW *et al.* (2001). Association of depressive symptoms and functioning in schizophrenia: A study in older outpatients. *Journal of Clinical Psychiatry*, 62, 797–803.

Kasckow JW, Mohamed S, Thallasinos A *et al.* (2001). Citalopram augmentation of antipsychotic treatment in older schizophrenia patients. *International Journal of Geriatric Psychiatry*, 16, 1163–1167.

Kay DWK and Roth M. (1961). Environmental and hereditary factors in the schizophrenias of old age ('late paraphrenia') and their bearing on the general problem of causation in schizophrenia. *Journal of Mental Science*, 107, 649–686.

Keefe RSE, Silva SG, Perkins DO and Liberman JA. (1999). The effects of atypical antipsychotic drugs on neurocognitive impairment in schizophrenia: A review and meta-analysis. *Schizophrenia Bulletin*, 25, 201–222.

Kennedy JS, Jeste DV, Kaiser CJ *et al.* (2003). Olanzapine vs. haloperidol in geriatric schizophrenia: Analysis of data from a double-blind controlled trial. *International Journal of Geriatric Psychiatry*, 18, 1013–1020.

McGurk SR. (1999). The effects of clozapine on cognitive functioning in schizophrenia. *Journal of Clinical Psychiatry*, 60, 24–29.

McGurk SR, Moriarty PJ, Harvey PD *et al.* (2000). The longitudinal relationship of clinical symptoms, cognitive functioning and adaptive life in geriatric schizophrenia. *Schizophrenia Research*, 42, 47–55.

McManus DQ, Arvanitis LA and Kowalcyk BB. (1999). Quetiapine, a novel antipsychotic: Experience in elderly patients with psychotic disorders. *Journal of Clinical Psychiatry*, 60, 292–298.

McQuaid JR, Granholm E, McClure FS *et al.* (2000). Development of an integrated cognitive-behavioral, social skills training intervention for older patients with schizophrenia. *Journal of Psychotherapy Practice and Research*, 9, 1–8.

Meltzer HY and McGurk SR. (1999). The effects of clozapine, risperidone, and olanzapine on cognitive function in schizophrenia. *Schizophrenia Bulletin*, 25, 233–255.

Owen PA and Castle DJ. (1999). Late-onset schizophrenia: Epidemiology, diagnosis, management and outcome. *Drugs and Aging*, 15, 81–89.

Patterson TL, McKibbin CL, Taylor MJ, *et al.* (2003). Functional Adaptation Skills Training (FAST): A pilot psychosocial intervention study in middle-aged and older patients with chronic psychotic disorders. *American Journal of Geriatric Psychiatry*, 11, 17–23.

Post F. (1966). *Persistent Persecutory States of the Elderly*, Pergamon Press, London.

Purdon SE. (1999). Cognitive improvement in schizophrenia with novel antipsychotic medications. *Schizophrenia Research*, 35, S51–S60.

Rabins P, Pauker S and Thomas J. (1984). Can schizophrenia begin after age 44? *Comprehensive Psychiatry*, 25, 290–293.

Radomsky ED, Haas GL, Mann J and Sweeney JA. (1999). Suicidal behavior in patients with schizophrenia and other psychotic disorders. *American Journal of Psychiatry*, 156, 1590–1595.

Rund BR and Borg NE. (1999). Cognitive deficits and cognitive training in schizophrenic patients: A review. *Acta Psychiatrica Scandinavica*, 100, 85–95.

Sable JA and Jeste DV. (2002). Antipsychotic treatment for late-life schizophrenia. *Current Psychiatry Reports*, 4, 299–306.

Sajatovic M, Ramirez LF, Garver D *et al.* (1998). Clozapine therapy for older veterans. *Psychiatric Services*, 49, 340–344.

Sciolla A and Jeste DV. (1998). Use of antipsychotics in the elderly. *International Journal of Psychiatry in Clinical Practice*, 2, S27–S34.

Seeman P, Corbett R, Nam D and Van Tol HH. (1996). Dopamine and serotonin receptors: amino acid sequences, and clinical role in neuroleptic parkinsonism. *Japanese Journal of Pharmacology,* 71, 187–204.

Twamley EW, Doshi RR, Nayak GV *et al.* (2002). Generalized cognitive impairments, everyday functioning ability, and living independence in patients with psychosis. *American Journal of Psychiatry,* 159, 2013–2020.

Twamley EW, Jeste DV and Bellack AS. (2003a). A review of cognitive training in schizophrenia. *Schizophrenia Bulletin,* 29, 359–382.

Twamley EW, Jeste DV and Lehman AF. (2003b). Vocational rehabilitation in schizophrenia: A literature review and meta-analysis of randomized controlled trials. *The Journal of Nervous and Mental Disease,* 191, 515–523.

Chapter 14

Treatment of cognitive deficits in first episode psychosis

Richard S. E. Keefe and Joseph W. Kang

Cognitive deficits in schizophrenia

Cognitive deficits are a core feature of schizophrenia. Compared to healthy controls, schizophrenia patients perform an average of two standard deviations below the mean of their healthy counterparts in several areas of cognition, especially attention, executive function, and memory (Addington and Addington 2002; Harvey and Keefe 1997). Impairment in these areas of cognition is an important factor in the long-term outcome and adaptive functioning of these patients (Green *et al.* 1996; Harvey *et al.* 1998; Velligan *et al.* 1997). Vigilance, memory, and card-sorting deficits have been found to be related to poor functional outcome in a large number of studies (see reviews by Green 1996, 2000). In elderly patients with schizophrenia, the severity of cognitive impairment predicts adaptive deficits independent of the severity of the illness or the site of care (Harvey *et al.* 1998), and is a far better predictor of adaptive functioning than positive and negative symptoms.

Cognitive deficits in first episode psychosis

Cognitive functioning is also severely impaired in patients experiencing their first episode of psychosis (Addington *et al.* 2003; Bilder *et al.* 2000; Hoff *et al.* 1992; Mohamed *et al.* 1999; Saykin *et al.* 1994; Sweeney *et al.* 1991). These deficits are independent of any potential deleterious effect of typical antipsychotic treatment, as patients with a first episode of schizophrenia who have never taken antipsychotic medication already exhibit cognitive impairment (Brickman *et al.* 2003; Mohamed *et al.* 1999; Saykin *et al.* 1994). Most importantly, cognitive deficits at first episode may herald a course of illness accompanied by functional deficits, as greater than 50 per cent of first episode patients with cognitive deficits are found to be on disability when followed up six months later (Ho *et al.* 1998).

Direct comparisons between first episode and chronic patients have suggested that both groups perform similarly, and both are clearly worse than healthy control subjects on neuropsychological tests (Hoff *et al.* 1990; Saykin *et al.* 1994). Individual test comparisons of the severity of impairment in schizophrenia reported in the Heinrichs and Zakzanis (1998) meta-analysis with a representative first episode sample from Bilder *et al.* (2000) support this conclusion (Gold 2003). However, chronic patients have been found to have a profile of slightly greater impairment on some domains such as processing speed and motor function (Bilder *et al.* 1992; Hoff *et al.* 1992; Saykin *et al.* 1994). For instance, in a study of cognitive functions in 37 never medicated patients with first-episode schizophrenia, 65 unmedicated, previously treated patients, and 131 healthy controls, the first-episode patients had a very similar severity and profile of deficits compared to the previously-treated patients (Saykin *et al.* 1994). While the first-episode patients were similarly impaired on those domains that traditionally show the greatest deficits in patients with schizophrenia (attention, verbal memory, and processing speed), they were slightly less impaired on tests of fine motor speed, spatial cognition, and visual memory. It is possible that greater impairment in these areas of cognition is associated with longer duration of illness and chronic treatment with typical antipsychotic medications (Saykin *et al.* 1994).

A longitudinal study with a follow-up of 10–12 years from baseline neuro-cognitive assessment in 24 first episode patients was recently reported by Stirling *et al.* (2003). Significant deterioration was seen over the follow-up period in three of nine subtests: WAIS object assembly and picture completion, and a visual memory test. Furthermore, change on these measures, as well as scores at follow-up, was significantly correlated with a global measure of functioning that included measures of independent living, time employed, and global assessment of functioning (GAF) scores.

These data, while equivocal, suggest that there may be some decline in cognitive function from onset through the longitudinal course of schizophrenia. However, one interpretation of the slightly more severe deficits in chronic patients compared with first-episode patients is that the increased severity may be attributable to the study samples (Keefe 2001). Longitudinal studies of schizophrenia are likely to take place at research settings in which patients are easily accessible over the course of time, such as state institutions. These patients may have a more chronic course of illness than those patients who receive treatment at the first episode of illness, and then are only seen as outpatients with occasional acute exacerbations through the course of their illness. Since treatment setting has been found to greatly differentiate the level of cognitive impairment in elderly patients (Harvey 1998), it may be that the cognitive differences between chronic and first episode patients are partially a reflection of the differences in good and poor outcome patient populations rather than a pure indication of the course of illness in all patients. Longitudinal studies of substantial duration, such as the Stirling *et al.* (2003) study are needed to address this issue further.

Neuroanatomical changes at first episode

A discussion of cognition in first episode psychosis must include a considera-tion of recent data suggesting neuroanatomical changes in the early phases of illness. Several studies using MRI technology (Gur *et al.* 1998; Thompson *et al.* 2001; Cahn *et al.* 2002) have suggested that gray matter reductions occur in patients in the early phases of psychosis. Patients in the first episode of illness, assessed at baseline while antipsychotic-naïve and then one year later, have been reported to have 20 cc of gray matter loss (Cahn *et al.* 2002). This loss was in contrast to healthy controls, who showed no change over the same interval. In younger adolescent patients studied after the onset of psychosis, annual gray matter losses of between 1–5 per cent were reported, especially in tempo-ral, parietal, and frontal regions (Thompson *et al.* 2001). Healthy controls showed no changes over the same period of time. Most importantly, these neuroanatomical reductions have been found to be related to an *absence* of improvement in cognitive function (Gur *et al.* 1998; Ho *et al.* 2003). However, other studies have shown no significant differences in gray matter volume change (DeLisi *et al.* 1995, 1997; James *et al.* 2002) over time. While these results remain controversial, and should be interpreted carefully (Weinberger and McClure 2002), they raise the question of whether early intervention in first episode psychosis may help to reduce any potential cognitive decline and neuroanatomical changes that may occur as part of the natural course of illness in these patients.

Cognitive decline and duration of untreated psychosis

Some researchers, assuming that the cognitive differences between first episode and chronic patients reflect an actual decline, have cited these data as support for the notion that psychosis may be neurotoxic in schizophrenia or that a neurodegenerative process is active (Lieberman 1999). The rationale is that if patients with schizophrenia have a downward course of illness, cognitive decline and corresponding neuroanatomical changes would be expected. It has also been suggested that proper treatment may interrupt this downward decline, and that an absence of treatment may prolong a patient's ability to respond once treatment is initiated (Wyatt 1991).

A meta-analysis of 22 different studies (Wyatt 1991) suggested a possible association between duration of untreated psychosis and patient outcome. Analysis of the duration of untreated psychosis in relation to time to remission or level of positive symptoms after a set period of treatment (typically one or two years), suggested that shorter duration of untreated psychosis is correlated with better outcome (Altamura *et al.* 2001; Black *et al.* 2001; Drake *et al.* 2000; Larsen *et al.* 2000; Loebel *et al.* 1992; Malla *et al.* 2002; Verdoux *et al.* 2001). However, other studies have reported no significant relationship between those variables (Ho *et al.* 2000; Craig *et al.* 2000).

One way to examine the possible neural toxicity of psychosis is to examine its effect on cognitive functioning. Several studies have investigated whether individuals who have experienced longer duration of untreated psychosis show more compromised cognitive functioning (Amminger *et al.* 2002; Barnes *et al.* 2000; Hoff *et al.* 2000; Norman *et al.* 2001). Two of these studies reported that a longer duration of untreated psychosis was associated with greater decline in cognitive functioning, as assessed by a worse post-onset cognitive functioning (Barnes *et al.* 2000) or a discrepancy between estimated premorbid and post-onset cognitive functioning (Amminger *et al.* 2002). In a separate study using a discrepancy index, this finding was not replicated (Norman *et al.* 2001).

Studies of the relationship between duration of untreated psychosis and brain structure have also been equivocal. Duration of untreated psychosis has been found to be positively related to enlargement of frontal sulci (Madsen *et al.* 1999) and inversely related to volume of the left superior temporal gyrus in males, but not females (Keshavan *et al.* 1998). However, no relationship of duration of untreated psychosis to lateral ventricular, temporal lobe, or cerebral hemisphere volumes in first-episode patients was found in a study by Hoff *et al.* (2000).

The possibility of a neurotoxic psychosis was supported by the results of several studies showing that patients had more difficulty responding to treatment after each subsequent episode of psychosis. First-episode patients have been found to respond significantly better the earlier that they are given medication and treatment (Malla *et al.* 1999). Responsiveness to antipsychotic medication was found to be less effective for subsequent episodes of psychosis (Lieberman *et al.* 1996).

One of the keys to better outcome may lie in the timing of intervention. Cognitive deficits may be part of the constellation of behavioral indications that an individual is at risk for developing schizophrenia later on in life.

Detecting, and possibly treating, these deficits even before psychosis transpires may allow a better outcome.

Cognitive deficits in premorbid phases of illness

Cognitive deficits appear to precede the onset of psychosis, and may help to predict the conversion to psychosis in individuals who are at ultra high risk for schizophrenia (Cornblatt 1999). Several studies have utilized a link between the Israeli Draft Board Registry, which contains measures of intellectual and language skills for the entire population of 16–17 year-olds in Israel, and the National Psychiatric Hospitalization Case Registry, which contains diagnostic information for all psychiatric hospitalizations in the country. Israeli law requires that all adolescents between the ages of 16–17 undergo pre-induction assessment to determine their intellectual, medical, and psychiatric eligibility for military service. This assessment is compulsory and is administered to the entire, unselected, population of Israeli adolescents. It includes individuals who will be eligible for military service, as well as those who will be excused from service based on medical, psychiatric, or social reasons.

The results of these studies suggest that cognitive functions are significantly impaired in those adolescents who are (N = 509) versus those who are not (N = 9,215) later hospitalized for schizophrenia. These deficits thus precede the onset of psychosis in young people destined to develop schizophrenia, and along with social isolation and organizational ability, cognitive deficits are a significant predictor of which young people will eventually develop a psychotic disorder (Davidson *et al.* 1999). One study from this series examined the cognitive performance of 44 patients with a first episode of schizophrenia who had previously undergone cognitive assessment as part of their registration with the Israeli Draft Board. Forty-four healthy subjects were also enrolled in the study and tested twice. The patients with schizophrenia performed worse than healthy subjects on both the first and second assessments. The schizophrenia patients did not demonstrate any significant change. Compared to the improvement in the healthy subjects, this absence of change suggested a significant deterioration on half of the tests administered. The stability of the deficits in these patients suggests that most of the cognitive impairment seen in patients with schizophrenia occurs prior to the first psychotic episode (Caspi *et al.* 2003).

Cognitive deficits are also found in individuals who are identified as being at 'ultra-high' risk (Yung and McGorry 1996) for schizophrenia by virtue of their family history of schizophrenia and/or the manifestation of mild signs and symptoms consistent with the prodromal symptoms of schizophrenia.

While several research groups are gathering data on this question, results have only recently begun to be reported (Brewer *et al.* 2003; Hawkins *et al.* 2003). Preliminary data from one study suggest that some cognitive impairments, namely olfactory identification deficits, predict which individuals at ultra-high risk will develop schizophrenia (Brewer *et al.* 2003). These studies are aimed in part to determine whether early intervention strategies targeting cognition, perhaps even before the onset of psychosis, may help reduce the likelihood that an individual at ultra-high risk will have a psychotic episode.

Treatment of cognitive deficits in first episode patients

The cognitive data reviewed above converge to raise a question of how early treatment should commence for patients experiencing their first episode of psychosis. Since cognitive functions appear to be related to long-term outcome, and since cognition may decline through the course of illness in schizophrenia, thus worsening outcome even further, it would seem that treatments targeted to improve cognition in the first episode of illness would be beneficial. Dozens of studies have investigated the impact of the newer antipsychotic medications on the cognitive deficits of schizophrenia, and many studies using adjunctive cognitive-enhancing co-treatments are underway. However, very few studies have investigated the impact of treatment on cognition in first episode psychosis. Preliminary data in this area will be reviewed below.

Typical antipsychotics

In general, typical antipsychotic medications such as haloperidol have not proven to be very effective in improving the cognitive deficits of schizophrenia (Blyler and Gold 2000). It appears as though typical antipsychotics may improve cognitive deficits to some extent in patients with first episode psychosis, but these improvements are directly related to changes in symptoms.

In a sample of 94 patients with first episode psychosis (Mohamed *et al.* 1999), significant impairment relative to 305 healthy controls was reported in 29 of 30 cognitive measures of various cognitive domains. The results for the 73 antipsychotic-naïve patients from this sample were identical to the 21 who had briefly (median, seven days) received antipsychotic medications prior to neurocognitive testing, supporting the notion that cognitive impairment in schizophrenia is not caused by antipsychotic treatment.

After treatment with typical antipsychotics, the cognitive deficits of schizophrenic patients in the first episode of psychosis appear do not worsen, yet remain severe. Patients with first-episode schizophrenia or schizoaffective illness who were given neurocognitive assessments after six months of treatment with typical antipsychotics, and who also met criteria for full symptom remission or stability of residual symptoms, demonstrated a very similar profile of cognitive impairments to antipsychotic-naïve patients (Bilder *et al.* 2000), with an average magnitude of impairment of 1.53 z-scores below the healthy control mean.

It appears as though these cognitive deficits do not change substantially through the course of treatment with typical antipsychotics in first episode patients. In a four-year longitudinal study (DeLisi *et al.* 1995) involving yearly cognitive assessments of first-episode patients treated with typical antipsychotics, very small (0.09 SDs per year) but statistically significant improvements were reported in global cognitive functions. Specific improvements in measures of motor and processing speed and 'right hemisphere' functions were also reported. A more comprehensive analysis of an extended sample from this study supported these data (Hoff *et al.* 1999). While healthy comparison subjects in this study improved substantially over time, the patients with schizophrenia did not. The patients had significantly less improvement on tests of verbal memory and sensory-perceptual functions. The authors concluded that the patients in this study did not benefit from repeated annual practice, yet the control subjects did (Hoff *et al.* 1999).

In a recent comparison of low doses of haloperidol to olanzapine on measures of cognition, haloperidol was found to have a mild cognitive benefit (Keefe *et al.* 2004). In this study, 167 patients in the first episode of schizophrenia, schizoaffective, or schizophreniform disorder were randomized to double-blind treatment with olanzapine or haloperidol for the 12-week acute phase of a two-year study. The statistical approach and design features of this study helped address the impact of dosing, side effects, and anticholinergic medication on neurocognition in patients receiving haloperidol. First, one of the most important features of this study design was the dosing strategy chosen for patients randomized to haloperidol. While previous studies of the impact of atypical antipsychotics suggested that risperidone, olanzapine, clozapine, and quetiapine improve neurocognitive performance in patients with schizophrenia, many of these studies have been criticized for the doses of typical antipsychotic medication (usually haloperidol) that was used, which averaged 736 mg per day when used in randomized studies as a comparator, and 924 mg when used as a baseline treatment (Harvey and Keefe 2001). In contrast to these previous studies, patients randomized to the haloperidol arm in the study by Keefe *et al.* (2004) received a mean modal dose of

5.21 mg per day (260.5 mg chlorpromazine-equivalents). The mean dose of haloperidol that patients received during the week of testing was slightly higher (5.54 mg, equivalent to 277.0 mg chlorpromazine). The effect sizes of neurocognitive change with haloperidol were 0.16 for an unweighted composite score and 0.26 for a weighted composite score. Although methodological differences between this study and the study of low-dose haloperidol by Green *et al.* (2002) limit direct comparison, the effect of low-dose haloperidol in the two studies was very similar between studies.

Even when lower doses of haloperidol are used, there is a significant relationship between treatment-related neurocognitive change, change in EPS, and the administration of anticholinergic medication in patients treated with haloperidol (Harvey *et al.* 2003; Keefe *et al.* 2004). These data suggest that the effect of typical antipsychotics may not be neutral (Carpenter and Gold 2002), but that some patients may have cognitive worsening and apparent negative symptom increases due to the side effects of these medications.

The significant improvement in overall cognition with low doses of haloperidol is supported by analyses of individual measures, which suggested specific improvement in visuospatial working memory and performance on the Wisconsin Card Sorting Test (Keefe *et al.* 2004). Although the working memory benefit was potentially explained by particularly severe baseline working memory impairments only in patients randomized to haloperidol, this finding parallels work completed in nonhuman primates, who, under stressful noise conditions, improve on measures of visuospatial working memory when haloperidol doses are low (0.005 mg/kg), but not when doses are higher (0.01 mg/kg) (Arnsten and Goldman-Rakic 1998), and worsen when doses are high (0.07–0.20 mg/kg) (Castner *et al.* 2000). One caveat to the overall cognitive benefit of haloperidol in this study was the fact that the most dramatic improvements (0.5 SD) were found on the California Verbal Learning Test. Alternate forms of this test were not used in the study, and substantial practice effects on verbal list learning tests have been reported in patients with schizophrenia (Hawkins and Wexler 1999). A conservative conclusion from this body of work is that low doses of haloperidol are less deleterious than high doses in their neurocognitive effects (Carpenter and Gold 2002; Green *et al.* 2002; Harvey and Keefe 2001; Keefe *et al.* 1999).

In sum, while patients in the first episode of schizophrenia have severe cognitive deficits that are present before treatment, initial treatment with typical antipsychotic medications does little to improve them. The severity of cognitive deficits may worsen slightly with illness progression, and may be related to deteriorated functioning, but this issue remains controversial. However, many of the previous studies have used doses of medication that are now considered to be too high to allow a cognitive benefit (Carpenter and Gold 2002; Harvey and Keefe 2001; Keefe *et al.* 1999). Recent efforts to improve cognition using lower doses of typical antipsychotic medications have yielded findings with less worsening, and potential improvement.

Atypical antipsychotics

Very few studies have compared the cognitive effects of atypical antipsychotic medications to low doses of a typical comparator. These studies have suggested that while lower doses of medication may be better than higher doses in improving cognition, atypical medications are slightly superior to even lower doses of typical medications.

One study (Keefe *et al.* 2004), discussed above, regarding the effects of lower doses of typical antipsychotics on cognition, compared the neurocognitive effects of olanzapine with low doses of haloperidol in patients with first-episode psychosis. Patients were assessed with a battery of neurocognitive tests at baseline and 12 weeks after treatment. An unweighted neurocognitive composite score composed of measures of verbal fluency, motor functions, working memory, verbal memory, and vigilance improved significantly with haloperidol or olanzapine treatment, with effect sizes of 0.16 and 0.24, respectively, which differed at a trend level of significance ($p = 0.082$). A principal components analysis of the same measures at baseline yielded a weighted composite score that was more sensitive to haloperidol and olanzapine treatment and to the difference between them. Using the first principal component as an outcome measure, patients treated with haloperidol showed a significant improvement in cognition from baseline, with an effect size of 0.26. However, patients treated with olanzapine improved to a significantly greater degree (effect size = 0.46) than those treated with haloperidol (p <0.02). It is important to note that the size of this effect is small relative to the severity of deficits found in patients with first-episode psychosis and schizophrenia, which range between 1.0 and 2.0 or more standard deviations from healthy controls (Bilder *et al.* 2000; Hoff *et al.* 1992). Thus, while olanzapine improves neurocognitive function in psychotic patients, the need for further improvement is substantial.

The neurocognitive measure that improved most in patients receiving olanzapine in this study was the response sensitivity measure (d-prime) obtained from the identical pairs version of the Continuous Performance Test (CPT-IP). This measure reflects patients' capacity to maintain vigilance in an effortful test of visual information processing with working memory components. This improvement was paralleled by substantial gains with olanzapine on another measure of information processing and speed, the Digit Symbol Test of the WAIS-R. The importance of deficits on CPTs has been demonstrated in cognitive, functional, and neurobiological studies of schizophrenia. This type of task has been found to correlate more strongly than other cognitive domains with various forms of functional outcome in patients with schizophrenia (Green 1996; Green *et al.* 2000). Very effortful CPTs, like the 4-digit version of the CPT-IP, have long been considered one of the fundamental impairments in schizophrenia (Seidman 1983), and reveal deficits in children at high-risk for schizophrenia (Cornblatt and Keilp 1994), especially those who develop schizophrenia as adults (Cornblatt *et al.* 1999), and impairments in patients with schizophrenia who perform normally in all other neurocognitive domains (Weickert *et al.* 2000). Finally, performance on similar tasks of active maintenance of visual information is mediated in part by activation of the dorsolateral prefrontal cortex (DLPFC) (Callicott *et al.* 1999; Cohen *et al.* 1997; Keilp *et al.* 1997), as well as other regions (Cohen *et al.* 1997; Hager *et al.* 1998; Keilp *et al.* 1997). The DLPFC tends to be less efficient in patients with schizophrenia (Barch *et al.* 2001; Callicott *et al.* 1998) while performing these tasks. Preliminary analyses from this study suggest that there is a significant relationship between the CPT improvement with olanzapine and gray matter changes in the frontal cortex (Lieberman *et al.* 2003). These data support the notion that cognitive changes with treatment in first episode psychosis may not only have neuroanatomical underpinnings, but may also reflect a healthy reduced neurotoxicity of psychosis (Lieberman 1999).

Whether neurocognitive improvement with atypical antipsychotics is secondary to other clinical changes, such as symptom improvement or release from the side effects of typical antipsychotics, is a matter of controversy (Carpenter and Gold 2002; Harvey and Keefe 2001; Keefe *et al.* 1999). The absence of significant correlation between neurocognitive change and symptom change in patients treated with olanzapine in this study (in contrast to patients treated with haloperidol) suggests that the cognitive benefit of olanzapine is not secondary to other clinical changes. In this study, the addition of other variables such as anticholinergic use, extrapyramidal symptoms, and estimated IQ, had little effect on the statistical differentiation of the medications, although duration of illness had a modest effect.

A study comparing the effects of low doses of haloperidol (mean modal dose = 2.8 mg) to risperidone (mean modal dose = 2.6 mg) in 555 first episode patients yielded slightly different findings. Preliminary reports from this study suggest that patients in each group demonstrated significant improvement in overall cognitive performance, and specific improvements in verbal and visual memory, attention, card sorting, and processing speed. Those patients treated with risperidone demonstrated cognitive improvements that were significantly greater than those found in patients treated with haloperidol, with specific improvements in verbal fluency and verbal delayed recall. As in the olanzapine first episode study, the changes in cognitive functions were correlated with changes in symptoms and side effects only in patients treated with haloperidol (Harvey *et al.* 2003). These data support the idea that atypical antipsychotics are superior to typicals in improving cognition, even in first episode patients treated with low doses of medication, and that this improvement is not limited to any one atypical antipsychotic medication.

One small-sample open-label study (N = 25) compared the cognitive effects of 13 weeks of treatment in drug-naïve first-episode schizophrenia patients randomized to comparable, low doses of a typical compound (zuclopenthixol; median dose = 8 mg [equivalent to 4 mg of haloperidol]) or an atypical compound (risperidone; median dose = 3 mg). Patients demonstrated severe deficits compared to controls on a battery of tests that included measures of executive functions, selective attention, motor speed and reaction time. The risperidone group showed significant within-group changes in reaction time, verbal fluency, selective attention, and planning time on a problem-solving task. The zuclopenthixol group showed significant within-group changes only in planning time on the problem-solving task. The only measure to improve significantly more in patients treated with risperidone than those treated with zuclopenthixol was motor speed. When extrapyramidal symptoms were accounted for statistically, the difference between the medications on this measure was no longer significant.

Clearly, further studies of the effects of olanzapine, risperidone and the other atypical antipsychotics in first episode patients are needed. The three studies completed to date, especially the two studies with substantial sample sizes, suggest that while low doses of typical antipsychotic medications may allow slight improvements in cognition, these improvements may be related to symptom improvement. In contrast to the effects of typical medications, the effect of olanzapine and risperidone appears to be significantly greater, and independent of the effects of these medications on symptoms or side effects.

An additional intriguing approach for improving the cognitive deficits of schizophrenia in first episode patients is cognitive enhancing, pharmacological co-treatments. While co-treatments such as donepezil and guanfacine in patients with schizophrenia have suggested mild improvements (Buchanan *et al.* 2003; Friedman *et al.* 2001), the impact of this strategy in first episode patients is unknown. This important area of research is just beginning.

Behavioral intervention

We were not able to find any studies on behavioral interventions to improve cognition in patients with first-episode psychosis. However, two lines of evidence suggested that this strategy might hold promise. First, cognitive rehabilitation treatment strategies to improve cognition have proven to be effective in patients with schizophrenia, especially in those patients treated with atypical antipsychotics (Wykes *et al.* 1999). These cognitive improvements following cognitive rehabilitation have been found to be associated with transient improvements in social functioning (Wykes *et al.* 2003) as well as increased activation of the dorsolateral prefrontal cortex consistent with improvement in brain functioning (Wykes *et al.* 2002). These studies suggest that cognitive rehabilitation treatment has social as well as neurobiological relevance. Second, cognitive-behavioral therapy targeted for reducing psychotic symptoms has been found to be more effective than routine care or supportive counseling in reducing psychotic symptoms of first episode patients, including auditory hallucinations (Lewis *et al.* 2002). This work demonstrates that first-episode patients can benefit from behavioral intervention. A potential avenue for future research would be the application of cognitive-behavioral or cognitive rehabilitation strategies targeted for improving cognition in first-episode patients.

Summary and conclusions

Cognitive deficits are a core feature of schizophrenia, and are present in first episode patients before treatment is initiated. Cognition has been shown to decline over time in first episode patients, particularly in those patients with structural brain changes. However, first episode patients may respond to treatment more effectively than patients that have experienced multiple episodes or have had long duration of untreated psychosis. The early detection of cognitive deficits and early intervention for cognitive impairment in first episode patients may help shape a better long term outcome.

Treatment studies of first episode patients have suggested the following:

- Initial treatment with standard doses of typical antipsychotic medications does little to change these cognitive deficits. Recent efforts to improve cognition using lower doses of typical antipsychotic medications have yielded more positive results. These cognitive improvements with typical medications appear to be found primarily in patients who have the greatest improvements in symptoms and/or the absence of deleterious side effects of typical antipsychotics and adjunctive treatments such as anticholinergic medications.

◆ In the two large-sample studies completed with olanzapine and risperidone, both of these medications improved cognition even more than low doses of typical antipsychotic medications. These improvements were of medium effect size, and were largely unrelated to any other symptom changes. Many more studies in this area have begun, and are needed for future research.

◆ Behavioral interventions utilizing methods such as cognitive behavioral therapy and cognitive rehabilitation, and pharmacological co-treatments, have not been completed on first episode patients. In schizophrenia, these interventions have shown promise, and possibly have a positive effect when used in conjunction with atypical antipsychotic medication.

References

Addington J and Addington D (2002). Cognitive functioning in first-episode schizophrenia. *Journal of Psychiatry and Neuroscience*, 27, 188–192.

Addington J, Brooks BL, Addington D (2003). Cognitive functioning in first episode psychosis. *Schizophrenia Research*, 62, 59–64.

Amminger GP, Edwards J, Brewer WJ, Harrigan S, McGorry PD (2002). Duration of untreated psychosis and cognitive deterioration in first-episode schizophrenia. *Schizophrenia Research*, 54, 223–230.

Altamura AC, Bassetti R, Sassella F, Salvadori D, Mundo, E (2001). Duration of untreated psychosis as a predictor of outcome in first-episode schizophrenia: A retrospective study. *Schizophrenia Research*, 52, 29–36.

Arnsten AF and Goldman-Rakic PS (1998). Noise stress impairs prefrontal cortical cognitive function in monkeys: evidence for a hyperdopaminergic mechanism. *Archives of General Psychiatry*, 55, 362–368.

Barch DM, Carter CS, Braver TS, Sabb FW, MacDonald A 3rd, Noll DC, Cohen JD (2001). Selective deficits in prefrontal cortex function in medication-naive patients with schizophrenia. *Archives of General Psychiatry*, 58, 280–288.

Barnes TRE, Hutton SB, Chapman H, Mutsatsa S, Puri BK, Joyce EM (2000). West London first episode study of schizophrenia: Clinical correlates of duration of untreated psychosis. *British Journal of Psychiatry*, 177, 201–211.

Bilder RM, Lipschutz-Broch L, Reiter G, Geisler SH *et al.* (1992). Intellectual deficits in first-episode schizophrenia: Evidence for progressive deterioration. *Schizophrenia Bulletin*, 18, 437–448.

Bilder RM, Goldman RS, Robinson D *et al.* (2000). Neuropsychology of first-episode schizophrenia: initial characterization and clinical correlates. *American Journal of Psychiatry*, 157, 549–559.

Black K, Peters L, Rui Q, Milliken H, Whitehorn D, Kopala L (2001). Duration of untreated psychosis predicts treatment outcome in an early psychosis program. *Schizophrenia Research*, 47, 215–222.

Blyler CR and Gold JM (2000). Cognitive effects of typical antipsychotic treatment: another look. In T Sharma and P Harvey (eds) *Cognitive Deficits in Schizophrenia*, pp. 241–265. Oxford, Oxford University Press.

Brewer WJ, Wood SJ, McGorry PD *et al.* (2003). Impairment of olfactory identification ability in individuals at ultra-high risk for psychosis who later develop schizophrenia. *American Journal of Psychiatry*, 160, 1790–1794.

Brickman AM, Buchsbaum MD, Bloom R, Bokhoven P, Paul-Odouard R, Haznedar MM, Dahlman KL, Hazlett EA, Aronowitz J, Heath D, Shihabuddin L (2003). Neuropsychological functioning in first-break, never-medicated adolescents with psychosis. *Schizophrenia Research*, 60, 126S.

Buchanan RW, Summerfelt A, Tek C, Gold, J (2003). An open-labeled trial of adjunctive donepezil for cognitive impairments in patients with schizophrenia. *Schizophrenia Research*, 59, 29–33.

Cahn W, Pol HE, Lems EB *et al.* (2002). Brain volume changes in first-episode schizophrenia: a 1-year follow-up study. *Archives of General Psychiatry*, 59, 1002–1010.

Callicott JH, Ramsey NF, Tallent K *et al.* (1998): Functional magnetic resonance imaging brain mapping in psychiatry: methodological issues illustrated in a study of working memory in schizophrenia. *Neuropsychopharmacology*, 18, 186–196.

Callicott JH, Mattay VS, Bertolino A *et al.* (1999). Physiological characteristics of capacity constraints in working memory as revealed by functional MRI. *Cerebral Cortex*, 9, 20–26.

Carpenter WT and Gold JM (2002). Another view of therapy for cognition in schizophrenia. *Biological Psychiatry*, 51, 969–971.

Caspi A, Reichenberg A, Weiser M *et al.* (2003). Cognitive performance in schizophrenia patients assessed before and following the first psychotic episode. *Schizophrenia Research*, 65, 87–94.

Castner SA, Williams GV, Goldman-Rakic PS (2000). Reversal of antipsychotic-induced working memory deficits by short-term dopamine D1 receptor stimulation. *Science*, 287, 2020–2022.

Cohen JD, Perlstein WM, Braver TS, Nystrom LE, Noll DC, Jonides J, Smith EE (1997). Temporal dynamics of brain activation during a working memory task. *Nature*, 386, 604–608.

Cornblatt BA and Keilp JG (1994). Impaired attention, genetics, and the pathophysiology of schizophrenia. *Schizophrenia Bulletin*, 20, 31–46.

Cornblatt BA, Obuchowski M, Roberts S, Pollack S, Erlenmeyer-Kimling L (1999). Cognitive and behavioral precursors of schizophrenia. *Development and Psychopathology*, 11(3), 487–508.

Craig TJ, Bromet EJ, Fennig S, Tanenberg-Karant M, Lavelle J, Galambos N (2000). Is there an association between duration of untreated psychosis and 24-month clinical outcome in a first-admission series? *American Journal of Psychiatry*, 157, 60–66.

Davidson M, Reichenberg A, Rabinowitz J, Weiser M, Kaplan Z, Mark, M (1999). Behavioral and intellectual markers for schizophrenia in apparently healthy male adolescents. *American Journal of Psychiatry*, 156, 1328–1335.

De Lisi LE, Tew W, Xie S-H *et al.* (1995). A prospective follow-up study of brain morphology and cognition in 1st episode schizophrenic patients. *Biological Psychiatry*, 38, 349–360.

De Lisi LE, Sakuma M, Tew W, Kushner M, Hoff AL, Grimson R (1997). Schizophrenia as a chronic active brain process: a study of progressive brain structural change subsequent to the onset of schizophrenia. *Psychiatry Research: Neuroimaging*, 74, 129–140.

Drake RJ, Haley CJ, Akhtar S, Lewis SW (2000). Causes and consequences of duration of untreated psychosis in schizophrenia. *British Journal of Psychiatry*, 177, 511–515.

Friedman JI, Adler DN, Temporini HD *et al.* (2001). Guanfacine treatment of cognitive impairment in schizophrenia. *Neuropsychopharmacology*, 25, 402–409.

Gold JM (14 April 2003). Cognitive deficits as core features of schizophrenia, presented at the Measurement and Treatment Research to Improve Cognition in Schizophrenia (MATRICS) Identifying Cognitive Targets and Establishing Criteria for Test Selection meeting. Potomac, MD.

Green MF (1996). What are the functional consequences of neurocognitive deficits in schizophrenia? *American Journal of Psychiatry*, 153, 321–330.

Green MF, Kern RS, Braff DL, Mintz J (2000). Neurocognitive deficits and functional outcome in schizophrenia: are we measuring the 'right stuff'? *Schizophrenia Bulletin*, 26, 119–136.

Green MF, Marder SR, Glynn SM, McGurk SR, Wirshing WC, Wirshing DA, Liberman RP, Mintz J (2002). The neurocognitive effects of low-dose haloperidol: a two-year comparison with risperidone. *Biological Psychiatry*, 51, 972–978.

Gur RE, Cowell P, Turetsky BI, Gallacher F, Cannon T, Bilker W, Gur RC (1998). A follow-up magnetic resonance imaging study of schizophrenia: relationship of neuroanatomical changes to clinical and neurobehavioral measures. *Archives of General Psychiatry*, 55, 145–152.

Hager F, Volz HP, Gaser C, Mentzel HJ, Kaiser WA, Sauer H (1998). Challenging the anterior attentional system with a continuous performance task: a functional magnetic resonance imaging approach. *European Archives of Psychiatry Clinical Neuroscience*, 248, 161–170.

Harvey PD and Keefe RSE (1997). Cognitive impairment in schizophrenia and implications of atypical neuroleptic treatment. *CNS Spectrums*, 2, 1–11.

Harvey PD, Howanitz E, Parrella M, White L, Davidson M, Mohs RC, Hoblyn J, Davis KL (1998). Symptoms, cognitive functioning, and adaptive skills in geriatric patients with lifelong schizophrenia: a comparison across treatment sites. *American Journal of Psychiatry*, 155, 1080–1086.

Harvey PD and Keefe RSE (2001). Studies of cognitive change in patients with schizophrenia following novel antipsychotic treatment. *American Journal of Psychiatry*, 158, 176–184.

Harvey PD, Bertisch HA, Friedman JI, Parrella M, White L, Davis KL (2003). Cognitive and functional changes in older patients with schizophrenia: evidence for cognitive threshold effects on functional decline? *Schizophrenia Research*, 60, 137S.

Hawkins KA and Wexler BE (1999). California Verbal Learning Test practice effects in a schizophrenia sample. *Schizophrenia Research*, 39, 73–78.

Hawkins KA, McGlashan, Keefe R *et al.* (2003). Neuropsychological status of the first-episode promodrome. *Schizophrenia Research*, 60, 4S.

Heinrichs RW and Zakzanis KK (1998). Neurocognitive deficit in schizophrenia: a quantitative review of the evidence. *Neuropsychology*, 12, 426–445.

Ho BC, Nopoulos P, Flaum M, Arndt S, Andreasen NC (1998). Two-year outcome in first-episode schizophrenia: predictive value of symptoms for quality of life. *American Journal of Psychiatry*, 155, 1196–1201.

Ho BC, Andreasen NC, Flaum, M, Nopoulos P, Miller D (2000). Untreated initial psychosis: its relation to quality of life and symptom remission in first episode schizophrenia. *American Journal of Psychiatry*, 157, 808–815.

Ho BC, Andreasen NC, Nopoulos P, Magnotta V, Arndt S, Flaum M (2003). Progressive structural brain abnormalities and their significance on outcome: A longitudinal MRI study early in the course of schizophrenia. *Archives of General Psychiatry*, 60, 585–594.

Hoff AL, Shukla S, Aronson TA, *et al.* (1990). Failure to differentiate bipolar disorder from schizophrenia on measures of neuropsychological function. *Schizophrenia Research*, 3, 253–260.

Hoff AL, Riordan H, O'Donnell DW, Morris L, DeLisi LE (1992). Neuropsychological functioning of first-episode schizophreniform patients. *American Journal of Psychiatry*, 149, 898–903.

Hoff AL, Sakuma M, Wieneke M, Horon R, Kushner M, DeLisi LE (1999). Longitudinal neuropsychological follow-up study of patients with first-episode schizophrenia. *American Journal of Psychiatry*, 156, 1336–1341.

Hoff AL, Sakuma M, Razi K, Heydebrand G, Csernansky JG, DeLisi LE (2000). Lack of association between duration of untreated illness and severity of cognitive and structural brain deficits at the first episode of schizophrenia. *American Journal of Psychiatry*, 157, 1824–1828.

James AC, Javaloyes A, James S, Smith DM (2002). Evidence for non-progressive changes in adolescent-onset schizophrenia: follow-up magnetic resonance imaging study. *British Journal of Psychiatry*, 180, 339–344.

Keefe RSE, Silva SG, Perkins DO, Lieberman JA (1999). The effects of atypical antipsychotic drugs on neurocognitive impairment in schizophrenia: a review and meta-analysis. *Schizophrenia Bulletin*, 25, 201–222.

Keefe RSE (2001). Neurocognition. In A Breier *et al.* (eds) *Current Issues in the Psychopharmacology of Schizophrenia*, pp. 192–205. Philadelphia, Lippincott, Williams & Wilkins.

Keefe RSE, Seidman, LJ, Christensen, BK *et al.* (2004). Comparative effect of atypical and conventional antipsychotic drugs on neurocognition in first-episode psychosis: A Randomized double-blind trial of olanzapine versus haloperidol. *American Journal of Psychiatry*, 161, 985–995.

Keilp JG, Herrera J, Stritzke P, Cornblatt BA (1997). The continuous performance test, identical pairs version (CPT-IP): III. Brain functioning during performance of numbers and shapes subtasks. *Psychiatry Research*, 74, 35–45.

Keshavan MS, Haas G, Kahn C, Aguilar E, Dick E, Schooler N, Sweeney J, Pettigrew J (1998). Superior temporal gyrus and the course of early schizophrenia: Progressive, static or reversible? *Journal of Psychiatric Research*, 32, 60–65.

Larsen, TK, Moe, LC, Vibe-Hansen, L, Johannessen, JO (2000). Premorbid functioning versus duration of untreated psychosis in one year outcome in first-episode psychosis. *Schizophrenia Research*, 45, 1–9.

Lewis S, Tarrier N, Haddock G, *et al.* (2002). Randomised controlled trial of cognitive-behavioural therapy in early schizophrenia: acute-phase outcomes. *British Journal of Psychiatry*, 181(suppl. 43), 91–97.

Lieberman JA, Alvir JM, Koreen A, Geisler S, Chakos M, Sheitman B, Woerner M (1996). Psychobiologic correlates of treatment response in schizophrenia. *Neuropsychopharmacology*, 14, 13S–21S.

Lieberman JA (1999). Is schizophrenia a neurodegenerative disorder? A clinical and neurobiological perspective. *Biol Psychiatry*, 46, 729–739.

Lieberman J, Chakos M, Wu H, Alvir J, Hoffman E, Robinson D, Bilder R (2001). Longitudinal study of brain morphology in first episode schizophrenia. *Biological Psychiatry*, 49, 487–499.

Lieberman JA, Charles HC, Sharma T *et al.* (2003). Antipsychotic treatment effects on progression of brain pathomorphology in first episode schizophrenia. *Schizophrenia Research*, 60, 293S.

Loebel AD, Lieberman JA, Alvir JM, Mayerhoff DI *et al.* (1992). Duration of psychosis and outcome in first-episode schizophrenia. *American Journal of Psychiatry*, 149, 1183–1188.

Madsen AL, Karle A, Rubin P, Cortsen M, Andersen HS, Henningsen R (1999). Progressive atrophy of the frontal lobes in first episode schizophrenia: Interaction with clinical course and neuroleptic treatment. *Acta Psychiatrica Scandinavica*, 100, 367–374.

Malla AK, Norman RMG, Voruganti LP (1999). Improving outcome in schizophrenia: the case for early intervention. *Canadian Medical Association Journal*, 160, 843–846.

Malla AK, Norman RMG, Manchanda R *et al.* (2002). One year outcome in first episode psychosis: Influence of DUP and other predictors. *Schizophrenia Research*, 54, 231–242.

Mohamed S, Paulsen JS, O'Leary D, Arndt S, Andreasen N (1999). Generalized cognitive deficits in schizophrenia: A study of first-episode patients. *Archives of General Psychiatry*, 56, 749–754.

Norman RMG, Townsend L, Malla AK (2001). Duration of untreated psychosis and cognitive functioning in first-episode patients. *British Journal of Psychiatry*, 179, 340–345.

Saykin AJ, Shtasel DL, Gur RE, Kester DB, Mozley LH, Stafiniak P, Gur RC (1994). Neuropsychological deficits in neuroleptic naive patients with first-episode schizophrenia. *Archives of General Psychiatry*, 51, 124–131.

Seidman LJ (1983). Schizophrenia and brain dysfunction: an integration of recent neurodiagnostic findings. *Psychological Bulletin*, 94, 195–238.

Stirling J, White C, Lewis S, Hopkins R, Tantam D, Huddy A, Montague L (2003). Neurocognitive function and outcome in first-episode schizophrenia: a 10-year follow-up of an epidemiological cohort. *Schizophrenia Research,* 65, 75–86.

Sweeney JA, Keilp JG, Haas GL, Hill J, Weiden PJ (1991). Relationships between medication treatments and neuropsychological test performance in schizophrenia. *Psychiatry Research,* 37, 297–308.

Thompson PM, Vidal C, Giedd JN *et al.* (2001). Mapping adolescent brain change reveals dynamic wave of accelerated gray matter loss in very early-onset schizophrenia. *Proceedings of the National Academy of Sciences,* 98, 11650–11655.

Velligan DI, Mahurin RK, Eckert SL, Hazleton BC *et al.* (1997). Relationship between specific types of communication deviance and attentional performance in patients with schizophrenia. *Psychiatry Research,* 70, 9–20.

Verdoux H, Lirand F, Bergey C, Assens F, Abalan F, Van Os J (2001). Is the association between duration of untreated psychosis and outcome confounded? A two-year follow-up study of first admitted patients. *Schizophrenia Research,* 49, 231–241.

Weickert TW, Goldberg TE, Gold JM, Bigelow LB, Egan MF, Weinberger DR (2000). Cognitive impairments in patients with schizophrenia displaying preserved and compromised intellect. *Archives of General Psychiatry,* 57, 907–913.

Weinberger DR and McClure RK (2002). Neurotoxicity, neuroplasticity, and magnetic resonance imaging morphometry. *Archives of General Psychiatry,* 59, 553–558.

Wyatt, RJ (1991). Neuroleptics and the natural course of schizophrenia. *Schizophrenia Bulletin,* 17, 325–351.

Wykes T, Reeder C, Corner J, Williams C, Everitt B (1999). The effects of neurocognitive remediation on executive processing in patients with schizophrenia. *Schizophrenia Bulletin,* 25, 291–308.

Wykes T, Brammer M, Mellers J, Bray P, Reeder C, Williams C, Corner J (2002). The effects of the brain of a psychological treatment, cognitive remediation therapy (CRT): An fMRI study. *British Journal of Psychiatry,* 181, 144–152.

Wykes T, Reeder C, Williams C, Corner J, Rice C and Everitt B (2003). Are the effects of cognitive remediation therapy (CRT) durable? Results from an exploratory trial. *Schizophrenia Research,* 2003 Jun 1;61(2-3):163–174.

Yung AR and McGorry PD (1996). The prodromal phase of first-episode psychosis: past and current conceptualizations. *Schizophrenia Bulletin,* 22, 353–370.

Index